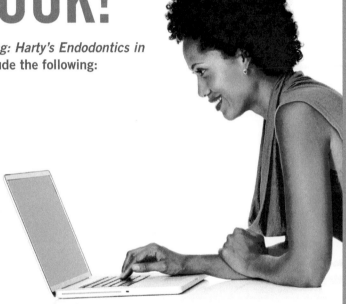

Harty's Endodontics in Clinical Practice

7th Edition

Harty's Endodontics in Clinical Practice

Edited by

Bun San Chong
BDS, MSc., PhD, LDS RCS(Eng), FDS RCS(Eng), FDS RCS(Edin),
MFGDP(UK), MRD, FHEA
Specialist in Endodontics,
Professor of Restorative Dentistry/Honorary Consultant,
Endodontic Lead and Director, Postgraduate Endodontics,
Barts and The London School of Medicine and Dentistry,
Queen Mary University of London,
London, UK

Illustrations by
Antbits

ELSEVIER
SAUNDERS

Edinburgh London New York Oxford Philadelphia St Louis Sydney Toronto 2017

ELSEVIER
SAUNDERS

ISBN 978-0-7020-5835-6

Notices

Knowledge and best practice in this field are constantly changing. As new research and experience broaden our understanding, changes in research methods, professional practices or medical treatment may become necessary.

Practitioners and researchers must always rely on their own experience and knowledge in evaluating and using any information, methods, compounds or experiments described herein. In using such information or methods they should be mindful of their own safety and the safety of others, including parties for whom they have a professional responsibility.

With respect to any drug or pharmaceutical products identified, readers are advised to check the most current information provided (i) on procedures featured or (ii) by the manufacturer of each product to be administered, to verify the recommended dose or formula, the method and duration of administration and contraindications. It is the responsibility of practitioners, relying on their own experience and knowledge of their patients, to make diagnoses, to determine dosages and the best treatment for each individual patient and to take all appropriate safety precautions.

To the fullest extent of the law, neither the Publisher nor the authors, contributors or editors assume any liability for any injury and/or damage to persons or property as a matter of products liability, negligence or otherwise, or from any use or operation of any methods, products, instructions or ideas contained in the material herein.

For Elsevier
Content Strategist: Alison Taylor
Content Development Specialist: Sally Davies
Project Manager: Andrew Riley
Designer/Design Direction: Miles Hitchen
Illustration Manager: Nichole Beard

your source for books,
journals and multimedia
in the health sciences

www.elsevierhealth.com

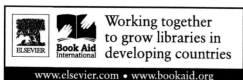

Working together
to grow libraries in
developing countries

www.elsevier.com • www.bookaid.org

The
publisher's
policy is to use
paper manufactured
from sustainable forests

Preface

The challenge of preparing a new, seventh edition of this long-established book is a valued opportunity to review the current state of the science and art of endodontics. It is also an occasion to reflect on my personal connection with, and to acknowledge, my predecessors. Fred Harty, whom this book is named after, was responsible for the first three editions and Tom Pitt Ford for the next two editions. Apart from academia, I have been a specialist in endodontics for over 25 years in the practice founded by Fred. Until the untimely loss of Tom, I had the privilege of working with him for over 20 years.

The aim of this book remains the same: to be an authoritative guide to proven, current clinical endodontic practice. Since it is imperative that practitioners keep up to date, this book is also intended for dental practitioners seeking to update or expand their knowledge – to help and support especially those who have chosen to embark on postgraduate education courses, or wishing to acquire extended skills, in endodontics.

Despite the recognition and the establishment of a specialist list in endodontics in the United Kingdom in 1998, there are still insufficient specialists available to treat all endodontic cases. Hence, endodontic treatment will continue to be carried out mostly in general dental practice, or other primary care settings. The demands of the recently introduced new undergraduate dental curriculum in the United Kingdom has meant that, in an increasingly crowded time-table, while time dedicated to learning activities related to theoretical knowledge may be unaltered, less is available for acquisition of practical, clinical skills. Nevertheless it is important to ensure that students and new graduates should not only be conversant in managing common endodontic problems but also be able to recognize, where appropriate, the need for referral to a specialist. A growing number of patients can continue to benefit from management of challenging or complex endodontic cases by specially trained practitioners and can expect to enjoy a favourable treatment outcome.

The international flavour of the list of contributors is recognition that there are no boundaries when it comes to improving patients' oral health and achieving equity in healthcare. However, given the international spectrum and the number of contributors, it is inevitable that there will be some duplication of material in this book. This should be viewed as beneficial reinforcement of relevant information. Different contributors will also have different writing styles and preferred terminology but, hopefully, not at the expense of clarity and cohesion.

I am grateful to the contributors for providing their perspective on, and for updating, the topics covered in this new edition. I wish to express my appreciation to contributors to the previous edition. I would also like to thank the team at Elsevier including Alison Taylor and Sally Davies. Once again, I acknowledge the patience and understanding of my family, Grace, James and Louisa.

B. S. Chong
2017

Contributors

Cecilia Bourguignon DDS, Cert Endo(UPenn), Foundation Fellow of IADT
Specialist in Endodontics,
Paris, France

Josette Camilleri BChD, MPhil, PhD, FIMMM, FADM
Associate Professor, Department of Restorative Dentistry,
Faculty of Dental Surgery, University of Malta,
Msida, Malta

Nicholas P. Chandler BDS, MSc., PhD, LDS RCS(Eng), FDS RCPS(Glas), FDS RCS(Edin), FFD RCSI
Associate Professor of Endodontics,
School of Dentistry, University of Otago,
Dunedin, New Zealand

Bun San Chong BDS, MSc., PhD, LDS RCS(Eng), FDS RCS(Eng), FDS RCS(Edin), MFGDP(UK), MRD, FHEA
Professor of Restorative Dentistry/Honorary Consultant,
Endodontic Lead & Director, Postgraduate Endodontics,
Barts and The London School of Medicine and Dentistry,
Queen Mary University of London,
London, UK

Paul R. Cooper BSc, PhD
Professor of Oral Biology,
School of Dentistry, University of Birmingham,
Birmingham, UK

Henry F. Duncan BDS, MClinDent, MRD RCS(Edin), FDS RCS(Edin)
Assistant Professor/Consultant in Endodontics,
Division of Restorative Dentistry,
Dublin Dental University Hospital, Trinity College Dublin, University of Dublin,
Dublin, Ireland

Michael P. Escudier MD, MBBS, BDS, FDS RCS(Eng), FDS(OM) RCS(Eng), FFGDP(UK), FHEA
Reader/Honorary Consultant in Oral Medicine,
King's College London Dental Institute,
London, UK

Massimo Giovarruscio DipDent(Rome)
Specialist in Endodontics/Clinical Teacher,
King's College London Dental Institute,
London, UK

James L. Gutmann DDS, Cert Endo, PhD, FICD, FACD, FADI, FAHD
Professor Emeritus,
Baylor College of Dentistry, Texas A&M University,
Dallas, Texas, USA

Michael Hülsmann Dr med dent, PhD
Professor, Department of Preventive Dentistry,
Periodontology and Cariology,
Dental School, University of Göttingen,
Göttingen, Germany

Francesco Mannocci MD, DDS, PhD
Professor of Endodontology/Honorary Consultant,
King's College London Dental Institute,
London, UK

Isabela N. Rôças DDS, MSc, PhD
Professor, Department of Endodontics and Head,
Molecular Microbiology Laboratory,
Faculty of Dentistry, Estácio de Sá University,
Rio de Janeiro, Brazil

Ilan Rotstein DDS
Professor/Associate Dean, Continuing Education and Chairman,
Endodontics, Orthodontics and General Practice Residency,
Herman Ostrow School of Dentistry of USC,
University of Southern California,
Los Angeles, California, USA

Edgar Schäfer Dr med dent, PhD
Professor/Head, Central Interdisciplinary Ambulance,
School of Dentistry, University of Münster,
Münster, Germany

Asgeir Sigurdsson Cand Odont, MS, Cert Endo(UNC)
Associate Professor/Chairman,
Department of Endodontics, New York University
    College of Dentistry,
New York, USA

José F. Siqueira Jr DDS, MSc, PhD
Professor/Director, Department of Endodontics,
Head, Molecular Microbiology Laboratory,
Faculty of Dentistry, Estácio de Sá University,
Rio de Janeiro, Brazil

Anthony J. Smith BSc, PhD
Emeritus Professor,
School of Dentistry, University of Birmingham,
Birmingham, UK

Simon J. Stone BDS, PhD, MFDS RCS(Edin), FHEA
Clinical Lecturer in Restorative Dentistry/Honorary
    StR in Endodontics,
School of Dental Sciences, Newcastle University,
Newcastle upon Tyne, UK

John M. Whitworth BChD, PhD, FDS RCS(Edin), FDS RCS(RestDent)
Professor of Endodontology/Honorary Consultant in
    Restorative Dentistry,
School of Dental Sciences, Newcastle University,
Newcastle upon Tyne, UK

Ferranti S. L. Wong BDS, MSc, PhD, FDS RCS(Edin), FDS RCS(Eng), FHEA
Professor/Honorary Consultant in Paediatric
    Dentistry,
Barts and The London School of Medicine and
    Dentistry,
Queen Mary University of London,
London, UK

Contributors to Previous Editions

The editor would like to acknowledge the great support and contributions made to the last edition by the following people, who made this book possible.

Philip J. C. Mitchell

Amanda L. O'Donnell

Dag Ørstavik

Shanon Patel

Heather E. Pitt Ford

John D. Regan

John S. Rhodes

James H. S. Simon

Andrew D. M. Watson

Contents

ⓔ To access your Evolve Resources visit:
http://evolve.elsevier.com/Harty/endodontics/

Register today and gain access to:
• Self-assessment section:
  ○ 140 MCQs
  ○ 16 Clinical cases with images

CHAPTER 1

Introduction and Overview

B. S. Chong

Chapter Contents

Summary

The science and art of endodontics have come a long way since its early days. A brief review of the history of endodontics is helpful in understanding its influence on current practice. The wider scope of modern endodontics encompasses a variety of procedures. Patients are no longer willing to accept tooth loss and expect better treatment and care. Microorganisms have an essential role in the pathogenesis of pulpal and periradicular diseases. The host defense response against root canal infection includes numerous inflammatory mediators and a range of cells. Continuing research has increased our knowledge of the root canal microbiota, which will hopefully result in dedicated strategies to manage the different types of root canal infection. Advances in endodontics are continuing, and many recent developments have been successfully translated into everyday clinical practice.

Introduction

Endodontology is the branch of dental sciences concerned with the form, function, health of, injuries to and diseases of the dental pulp and periradicular region, as well as their relationship with systemic well-being and health. Endodontic treatment can be defined as the prevention or treatment of apical periodontitis, the principal disease. The concept of treating the pulp of the tooth to preserve the tooth itself is a relatively modern development in the history of dentistry. It may be useful to very briefly review the history of pulp treatment to better appreciate modern views on endodontic treatment.

Toothache has been a scourge of mankind from the earliest times. Both the Chinese and Egyptians left records describing caries and alveolar abscesses. The Chinese believed that abscesses were caused by a white worm with a black head, which lived within the tooth. The 'worm theory' was accepted until the middle of the eighteenth century. When doubts were raised, they could not be expressed forcibly because those in authority still believed in the worm theory.[1] The Chinese treatment for an abscessed tooth was aimed at killing the worm with a preparation that contained arsenic. The use of this drug was taught in most dental schools as recently as the 1950s in spite of the realization that it was self-limiting and that extensive tissue destruction occurred if even minute amounts of the drug leaked into the soft tissues. Pulp treatment during Greek and Roman times was aimed at destroying the pulp by cauterization with a hot needle or boiling oil or with a preparation containing opium and hyoscyamus. Near the end of the first century AD, it was realized that drilling into the pulp chamber to obtain drainage could relieve pain. In spite of modern antibiotics, there is still no better method of relieving the pain of an abscessed tooth than drainage.

Endodontic knowledge remained static until the sixteenth century when pulpal anatomy was described. Until the latter part of the nineteenth century, 'root canal therapy' consisted of alleviating pulpal pain, and the main function of the opened root canal was to provide retention for a dowel crown.[2,3] At the same time, bridgework became popular, and many dental schools taught that no tooth should be used as an abutment unless it was first devitalized.[4] Root canal therapy became commonplace partly for these reasons and also because the discovery of cocaine led to painless pulp extirpation. Injecting 4% cocaine as a mandibular nerve block was first reported in 1884[3,5]; 20 years later the first synthetic local anaesthetic, procaine, was produced. Around this time, the first reports of endodontic surgery appeared.[6] The first radiograph of teeth was taken in 1896,[2,7,8] shortly after the discovery of X-rays by Roentgen in 1895.[9] This further popularized 'root canal therapy' and gave it some credibility. About the same time, dental manufacturers began to produce special instruments which were used primarily to remove pulp tissue or clean debris from the canal. There was no concept of filling the root canals since the objective of the procedure was to provide retention for a post crown.

By 1910, 'root canal therapy' had reached its zenith, and no self-respecting dentist would extract a tooth.

Every root stump was retained and a crown constructed. Sinus tracts often appeared in these stumps and were treated by various ineffective methods for many years.[10] The connection between the sinus tract and pulpless tooth was known but not acted upon. In 1911, William Hunter[11,12] attacked the 'American dentistry' and blamed the bridgework for several diseases of unknown aetiology. He reported recovery from these conditions in a few patients after the extraction of their teeth. It is interesting to note that he did not condemn 'root canal therapy' itself but rather the ill-fitting bridgework and the sepsis that surrounded it. Around this time, microbiology became established and the findings of microbiologists added fuel to the fire of Hunter's condemnations. Radiography, which at first helped the dentist, now provided irrefutable evidence of apical periodontitis surrounding the roots of pulpless teeth.

While the theory of 'focal infection' was not enunciated by Billings[13] until 1918, Hunter's condemnations started a reaction to 'root canal therapy', and there began the wholesale removal of both nonvital and perfectly healthy teeth. The blame for obscure diseases was placed on the dentition,[14] and as dentists could not refute this theory, countless mouths were mutilated. Naturally, not all dentists accepted this wholesale dental destruction. Some, particularly in continental Europe, continued to save teeth in spite of the focal sepsis theory. It is difficult to know why dentists in continental Europe disregarded this theory, but one explanation may be that their patients equated the loss of teeth with a loss of virility, and therefore, did not allow their dentists to mutilate their dentitions. Alternatively, it could be that these practitioners were not so readily swayed by vanity as were their British colleagues.

Modern Endodontics

The re-emergence of endodontics as a respectable branch of dental science began in the 1930s.[15,16] The occurrence and degree of bacteraemia during tooth extraction were shown to depend on the severity of periodontal disease and the amount of tissue damage during the operation. The incongruity between the microbiological findings in the treatment of chronic oral infection and the histological picture was demonstrated. When the gingival sulcus was disinfected by cauterization before extraction, microorganisms could not be demonstrated in the bloodstream immediately postoperatively.

Gradually, the concept that a 'dead' tooth, one without a pulp, was not necessarily infected began to be accepted. Furthermore, it was realized that the function and usefulness of the tooth depended on the integrity of the periodontal tissues and not on the vitality of the pulp.[17] Another significant advance was clarification of the 'hollow tube' theory[18] by research using sterile polyethylene tube implants in rats.[19,20] The tissue surrounding the lumina of clean, disinfected tubes, which were closed at one end, was relatively free of inflammation and displayed a normal capacity for repair. When such tubes were filled with muscle, the inflammatory reaction was only severe around the openings of the tubes that contained tissue contaminated with gram-negative cocci. These findings stress on the microbial contents of the tube; if the tube contains microorganisms, the potential for repair is far less favourable than when the lumen of the tube is clean and sterile.[21] This infected situation is likely to be found in most root canals requiring treatment.

Until relatively recently, practitioners were preoccupied with a mechanistic approach to root canal treatment and to the perceived effects of various potent drugs on the microorganisms within the root canal, rather than a total antimicrobial approach of effective cleaning, adequate shaping and complete filling of the root canal space.[22] This preoccupation diverted attention from the effects of such drugs on periradicular tissues. Medicaments that kill microbes may also be toxic to living tissue.[23] The consequences of such materials passing out of the tooth into the surrounding vital tissues can be localized tissue necrosis. These avoidable problems cause distress to patients and can lead to litigation. Effective elimination of microorganisms from the root canal system is best achieved by instrumentation combined with irrigation.

The concept that an 'apical seal' was important led to the search for filling and sealing materials that were stable, nonirritant and provided a perfect seal at the apical foramen. With the realization of the negative impact of coronal leakage[24,25] and the biodegradation of root canal fillings, total filling of the root canal space, including lateral and accessory canals, has assumed a much greater importance. This is facilitated by the use of adhesive materials where appropriate and the placement of suitable bases and well-sealed restorations. Despite arguments about the relative importance between the quality of the root filling and the coronal restoration on treatment outcome, there can be no disagreement that both should be performed well[26–29] and are mutually beneficial to the long-term prognosis of the root-treated tooth.[30,31]

Scope of Endodontics

The extent of the subject has altered considerably in the last 60 years. Formerly, endodontic treatment confined itself to root canal filling techniques by conventional methods; even endodontic surgery, which is an extension of these methods, was considered to be in the field of oral surgery. Modern endodontics has a much wider field[32,33] and includes the following:

- the differential diagnosis and treatment of orofacial pain of pulpal and periradicular origin;
- prevention of pulpal disease and vital pulp therapy;
- root canal treatment;
- management of post-treatment endodontic disease;
- surgical endodontics;
- bleaching of endodontically treated teeth;
- treatment procedures related to coronal restorations using a core and/or a post involving the root canal space;
- endodontically related measures in connection with crown-lengthening and forced eruption procedures;
- treatment of traumatized teeth.

Role of Microorganisms

The Chinese belief that dental abscesses were caused by small worms persisted until the eighteenth century. At the end of the nineteenth century, Miller[34] demonstrated the role of bacteria in root canal infections and noted that different microorganisms were found in the root canal compared with the open pulp chamber. Shortly afterward, systematic culturing of root canals was undertaken.[35] Unfortunately, these methods, which were potentially so valuable for improving the outcome of root canal treatment, were used to condemn much of the dentistry carried out at the time.[12] During the 1930s, microbiological techniques were used to re-establish the scientific basis of root canal treatments. However, techniques at that time only readily identified aerobic bacteria, which led to confusing results in clinical studies.[36,37] Consequently, clinicians became complacent about the role of microorganisms and performed treatment simply as a technical exercise.

The development of anaerobic culturing allowed the identification of many previously unknown microorganisms present in root canals.[38] This led rapidly to the demonstration that the majority of these microorganisms were anaerobes,[39,40] and the realization that canals previously considered sterile contained anaerobes alone. Furthermore, when traumatized teeth were examined, there was a close correlation between the presence of anaerobic bacteria in the root canal and a periradicular radiolucency[40]; in the absence of infection, the necrotic pulp and stagnant tissue fluids cannot induce or perpetuate a periradicular lesion. This was later demonstrated experimentally in teeth where the pulp tissue had been removed; only in those where the pulp was infected did periradicular inflammation occur.[41] Although microbial analysis of root canals may not be a technique applicable to everyday clinical practice, the results of research have provided rational explanations for pulp and periradicular diseases and its treatment.[42] Microorganisms, which previously could not be cultured, and thus, were mistakenly considered absent can now be identified. Currently, over 50% of the oral microbiota remains uncultivable.[43–45] However, the use of molecular biology and culture-independent techniques has enabled the identification of microbes that would be undetectable by conventional culturing techniques.[43,45–47] As knowledge in this area expands, our understanding of the root canal microbiota also expands. The presence of specific or a combination of microorganisms, symbiotic and dysbiotic microbiota, and their implications remain to be fully appreciated. It is expected that molecular microbiology and culture-independent methods will continue to help elucidate the microbial diversity of endodontic infections.[45]

Most root canal infections contain a mixture of microorganisms, with bacteria being the main candidate pathogen.[45] It has also been shown that the relative proportions of different microorganism are determined by the local environmental conditions.[48] Endodontic pathogens do not occur at random but are found in specific combinations.[49] If a selection of microorganisms is inoculated into root canals in fixed proportions, their relative numbers will change over time, with a decline in aerobes and an increase in anaerobes.[48] It has also been established that combinations of microorganisms are more likely to survive than inocula of single species[50]; to survive, different species of microorganisms form complex ecological and nutritional relationships.

Microorganisms are normally confined to the root canal system in pulpless teeth and exist in two forms:
- planktonic—loose collections or suspensions within the root canal lumen;
- biofilm—dense aggregates that form plaques on and within the root canal wall.

The intraradicular infection may be divided into three categories:
- primary—caused by microorganisms that initially invaded and colonized the necrotic pulp;
- secondary—caused by microorganisms that were not present in the primary infection but were introduced into the root canal system after dental intervention;
- persistent infection—caused by microorganisms associated with the primary or secondary infection that managed to survive treatment procedures and nutritional deprivation.

It is unusual for microorganisms to be present in periradicular lesions; the host defenses prevent them from invading the periradicular tissues. However, in certain circumstances and with some species, microorganisms may establish an extraradicular infection, which may be dependent or independent of the intraradicular infection but the incidence of independent extraradicular infection in untreated teeth is low.[45,51]

Tissue Response to Root Canal Infection

The role of an infection in the demise of damaged pulps was demonstrated in a classic study by Kakehashi and co-workers in the 1960s[52] and eventually led to a biological approach to operative dentistry.[53] The presence of microorganisms, their byproducts or damaged tissue in the root canal can cause apical periodontitis, typically at the apical foramen but also around the foramina of any lateral or accessory canals, or at a fracture site. The periradicular inflammation prevents the spread of infection from the tooth to the alveolar bone; otherwise, osteomyelitis would occur. The inflammatory lesion contains inflammatory mediators and numerous inflammatory cells. The interaction between these cells and the antigenic substances from the root canal results in the release of a large number of inflammatory mediators which play a major role in the development of periradicular lesions.[54,55]

As long as antigens emerge from the canal foramina, there will be a continuing inflammatory response, mediated in a number of different ways. This is a very dynamic response to rapidly multiplying microorganisms in the root canal and may not be readily apparent to the clinician observing a radiograph or a histologist examining a slide of fixed cells. Endodontic treatment is primarily directed at the effective elimination of the microorganisms, allowing inflammation to subside and healing to occur.

Evidence-based Practice and Quality Assurance

Evidence-based treatment requires the integration of the best evidence with the patient's values, aspirations and preferences, combined with the practitioner's own clinical proficiency and judgement to offer more effective ways of managing clinical problems.[56,57] The general public across the world now expect healthcare professionals to deliver a high standard of service; dentistry, and endodontic treatment is no exception. In the United Kingdom, guidance has been published by the regulatory body on the standards[58] expected of, and the scope of practice[59] for, the whole dental team. The European Society of Endodontology has issued quality guidelines for endodontic treatments.[60] It is essential that dental practices have a quality control system to ensure that each step in history, diagnosis and treatment is carried out in a logical and consistent manner; this is to ensure a high standard of care and treatment, known as clinical governance. Patients are increasingly well informed and will not tolerate poor standards, for example, out-of-date views or empirical practices.[61] In the United Kingdom and in line with many other countries, one of the largest source of

dental negligence claims relate to endodontics[62]; the requirement for all registered healthcare professionals to have indemnity is no longer an ethical but rather a legal requirement. The dramatic rise in litigation is a reflection that patients are increasingly prepared to seek redress for any failures regarding their care or treatment.[63,64]

In a survey in England of newly qualified dentists in vocational training to join the National Health Service, most expressed a lack of preparedness with regard to complex/molar endodontics, with 66% rating their preparedness as 'poor' and 3% as 'very poor'.[65] The technical challenges of root treating a molar tooth have been described as involving 'preparation to tenths of millimetres of accuracy in a root canal narrower than a pin and in a place the dentist cannot see'.[66] Treatment failures invariably drain valuable and limited financial resources from public health services such as the National Health Service.[29]

Those dentists who have undertaken further training to become specialists[67] are expected to achieve consistently high standards in diagnosis and treatment. However, general practitioners cannot continue to practise in the way that they were taught at dental school many years ago; they must keep up to date[68] and offer referral to an appropriate specialist when the treatment required is beyond their skill. This change has already occurred in the United States and is spreading to other countries. In the United Kingdom, continuing professional development is now mandatory for recertification with the regulatory body and practitioners are also required to refer patients for further advice or treatment when it is necessary or if requested by the patient.[58] Almost all endodontic procedures can be carried out with a predictable outcome. Root canal treatment has a reported a favourable outcome rate of over 90%,[31,69] even though closer analysis reveals that retreatment of teeth with apical periodontitis is less favourable than initial treatment in teeth without apical periodontitis.[70-72] Unfortunately, this is not reflected in the cross-sectional studies of the general population that report high rates of root-filled teeth with concomitant apical periodontitis because of poor technical quality root canal treatment.[29] Therefore, it is essential that individual practitioners monitor their outcomes against accepted criteria[73] and that their treatment protocols conform to published guidelines.[60]

Treatment outcomes can be assessed in different ways[74,75] and should encompass not only clinical but also other evidence such as radiological evidence.

Developments in Endodontics

In the last 30 years, there have been significant advances in our knowledge and understanding of the dental pulp, including its response to injury, inflammation, immunity, infection and nociceptive mechanisms.[55] The dental pulp may be damaged as a result of caries or infection consequent to trauma or operative dentistry. It is recognized that current clinical methods of assessing pulpal and periradicular health have limitations. As a result, molecular assessment methods have received attention. However, more research into molecular diagnostics in endodontics is needed before it becomes a clinical tool.[76]

With a reduced incidence of dental caries, a greater emphasis on preventing sports injuries and minimal intervention dentistry,[77] the ultraconservative management of caries and the preparation of smaller cavities combined with better restorative materials in operative dentistry, the expectation is a decline in the number of teeth with damaged pulps. However, the trend and popularity of 'cosmetic' dentistry potentially risks irreversibly compromising the pulp.[78] The degree to which adhesive restorative materials will be successful in preventing pulp damage[79] in clinical practice is another unquantifiable variable.

Progress in the understanding of the cellular and molecular processes involved in the dentine/pulp complex has heralded a new era of regenerative dentistry.[55,80] The media trumpeted research in this field with the assertion that one day everyone will be able to grow a completely new set of teeth. The identification of stem cells in the dental pulp, the bioactive molecules within the dentine matrix, and specific processes promoting tissue regeneration will hopefully translate into biologically based therapies in everyday clinical practice.[55,81,82] The ability to control tissue injury, microbial infection and inflammation will tip the balance, so that instead of necrosis, there will be regeneration and maintenance of pulpal vitality. The ultimate goal of regenerative endodontics is to replace diseased, damaged or missing pulp tissues with healthy tissues to revitalize teeth.[83,84]

The management of persistent infection in previously endodontically treated teeth is challenging.[45,85] Endodontic pathogens have the capability to adapt, including the formation of biofilms, in response to changes in the root canal environment.[86–88] As the breadth of microbial diversity in the oral cavity has been revealed by molecular, culture-independent techniques,[43,45] several newly identified species/phylotypes have emerged as potential pathogens.[45] Findings have revealed new candidate endodontic pathogens, including as-yet-uncultivated bacteria and taxa, which may participate in the mixed infections associated with apical periodontitis in previously treated teeth.[44,45] Improved knowledge of the microbiota should eventually lead to dedicated strategies for managing different types of root canal infection, including those that are recalcitrant. This is of paramount significance because as with periodontal disease,[89,90] the question has been raised as to the likelihood of endodontic infections affecting systemic health[91,92]; for example, the association with diabetes mellitus[93] and the risk of coronary artery disease.[94]

Images captured on X-ray films or via digital sensors are two-dimensional 'shadowgraphs' with inherent problems of geometric distortions and anatomical noise.[95] Cone beam computed tomography (CBCT) is a newer imaging technique which is designed to overcome some of the deficiencies of conventional radiography.[96] CBCT produces undistorted and accurate images of the area under investigation, enhancing diagnosis and in the process aiding, for example, the planning of endodontic surgery and the management of resorption lesions. Since CBCT is able to detect lesions that are not easily discernible on conventional radiographs, it should also enable more objective assessment of healing after endodontic treatment.[8,29] However, in keeping with radiation safety principles, to ensure prudent clinical application and to prevent misuse, the benefits of a CBCT scan must be justified and outweighed by any associated risks.[97] It is expected that there will be continuing advancement and development of dental imaging technologies.[9]

Since its introduction, use of the operating microscope in endodontics has increased[98] and it has become an invaluable tool.[99] From diagnosis to canal location through canal preparation and filling, the improved vision and illumination afforded by the operating microscope is immensely beneficial. Although it is difficult to know the effects of magnification devices on treatment outcomes,[100] the need for a microscope for optimum vision in endodontics is not in doubt.[101]

Techniques, in particular instruments, for the preparation of root canals have altered substantially in recent years.[102,103] A crown-down concept is now the main approach to shaping and cleaning root canals.[104] Manufacturers are always introducing newer instruments for the preparation of root canals. The development of nickel–titanium instruments continues unabated and now includes, apart from rotary, reciprocating and single-file systems that are coupled with the promise of speed, ease and efficiency. However, not all claims can be substantiated, and any instrument or technique is only as good as the operator. Endodontic treatment should always be guided by biological and evidence-based principles. Speed, expediency and technical wizardry do not guarantee a favourable treatment outcome.

There has been a quiet revolution in endodontic surgery.[6] This treatment modality is no longer a substitute for failure to manage properly the root canal system nonsurgically. The indications for endodontic surgery have decreased, and nonsurgical retreatment should first be considered. Newer root-end filling materials, among other advances, including developments in the surgical armamentarium, the implementation of microsurgical techniques and enhanced illumination and magnification, have helped improve the predictability and outcome of endodontic surgery.[105,106] The use of amalgam as a root-end filling material is confined to history, with zinc oxide-eugenol materials and mineral trioxide aggregate (MTA) now being widely used.[105] In the first prospective clinical study on the use of MTA as a root-end filling material, a high rate of success (92%) was achieved.[107] Extended applications of MTA with the ability to encourage hard tissue deposition has helped promote the use of this material not only as a root-end filling but also a perforation sealant, pulp capping agent and apical plug for teeth with an opened apex. Further development of MTA, considered the first endodontic 'bioceramic' material,[108,109] and other tricalcium silicate cement-based materials for a variety of clinical applications are continuing.[109–111]

The advent of implants has led to clinicians being confronted with the decision to either extract a tooth and place an implant or preserve the natural tooth by root canal treatment. There are debates about the advantages of implants versus endodontics[112–114] that are fuelled by the myopic perception within both camps that one discipline is a threat to the other. This has led to the movement to incorporate implant placement into endodontic surgery. In reality, both disciplines are complementary to each other. Endodontic treatment of a tooth represents a feasible, practical and economical way[115] to preserve function in a vast array of cases, and in selected situations in which prognosis is poor, a dental implant may be a suitable alternative.[112–114]

A majority of endodontic treatments is within the capability of general practitioners or may be carried out in other primary care settings, but there will inevitably be cases that are best managed by specialists.[29,116] Endodontic referral practices undertake more root canal retreatments because of technical deficiencies in the original treatment. In many cases, this is difficult and challenging, but success can be very rewarding, particularly when in the past, the alternative would have been extraction. Although after tooth loss a replacement in the form of an implant is available, the retention of the natural tooth remains ideal as the occurrence of peri-implant diseases (peri-implant mucositis and peri-implantitis) is not uncommon.[117] Therefore, it is encouraging that many more patients are refusing to allow a tooth with an exposed or infected pulp to be extracted, but instead ask for it to be saved by root canal treatment.[118] High-quality endodontic treatment will make a significant contribution to good oral health.

Learning Outcomes

At the end of this chapter, readers will be able to explain and discuss the:

- history of endodontics and its influence on current practice;
- scope of modern endodontics;
- essential role of microorganisms in the pathogenesis of pulpal and periradicular diseases;
- tissue response to root canal infection;
- high standard of endodontic care and treatment expected by patients;
- recent developments in endodontics.

REFERENCES

1. Curson I. History and endodontics. Dental Practitioner and Dental Record 1965;15:435–9.
2. Cruse WP, Bellizzi R. A historic review of endodontics, 1689–1963, I. Journal of Endodontics 1980;6:495–9.
3. Cruse WP, Bellizzi R. A historic review of endodontics, 1689–1963, II. Journal of Endodontics 1980;6:532–5.
4. Prinz H. Dental chronology. A record of the more important historic events in the evolution of dentistry. London: Kimpton; 1945.
5. Chong BS, Miller JE, Sidhu SK. Alternative local anaesthetic delivery systems, devices and aids designed to minimise painful injections – a review. ENDO (Lond Engl) 2014;8: 7–22.
6. Gutmann JL. Surgical endodontics: past, present, and future. Endodontic Topics 2014;30:29–43.
7. Grossman LI. Endodontics 1776–1976: a bicentennial history against the background of general dentistry. Journal of the American Dental Association 1976;93:78–87.
8. Todd R. Dental imaging – 2D to 3D: a historic, current, and future view of projection radiography. Endodontic Topics 2014;31:36–52.
9. Chong BS. Without a shadow of doubt. ENDO (Lond Engl) 2009;3:251.
10. Gutmann JL. On the management of root canals in teeth that exhibit a draining 'fistulous' tract. Journal of the History of Dentistry 2014;62:69–72.
11. Cruse WP, Bellizzi R. A historic review of endodontics, 1689–1963, III. Journal of Endodontics 1980;6:576–80.
12. Hunter W. The role of sepsis and antisepsis in medicine. Lancet 1911;1:79–86.
13. Billings F. Focal infection. New York: Appleton; 1918.
14. Pallasch TJ, Wahl MJ. Focal infection: new age or ancient history? Endodontic Topics 2003;4:32–45.
15. Fish EW, MacLean I. The distribution of oral streptococci in the tissues. British Dental Journal 1936;61:336–62.
16. Okell CC, Elliott SD. Bacteraemia and oral sepsis with special reference to the aetiology of subacute endocarditis. Lancet 1935;2:869–72.
17. Marshall JA. The relation to pulp-canal therapy of certain anatomical characteristics of dentin and cementum. Dental Cosmos 1928;70:253–63.
18. Rickert UG, Dixon CM. The controlling of root surgery. Paris: Eighth International Dental Congress. IIIa; 1931. p. 15–22.
19. Torneck CD. Reaction of rat connective tissue to polyethylene tube implants, I. Oral Surgery, Oral Medicine, Oral Pathology 1966;21:379–87.
20. Torneck CD. Reaction of rat connective tissue to polyethylene tube implants, II. Oral Surgery, Oral Medicine, Oral Pathology 1967;24:674–83.
21. Wu MK, Moorer WR, Wesselink PR. Capacity of anaerobic bacteria enclosed in a simulated root canal to induce inflammation. International Endodontic Journal 1989;22:269–77.
22. Kawashima N, Wadachi R, Suda H, et al. Root canal medicaments. International Dental Journal 2009;59:5–11.
23. Chong BS, Pitt Ford TR. The role of intracanal medication in root canal treatment. International Endodontic Journal 1992;25:97–106.
24. Chong BS. Coronal leakage and treatment failure. Journal of Endodontics 1995;21:159–60.
25. Saunders WP, Saunders EM. Coronal leakage as a cause of failure in root-canal therapy: a review. Endodontics and Dental Traumatology 1994;10:105–8.
26. Chugal NM, Clive JM, Spångberg LS. Endodontic infection: some biologic and treatment factors associated with outcome. Oral Surgery, Oral Medicine, Oral Pathology, Oral Radiology, and Endodontics 2003;96:81–90.
27. Chugal NM, Clive JM, Spångberg LS. Endodontic treatment outcome: effect of the permanent restoration. Oral Surgery, Oral Medicine, Oral Pathology, Oral Radiology and Endodontology 2007;104:576–82.
28. Kirkevang L-L, Væth M, Hörsted-Bindslev P, et al. Risk factors for developing apical periodontitis in a general population. International Endodontic Journal 2007;40:290–9.
29. Di Filippo G, Sidhu SK, Chong BS. Apical periodontitis and the technical quality of root canal treatment in an adult sub-population in London. British Dental Journal 2014;216:E22.
30. Ng Y-L, Mann V, Rahbaran S, et al. Outcome of primary root canal treatment: systematic review of the literature – Part 1. Effects of study characteristics on probability of success. International Endodontic Journal 2007;40:921–39.
31. Ng Y-L, Mann V, Rahbaran S, et al. Outcome of primary root canal treatment: systematic review of the literature – Part 2. Influence of clinical factors. International Endodontic Journal 2008;41:6–31.
32. American Association of Endodontists. Glossary of endodontic terms. 8th ed. Chicago: American Association of Endodontists; 2012.
33. European Society of Endodontology. Undergraduate curriculum guidelines for endodontology. International Endodontic Journal 2013;46:1105–14.
34. Miller WD. An introduction to the study of the bacteriopathology of the dental pulp. Dental Cosmos 1894;36: 505–28.
35. Onderdonk TW. Treatment of unfilled root canals. International Dental Journal 1901;22:20–2.
36. Bender IB, Seltzer S, Turkenkopf S. To culture or not to culture? Oral Surgery, Oral Medicine, Oral Pathology 1964; 18:527–40.
37. Seltzer S, Turkenkopf S, Vito A, et al. A histologic evaluation of periapical repair following positive and negative root canal cultures. Oral Surgery, Oral Medicine, Oral Pathology 1964;17:507–32.
38. Möller AJR Microbiological examination of root canals and periapical tissues of human teeth. Thesis, Akademiforlaget, Gothenberg, Sweden; 1966. p. 1–380.
39. Kantz WE, Henry CA. Isolation and classification of anaerobic bacteria from intact chambers of non-vital teeth in man. Archives of Oral Biology 1974;19:91–6.
40. Sundqvist G Bacteriological studies of necrotic dental pulps. Thesis. University of Umea, Sweden; 1976. p. 1–94.
41. Möller AJR, Fabricius L, Dahlén G, et al. Influence on periapical tissues of indigenous oral bacteria and necrotic pulp tissue in monkeys. Scandinavian Journal of Dental Research 1981 ;89:475–84.
42. Sundqvist G. Taxonomy, ecology, and pathogenicity of the root canal flora. Oral Surgery, Oral Medicine, Oral Pathology 1994;78:522–30.
43. Munson MA, Pitt-Ford T, Chong B, et al. Molecular and cultural analysis of the microflora associated with endodontic infections. Journal of Dental Research 2002;81:761–6.
44. Siqueira JF, Rôças IN. As-yet-uncultivated oral bacteria: breadth and association with oral and extra-oral diseases.

Journal of Oral Microbiology 2013;5:doi:10.3402/jom. v5i0.21077.

45. Siqueira JF, Rôças IN. Present status and future directions in endodontic microbiology. Endodontic Topics 2014;30:3–22.

46. Siqueira JF Jr, Rôças IN. Exploiting molecular methods to explore endodontic infections: Part 1 – Current molecular technologies for microbiological diagnosis. Journal of Endodontics 2005;31:411–23.

47. Siqueira JF Jr, Rôças IN. Exploiting molecular methods to explore endodontic infections: Part 2 – Redefining the endodontic microbiota. Journal of Endodontics 2005;31:488–98.

48. Fabricius L, Dahlén G, Holm SE, et al. Influence of combinations of oral bacteria on periapical tissues of monkeys. Scandinavian Journal of Dental Research 1982;90:200–6.

49. Peters LB, Wesselink PR, van Winkelhoff AJ. Combinations of bacterial species in endodontic infections. International Endodontic Journal 2002;35:698–702.

50. Fabricius L, Dahlén G, Öhman AE, et al. Predominant indigenous oral bacteria isolated from infected root canals after varied times of closure. Scandinavian Journal of Dental Research 1982;90:134–44.

51. Siqueira JF Jr, Rôças IN. Update on endodontic microbiology: candidate pathogens and patterns of colonisation. ENDO (Lond Engl) 2008;2:7–20.

52. Kakehashi S, Stanley HR, Fitzgerald RJ. The effects of surgical exposures of dental pulps in germ-free and conventional laboratory rats. Oral Surgery, Oral Medicine, Oral Pathology 1965;20:340–9.

53. Bergenholtz G, Cox CF, Loesche WJ, et al. Bacterial leakage around dental restorations: its effect on the pulp. Journal of Oral Pathology 1982;11:439–50.

54. Kiss C. Cell-to-cell interactions. Endodontic Topics 2004;8:88–103.

55. Holland GR, Botero TM. Pulp biology: 30 years of progress. Endodontic Topics 2014;31:19–35.

56. Bergenholtz G, Kvist T. Evidence-based endodontics. Endodontic Topics 2014;31:3–18.

57. Hurst D, Chong BS. Evidence-based dentistry: an introduction. ENDO (Lond Engl) 2012;6:283–8.

58. General Dental Council. Standards for the dental team. London: General Dental Council; 2013.

59. General Dental Council. Scope of practice. London: General Dental Council; 2013.

60. European Society of Endodontology. Quality guidelines for endodontic treatment: consensus report of the European Society of Endodontology. International Endodontic Journal 2006;31:921–30.

61. Chong BS. Absence of evidence is not evidence of absence. ENDO (Lond Engl) 2012;6:247.

62. Nehammer CF, Chong BS, Rattan R. Endodontics. Clinical Risk 2004;10:45–8.

63. Chong BS. No win, no fee. ENDO (Lond Engl) 2015;9:155–6.

64. Chong BS, Quinn A, Pawar RR, et al. The anatomical relationship between the roots of mandibular second molars and the inferior alveolar nerve. International Endodontic Journal 2015;48:549–55.

65. Patel J, Fox K, Grieveson B, et al. Undergraduate training as preparation for vocational training in England: a survey of vocational dental practitioners' and their trainers' views. British Dental Journal 2006;201:9–15.

66. Department of Health. NHS dental services in England. An independent review led by Professor Jimmy Steele. London: Department of Health Publications; 2009.

67. European Society of Endodontology. Accreditation of postgraduate speciality training programmes in Endodontology. Minimum criteria for training Specialists in Endodontology within Europe. International Endodontic Journal 2010;43:725–37.

68. Chong BS. Education is not the filling of a pail, but the lighting of a fire. ENDO (Lond Engl) 2014;8:175.

69. Ng YL, Mann V, Gulabivala K. Tooth survival following nonsurgical root canal treatment: a systematic review of the literature. International Endodontic Journal 2010;43:171–89.

70. Ng YL, Mann V, Gulabivala K. Outcome of secondary root canal treatment: a systematic review of the literature. International Endodontic Journal 2008;41:1026–46.

71. Ng YL, Mann V, Gulabivala K. A prospective study of the factors affecting outcomes of non-surgical root canal treatment: II: tooth survival. International Endodontic Journal 2011;44:610–25.

72. Ng YL, Mann V, Gulabivala K. A prospective study of the factors affecting outcomes of nonsurgical root canal treatment: I: periapical health. International Endodontic Journal 2011;44:583–609.

73. Chong BS. Highlighting deficiencies. British Dental Journal 2008;204:596–7.

74. Chong BS. Managing endodontic failure in practice. London: Quintessence Publishing Co. Ltd; 2004. p. 1–10.

75. Chong BS. A rose by any other name would smell as sweet. ENDO (Lond Engl) 2011;5:239–40.

76. Rechenberg D-K, Zehnder M. Molecular diagnostics in endodontics. Endodontic Topics 2014;30:51–65.

77. Banerjee A. Minimal intervention dentistry: VII: minimally invasive operative caries management: rationale and techniques. British Dental Journal 2013;214:107–11.

78. Kelleher M. Porcelain pornography. Faculty Dental Journal 2011;2:134–41.

79. Dawson VS, Amjad S, Fransson H. Endodontic complications in teeth with vital pulps restored with composite resins: a systematic review. International Endodontic Journal 2015;48:627–38.

80. Smith AJ, Smith JG, Shelton RM, et al. Harnessing the natural regenerative potential of the dental pulp. Dental Clinics of North America 2012;56:589–601.

81. Chong BS. Regenerative endodontics – fact or pulp fiction? ENDO (Lond Engl) 2010;4:251–2.

82. Mao JJ, Kim SG, Zhou J, et al. Regenerative endodontics: barriers and strategies for clinical translation. Dental Clinics of North America 2012;56:639–49.

83. Goodis HE, Kinaia BM, Kinaia AM, et al. Regenerative endodontics and tissue engineering: what the future holds? Dental Clinics of North America 2012;56:677–89.

84. Albuquerque MTP, Valera MC, Nakashima M, et al. Tissue-engineering-based strategies for regenerative endodontics. Journal of Dental Research 2014;93:1222–31.

85. Wu M-K, Dummer PMH, Wesselink PR. Consequences of and strategies to deal with residual post-treatment root canal infection. International Endodontic Journal 2006;39:343–56.

86. Chávez de Paz LE, Davies JR, Bergenholtz G, et al. Strains of *Enterococcus faecalis* differ in their ability to coexist in biofilms with other root canal bacteria. International Endodontic Journal 2015;48:916–25.

87. Svensäter G, Bergenholtz G. Biofilms in endodontic infections. Endodontic Topics 2004;9:27–36.

88. Di Filippo G, Sidhu SK, Chong BS. The role of biofilms in endodontic treatment failure. ENDO (Lond Engl) 2014;8:87–103.

89. Otomo-Corgel J, Pucher JJ, Rethman MP, et al. State of the science: chronic periodontitis and systemic health. Journal of Evidence-Based Dental Practice 2012;12:20–8.

90. Ide M, Linden GJ. Periodontitis, cardiovascular disease and pregnancy outcome – focal infection revisited? British Dental Journal 2014;217:467–74.

91. Tjäderhane L. Endodontic infections and systemic health – where should we go? International Endodontic Journal 2015;48:911–12.

92. van der Waal SV, Lappin DF, Crielaard W. Does apical periodontitis have systemic consequences? The need for well-planned and carefully conducted clinical studies. British Dental Journal 2015;218:513–16.

93. Segura-Egea JJ, Martín-González J, Castellanos-Cosano L. Endodontic medicine: connections between apical periodontitis and systemic diseases. International Endodontic Journal 2015;48:933–51.

94. Cotti E, Mercuro G. Apical periodontitis and cardiovascular diseases: previous findings and ongoing research. International Endodontic Journal 2015;48:926–32.

95. Patel S, Dawood A, Whaites E, et al. New dimensions in endodontic imaging: Part 1. Conventional and alternative radiographic systems. International Endodontic Journal 2009;42:447–62.

96. Patel S. New dimensions in endodontic imaging:II. Cone beam computed tomography. International Endodontic Journal 2009;42:463–75.

97. Chong BS. 'VOMIT' and 'Incidentaloma'. ENDO (Lond Engl) 2015;9:3–4.

98. Kersten DD, Mines P, Sweet M. Use of the microscope in endodontics: results of a questionnaire. Journal of Endodontics 2008;34:804–7.

99. Kim S, Baek S. The microscope and endodontics. Dental Clinics of North America 2004;48:11–18.

100. Del Fabbro M, Taschieri S, Lodi G, et al. Magnification devices for endodontic therapy. Cochrane Database of Systematic Reviews 2009;(3):Art. No.:CD005969,doi:10.1002/14651858.CD005969.pub2.

101. Perrin P, Neuhaus KW, Lussi A. The impact of loupes and microscopes on vision in endodontics. International Endodontic Journal 2014;47:425–9.

102. Hülsmann M, Peters OA, Dummer PMH. Mechanical preparation of root canals: shaping goals, techniques and means. Endodontic Topics 2005;10:30–76.

103. Young GR, Parashos P, Messer HH. The principles of techniques for cleaning root canals. Australian Dental Journal 2007;52:S52–63.

104. Peters OA. Current challenges and concepts in the preparation of root canal systems: a review. Journal of Endodontics 2004;30:559–67.

105. Chong BS, Pitt Ford TR. Root-end filling materials: rationale & tissue response. Endodontic Topics 2005;11:114–30.

106. Chong BS, Rhodes JS. Endodontic surgery. British Dental Journal 2014;216:281–90.

107. Chong BS, Pitt Ford TR, Hudson MB. A prospective clinical study of Mineral Trioxide Aggregate and IRM when used as root-end filling materials in endodontic surgery. International Endodontic Journal 2003;36:520–6.

108. Haapasalo M, Parhar M, Huang X, et al. Clinical use of bioceramic materials. Endodontic Topic 2015;32:97–117.

109. Wang Z. Bioceramic materials in endodontics. Endodontic Topics 2015;32:3–30.

110. Camilleri J. Mineral trioxide aggregate: present and future developments. Endodontic Topics 2015;32:31–46.

111. Trope M, Bunes A, Debelian G. Root filling materials and techniques: bioceramics a new hope? Endodontic Topics 2015;32:86–96.

112. Zitzmann NU, Krastl G, Hecker H, et al. Endodontics or implants? A review of decisive criteria and guidelines for single tooth restorations and full arch reconstructions. International Endodontic Journal 2009;42:757–74.

113. Zitzmann NU, Krastl G, Hecker H, et al. Strategic considerations in treatment planning: deciding when to treat, extract, or replace a questionable tooth. Journal of Prosthetic Dentistry 2010;104:80–91.

114. Silvestrin T. The role of implant dentistry in the specialty of endodontics. Endodontic Topics 2014;30:66–74.

115. Pennington MW, Vernazza CR, Shackley P, et al. Evaluation of the cost-effectiveness of root canal treatment using conventional approaches versus replacement with an implant. International Endodontic Journal 2009;42:874–83.

116. Chong BS, Miller J, Sidhu S. The quality of radiographs accompanying endodontic referrals to a health authority clinic. British Dental Journal 2015;219:69–72.

117. Derks J, Tomasi C. Peri-implant health and disease. A systematic review of current epidemiology. Journal of Clinical Periodontology 2015;42:S158–71.

118. Vernazza CR, Steele JG, Whitworth JM, et al. Factors affecting direction and strength of patient preferences for treatment of molar teeth with nonvital pulps. International Endodontic Journal 2015;48:1137–46.

CHAPTER 2

General and Systemic Aspects of Endodontics

M. P. Escudier

Chapter Contents

Summary

A patient's general health may have an effect on endodontic treatments. In addition, pain is the predominant complaint associated with endodontic disease. This chapter will cover the potential effects of several systemic conditions and disorders, as well as medications, on the treatment planning and management of endodontic patients; the diagnosis of orofacial pain of both odontogenic and nonodontogenic origin and the use of antibiotics and analgesics in endodontic cases.

Introduction

The treatment of pulpal and periradicular infections with the use of modern endodontic techniques is safe and effective provided they are appropriately applied and undertaken by competent clinicians. In line with this, a full assessment of both the medical history and clinical presentation should be undertaken before commencing treatment. Comprehensive and sensible treatment planning based on a careful analysis of the information gathered will help to protect the patient from harm and the clinician from criticism, legal or otherwise.

The clinician largely depends on the medical history to identify systemic disease or treatment that may affect patient management. Therefore, it is vital that the medical history is comprehensive and regularly updated. In addition, any areas of uncertainty or concern should, if possible, be discussed with the patient's physician before commencing active treatment. Many patients have systemic disorders which are well controlled and managed medically; they are unlikely to influence the outcome of the dental treatment. However, the medical treatment itself may influence the management, for example, patients taking prednisolone or warfarin.

The assessment will initially consist of the history and a clinical examination, which together will provide a differential diagnosis. It should be remembered that the history is the single most important factor in arriving at a diagnosis.[1] However, the clinical examination and subsequent investigations will increase the confidence of the clinician in reaching a diagnosis, even though they may contribute relatively few new facts.[2]

The fear of transmission of human immunodeficiency virus (HIV) or hepatitis viruses, as well as prions, has highlighted the importance of applying the current guidelines for infection control and decontamination in endodontics, as in any other aspect of clinical dentistry.[3]

Differential Diagnosis of Dental Pain

The commonest cause of pain in the orofacial region is dental disease leading to pulpal pain (see also Chapter 5). As such, dental surgeons should be experienced and competent in the diagnosis and management of odontogenic pain. However, the differential diagnosis of pain in the teeth, jaws and face is far wider than is sometimes appreciated. Pain may be nonodontogenic:

- referred from a distant origin (e.g. cardiac);
- have an unusual local cause (e.g. osteomyelitis);
- psychogenic in origin (e.g. atypical (persistent) facial pain);
- neurologic (e.g. trigeminal neuralgia);
- modified by apparently unrelated factors (e.g. previous cerebrovascular accident).

A broader diagnostic sieve should be remembered,[4] particularly if the pattern of presentation is unusual, the examination findings are sparse or conflicting or if pain persists or develops in spite of apparently successful treatment.[5]

The essence of good clinical practice is a methodical and disciplined approach: a history, followed by examination, special investigations (usually radiographic), analysis and conclusion. Orofacial pain has been extremely well dealt with in other texts.[6,7]

TABLE 2-1	**Pain History**	
Duration	When did your pain start? Have you ever experienced pain like this before?
Character	What type of pain is it?
Periodicity	When do you get the pain? Does it come and go? Is there any particular pattern to the pain?
Severity	How severe is your pain?
Site	Where is your pain?
Radiation	Does your pain spread to other areas?
Provoking factors	Does anything make your pain worse?
Relieving factors	Does anything make your pain better?
Associated factors	Have you noticed anything else about your pain?

PAIN HISTORY

A thorough, structured pain history will provide a diagnosis in the majority of cases and will help to identify those areas in need of further investigation. This should commence with the patient being asked to describe the pain in their own words, before being asked direct questions. Certain core information should be elicited in all cases (Table 2-1).[6,7]

EXAMINATION

The assessment of a patient starts with their entry into the clinical setting. This will enable observation of the patient's general demeanour, as well as any locomotor problems such as walking aids or possible neurological deficits. It may also enable identification of a facial swelling, and particular attention should be paid to facial symmetry, notably that of the cheeks, mandibular angle region and nasolabial folds. Observation of the patient's face during history taking may reveal a subtle neurological feature requiring a formal assessment of cranial nerve function. An assessment of the level of pain can be made using the facial expression,[8] although it is important to remember that facial expressions can be manipulated. Hence, avoiding or flinching from an examination may be a more accurate indicator of a trigger spot or tenderness than responses to questioning during examination. The observation of mandibular movements is the essential preliminary to examination of temporomandibular joint function.[9]

The features of a comprehensive examination of the teeth and jaws are described in Chapter 3. The soft tissues of the cheeks, palate, tongue and floor of the mouth may also yield vital and relevant information. The necessity of a detailed occlusal examination depends on the history and clinical setting. Similarly, the history will determine the necessity or desirability of a formal assessment of the temporomandibular apparatus. The maxillary sinus as a cause of pain is considered later in this chapter. Thermal or electrical stimulation of suspect teeth, differential local anaesthetic injections and removal of restorations all have their place in diagnosis. In addition, radiography is usually essential, but all these techniques must supplement, but never replace, the history and clinical examination.

PERSISTENT OROFACIAL PAIN

The orofacial region, including the teeth, is a common site for the expression of pain or discomfort as a manifestation of underlying psychosocial disharmony. It may represent anything from a plea for help to a symptom of frank psychosis. The dental surgeon should avoid being manipulated by the patient or their relatives into undertaking treatment when the diagnosis is uncertain or the evidence is conflicting. In such circumstances, it is better to defer active, irreversible treatment until a definitive diagnosis can be obtained. In many such cases, the pain will either resolve spontaneously or there will be further evidence to assist in the diagnosis in due course (e.g. the development of a hemifacial rash of herpes zoster). A review appointment should be arranged with the caveat that the patient may return sooner should the need arise. The dental practitioner also has the opportunity to refer the patient for a second opinion at any time, particularly if the diagnosis continues to remain unclear.

Certain features in the history often help in the diagnosis of persistent (idiopathic) facial pain. The pain is often unremitting and may have been present for months or even years. The stated severity may be out of proportion to the observed level of distress,

disturbance of life or self-therapy. The pain may not follow anatomical boundaries and may be described as throbbing, nagging, aching, miserable or cruel in nature. It does not usually disturb sleep, although there may be coincident disturbance of sleep pattern, and simple analgesics, such as ibuprofen, are classically reported to only 'take the edge off' the pain. In addition, other chronic pain conditions, such as headache, low back pain and abdominal or pelvic pain, are often present. There may also be obvious secondary gain (family or social) for the sufferer. In such cases, it is important to seek further information in relation to the patient's social history and family circumstances. There is often a history of long-term or recent distressing life events such as bereavement, divorce or job loss.[6,7]

Depression is common in patients with chronic pain and may be effectively detected by two simple questions[10]: (1) During the last month have you often been bothered by feeling down, depressed or hopeless? and (2) During the past month have you been bothered by having little interest or pleasure in doing things? Psychiatric treatment or psychotherapy is often beneficial and may be curative. Such cases are often best referred to an oral physician as direct referral to a psychiatrist may be met with difficulties.

Recently, the International Research Diagnostic Criteria for Temporomandibular Disorders (RDC/TMD) Consortium of the International Association of Dental Research (IADR) proposed an ontological approach to reclassify persistent pain perceived within the dentoalveolar region as persistent dentoalveolar pain disorder (PDAP).[11] The diagnostic criteria for PDAP, a subset of chronic orofacial pain, were formulated to model the taxonomical structure of all orofacial pain conditions. The aim of the RDC/TMD Consortium is to foster evidence-based diagnosis and management of orofacial pain and jaw disorders.

Maxillary Sinus

The close proximity of the maxillary sinuses to the maxillary teeth can make the diagnosis of pain difficult. The distinction between pain of dental origin and sinusitis may be helped by the presence of obvious dental disease or a typical acute or recurrent sinusitis with nasal discharge. Acute sinusitis rarely occurs without preceding symptoms of 'a cold' and tenderness to pressure of a whole quadrant of teeth is characteristic. In such cases, the use of broad-spectrum antibiotics (e.g. amoxicillin 500 mg for 7–14 days) may be of benefit.[12] However, the clinician will need to weigh the small benefits of the antibiotic treatment against the potential for adverse effects at both the individual and general population levels.[12] Periradicular infection of premolar or molar teeth may lead to purulent discharge into the sinus with associated pain. A further consideration is the risk of penetration of the sinus wall or even the sinus lining by endodontic instruments or during periradicular surgery. This may result in acute sinusitis from bacterial contamination of the sinus. The condition may resolve spontaneously, but the prescription of a broad-spectrum antibiotic and nasal decongestant is usual practice.

Small oro-antral communications usually heal spontaneously, and in the case of periradicular surgery, the replacement of the surgical flap is sufficient to seal the opening. The identity of microorganisms involved in a sinus infection is often unclear, and broad-spectrum antibiotics (amoxicillin 500 mg three times a day) may be required. It is typical to continue therapy for 5 days, although a one-off 3 g dose of amoxicillin is equally effective. If there is a poor drainage of the sinus (e.g., a history of chronic sinusitis), nasal drops (0.5% ephedrine) should be prescribed. In addition, the inhalation of relieving agents, such as menthol and eucalyptus, can have a soothing effect and may be of benefit.

A connection between sinus disease and root canal treatment has been reported[13]; aspergillosis of the maxillary antrum resulted after root canal treatment with zinc oxide-based cements, which are known to promote cultures of aspergillus.

Systemic Disease and Endodontics

Disabled or debilitated patients cannot be expected to readily tolerate complex and lengthy treatment procedures. However, even in cases of severe ill health, some patients have a strong desire to retain their natural teeth. It is the dentist's duty to try to accommodate the patient's request. Even in terminal illness, simple treatment can greatly aid comfort, masticatory function and morale. Good decision-making is dependent on frank and thoughtful discussion with the patient and health team involved in the patient's care. In conditions such as cardiac abnormalities, endodontic treatment should only be conducted if a high standard of treatment can be achieved, which may involve referral to a specialist.

Both the patient's general health prognosis and the prognosis of the tooth being treated must be considered; this may lead to the decision to extract the tooth rather than undertake complex root canal treatment. In chronic diseases that are subject to cyclical remission, either spontaneous or facilitated by treatment, it is sensible to defer dental intervention until optimum physical health is achieved. This is particularly true of haematological disorders such as leukaemia, especially if the patient receives periodic transfusion or cycles of chemotherapy. Sufferers from haemorrhagic diatheses will not require factor replacement or antifibrinolytic therapy for nonsurgical root canal treatment, but they may be required if local anaesthetic is needed or endodontic surgery is to be undertaken. In all such cases, the patient's haematologist should be consulted to discuss any necessary preoperative and perioperative measures.

The evidence demonstrating that the presence of systemic disease has a major influence on the healing of periradicular lesions has been inconclusive.[14] However, there is evidence that patients with diabetes mellitus have a higher prevalence of periradicular lesions, more significant-sized osteolytic lesions, an increased risk of asymptomatic infections and poorer prognosis for root-filled teeth.[15] The pulps of patients with diabetes mellitus tend to have limited collateral circulation, impaired immune response and a higher risk of becoming infected.[16]

Progressive narrowing of pulp chambers and root canals due to excessive dentine formation in patients receiving substantial doses of corticosteroids after renal transplantation has also been observed.[17] There is no need for antibiotic prophylaxis when undertaking dental treatment in these patients, although some renal transplant units still advise the need for prophylaxis. In such circumstances, it would be advisable to discuss the individual case with the renal unit concerned.

ENDODONTICS AND INFECTIVE ENDOCARDITIS

Infective endocarditis (IE) is an uncommon but life-threatening condition with an overall mortality of

20%. Since 1955, antibiotic prophylaxis has been recommended for at-risk individuals on the basis that endocarditis usually followed bacteraemia arising from certain dental procedures and the bacteria responsible were usually sensitive to antibiotics.[18] However, the British Society for Antimicrobial Chemotherapy[19] and the American Heart Association[20] have challenged this dogma by highlighting the common occurrence of bacteraemias that arise from everyday activities such as toothbrushing, the lack of association between episodes of IE and prior interventional procedures and the questionable efficacy of antibiotic prophylaxis regimens. Against this background, in the UK, the Department of Health asked the National Institute for Health and Care Excellence (NICE) to assess the evidence. After conducting a review of the available scientific evidence, in 2008, NICE recommended that people at risk of developing IE undergo dental procedures[21]:

- antibiotic prophylaxis is not recommended;
- chlorhexidine mouthwash should not be offered;
- any episodes of infection should be investigated and treated promptly to reduce the risk of endocarditis developing.

NICE also recommended that healthcare professionals should offer people at risk of IE clear and consistent information about prevention; these include the following:

- benefits and risks of antibiotic prophylaxis, and an explanation as to why antibiotic prophylaxis is no longer routinely recommended;
- importance of maintaining good oral health;
- symptoms that may indicate IE and when to seek expert advice;
- risks of undergoing invasive procedures, including nonmedical procedures such as body piercing or tattooing.

Since the introduction of the NICE guidelines,[21] several studies have analyzed the changes in IE epidemiology; the results have shown no increase in the incidence of infective endocarditis.[22-24] An analysis of hospital discharge episode statistics and prescribing patterns[25] recently showed a small but significant increase in the incidence of IE since 2008; 0.11 cases per 10 million people per month (95% CI 0.05–0.16) over the projected historical trend, which by March 2013 would account for an excess of 35 cases per month. This increase was seen in all patients at risk of IE and corresponded to a decrease in the use of antibiotic prophylaxis of almost 90% over the same period. In the absence of any prospective randomized clinical trials, the implications of the various studies remain unclear.[26] NICE recently conducted a review and concluded that any increase in the incidence of IE has not been well understood and may be due to a number of factors; hence, no new recommendations have been added.[27]

ENDODONTICS IN PATIENTS WITH PROSTHETIC JOINTS

There is no special risk to patients with hip or knee prostheses from any form of dental treatment and certainly not from endodontic procedures.[28] However, some orthopaedic patients are still advised regarding the need for antibiotic prophylaxis; in such cases, it would be advisable to discuss the individual situation with the orthopaedic surgeon concerned.

ENDODONTICS IN PATIENTS TAKING ANTICOAGULANT OR ANTIPLATELET MEDICATIONS

Newer oral anticoagulant and antiplatelet drugs are currently available[29,30]; they are increasingly being prescribed, and therefore, more likely to be encountered in patients presenting for dental treatment. These patients can have a higher risk of bleeding after invasive dental procedures.

Oral Anticoagulants

Vitamin K Antagonists. These include warfarin, adenocoumarol and phenindione, which have an indirect effect on the production of clotting factors. The anticoagulant effect of these drugs is measured by the International Normalized Ratio (INR), which due to the nature of the action of these drugs, takes several days to alter after a change in dosage. As these drugs interact with many other medications, it is sensible to check for any possible interactions before prescribing any drugs for patients taking a Vitamin K antagonist.

Of these, warfarin is the most commonly used oral anticoagulant and the desired therapeutic range (deep vein thrombosis INR 2.0–3.0, prosthetic heart valve INR 3.0–4.0) and duration of treatment varies depending on the medical condition. In such patients, the first question to ask is whether the warfarin therapy is to be discontinued at any time. If so, then a decision can be made as to whether the proposed treatment can be deferred until that time. However, if treatment is required or the warfarin therapy is ongoing, altering the INR will need to be considered. Warfarin therapy should not be stopped or altered before dental treatment without the agreement of the anticoagulant team. Endodontic treatment with or without local anaesthesia (except inferior alveolar nerve blocks) can safely be undertaken with an INR of 4.0 or less and provided that the INR is stable.[31,32] Periradicular surgery, involving raising a mucoperiosteal flap and bone removal, is best avoided in cases with an INR of 2.5, as are inferior alveolar nerve blocks. In all cases, the INR should be formally checked within 24 hours, before the procedure and ideally on the day of treatment.[31] Patients presenting with an INR much higher than their normal value, even if it is less than 4.0, should have their procedure postponed and should be referred back to the clinician maintaining their anticoagulant therapy.[31]

There are now anticoagulants that do not require regular blood test monitoring of the INR.

Factor X Inhibitors. The drugs rivaroxaban and apixaban are both administered orally and act by directly inhibiting activated Factor X. It is useful to clarify the anticipated duration of treatment as where this is likely to be of a short duration, such as after orthopaedic surgery, it may be possible to defer dental intervention until the medication has been stopped. However, in a dental emergency or in cases in which the medication is being used on a longer-term basis, such as in the management of deep vein thrombosis, pulmonary embolism or atrial fibrillation, its effect on coagulation will need to be considered. Fortunately, its anticoagulant effect is equivalent to a patient on warfarin with a target INR of 2.0 to 3.0. In view of this, the predictable nature of the medication and the absence of a routine blood test to monitor anticoagulant activity, these patients do not require preoperative blood tests and can be safely managed with local measures. However, where practical, the number of teeth to be extracted at a single visit should be limited to 3 to 4, and it is advisable to assess the extent of bleeding after the extraction of the first tooth.

Thrombin Inhibitors. Dabigatran etexilate is a direct thrombin inhibitor administered orally and is generally used in atrial fibrillation. Its anticoagulant effect is similar to that of the Factor X inhibitors, and hence, patients taking this medication can be managed in the same manner.

Antiplatelet Medications

These medications inhibit the aggregation of platelets and so suppress the first phase of haemostasis.[33] As cessation, or modification, of the antiplatelet therapy is associated with an increased risk of thromboembolic events, it should be avoided unless conducted under medical supervision.

The original antiplatelet medication was aspirin, the use of its low doses is unlikely to pose significant problems provided appropriate local measures are used.[34] In recent years, a number of other medications have become more common and include clopidogrel, dipyridamole, prasugrel and ticagrelor. These may all be used alone or in combination, usually with aspirin or sometimes with coumarin.

Patients on a single antiplatelet drug or dual antiplatelet therapy (DAPT) such as aspirin/dipyridamole, have an increased risk of bleeding, but this may not be clinically significant. Hence, treatment can proceed with appropriate local measures.[35]

Patients taking aspirin in combination with clopidogrel or prasugrel have an increased risk of postoperative bleeding.[36] They may also have an unstable cardiac problem and/or have recently undergone cardiology interventions such as 'stenting'. In these cases, the medical status and need to continue the antiplatelet therapy may mean that the dental treatment is best postponed, at least until the period of DAPT is over.

ENDODONTICS IN PATIENTS TAKING CORTICOSTEROIDS

Corticosteroids may be administered topically, via an inhaler or systemically. Systemic corticosteroids taken at a dose higher than 7.5 mg (10 mg in some guidelines) daily for over a month or in high doses (>40 mg per day) for periods as short as a week, may cause adrenocortical suppression. In the case of high doses for short periods ('pulsed'), the effects are not clinically significant after a month off treatment. Therefore, deferral of treatment until after this time would be prudent. In the case of long-term corticosteroid therapy, prophylaxis is required and is best administered either orally or intravenously. Two regimes may be used depending on the preference of the patient and clinician. The first requires that the patient double the normal daily dose on the day before, the day of, and the day after treatment. The second is a one-off dose of 100 mg hydrocortisone administered orally 1 h before treatment or intravenously a few minutes before treatment.

It should also be noted that some inhaled corticosteroids (e.g. fluticasone) may cause adrenal suppression. Similarly, potent topical corticosteroids (e.g. Eumovate (clobetasone butyrate)) prescribed by dermatologists and applied to large areas, particularly if ulcerated, may also produce suppression and require corticosteroid prophylaxis before dental treatment.

ENDODONTICS IN PATIENTS TAKING ANTIRESORPTIVE AGENTS

The relevance of these drugs to the dental surgeon is their association with osteonecrosis of the jaws after dental intervention. It was originally termed *bisphosphonates osteonecrosis of the jaw (BRONJ)* due to its association with the drug commonly used to reduce the morbidity associated with osteoporosis, as well as other osteoclast-mediated bone diseases such as osteopenia, fibrous dysplasia, Paget's disease, multiple myeloma and metastatic bone cancer. More recently, osteonecrosis has been seen in association with non-bisphosphonate antiresorptives (e.g. denosumab), for which the term *antiresorptive osteonecrosis of the jaw (ARONJ)* was introduced.[37] The overarching term of *medication-related osteonecrosis of the jaw (MRONJ)* has been suggested.[38]

The diagnosis of MRONJ requires that there is a history of exposure to bisphosphonates/antiresorptive medications, that there is an exposed bone within the oral cavity for at least 6 to 8 weeks, and that there is no history of prior radiation therapy to the jaws.

The current view that the condition is caused by the effect of the medication on osteoclast function is based on two facts:

- the predilection of the condition for the jaws where bisphosphonate-mediated suppression of bone remodelling is most profound due to greater bone turnover rates[39,40];

- that denosumab, a completely humanized antibody, which inhibits the receptor activator of nuclear factor kappa-B ligand (RANKL), found on the surface of osteoblasts, profoundly suppresses osteoclast function and bone remodeling.[37]

The risk of bisphosphonate-associated osteonecrosis (BON) is related to the type, dose and duration of bisphosphonate therapy and the nature of the dental intervention. Intravenous bisphosphonate therapy (pamidronate and zoledronate) confers a much higher risk of BON (up to 20%) than oral therapy (alendronate, risedronate and ibandronate) where the risk is 0 to 0.04%.[41]

The risk of developing BRONJ after dental intervention is associated with:
- Recent dento-alveolar trauma[42]
- Duration of bisphosphonate therapy[43]
  - Oral: >3 years with a linear increase thereafter
  - Intravenous: mean 9 months
- Potency of bisphosphonate[41]
  Oral (alendronate, risedronate, ibandronate): 0.0–0.04%
  Intravenous (pamidronate, zoledronate): up to 20%
- Concomitant corticosteroid therapy or chemotherapy

Denosumab has been reported to be equally problematic as intravenous bisphosphonates.[37]

Therefore, with patients on antiresorptive agents, endodontic treatment is preferred over extraction if a tooth is restorable. Routine endodontic technique should be used, although manipulation beyond the apex is to be avoided[41]; it is important to maintain length control with all endodontic procedures.

If extractions or bone surgery are necessary, the patient should be stratified as either low or high risk and managed according to appropriate guidelines,[38,44,45] which will involve informing the patient of the risk of MRONJ and consideration of alternative treatment options. In some situations, depending on risk, removal of the clinical crown and endodontic treatment to allow passive exfoliation of the remaining root may be appropriate. In all cases, a conservative surgical technique should be adopted with primary closure, if possible.[41] In addition, immediately before and after any surgical procedures involving bone, the patient should be instructed to rinse gently with a chlorhexidine-containing mouthwash until the wound has healed. The regimen may be extended depending on the progress of healing. The use of prophylactic antibiotics after a surgical procedure should be based on the risk of developing an infection and not on the patient's bisphosphonate therapy. There is no evidence that the use of antibiotics is effective in preventing MRONJ.[41]

Use of Antibiotics in Endodontics

Antibiotics or other antimicrobial drugs are either bactericidal (kill susceptible bacteria) or bacteriostatic (arrest their multiplication), thereby allowing the natural defense processes to combat infection and healing to progress (Table 2-2). They do not relieve pain or reduce swelling, and given the lack of sufficient evidence of effectiveness, antibiotics should not be used to treat irreversible pulpitis.[46,47] There is only very low-quality evidence, which is considered insufficient to determine the effects of systemic antibiotics on adults with symptomatic apical periodontitis or acute apical abscess.[48] Hence, antibiotics should be reserved for controlling a spreading cellulitis or if there are signs of systemic involvement of infection. Overuse should be avoided to prevent further increase in resistant strains of microorganisms,[49] and adherence to clinical guidelines is recommended.[50] The *Antibiotic Guardian* campaign was launched recently by Public Health England (PHE) as part of activities to support *European Antibiotic Awareness Day,* a public health initiative aimed at encouraging the responsible use of antibiotics. This is further reinforced by antimicrobial stewardship guidelines recently released by both PHE and NICE.[51,52]

Ideally, apart from a history of allergy, the choice of antibiotic should be based on the results of identification and sensitivity testing of the microorganisms responsible for the infection. This is seldom feasible in practice and requires culture techniques in a laboratory setting, as simple Gram staining and microscopy are often of little help. However, most bacteria associated with dentoalveolar infection are still sensitive to penicillins and hence, if not allergic, phenoxymethylpenicillin 250 mg or 500 mg, four times a day for 5 days, depending on the severity of the infection, is appropriate.[50] Amoxicillin 250 mg, three times a day for 5 days, may be preferred because of its efficient absorption. Metronidazole 200 mg or 400 mg, three times a day for 3 to 5 days, will assist in the elimination of anaerobes and may be used alone or in combination with a penicillin. The newer penicillinase-resistant antibiotic Augmentin (amoxicillin 250 mg and clavulanic acid 125 mg) may be preferred for ease of use and patient compliance. A potential unwanted side effect of the use of broad-spectrum antibiotics is interference with the absorption of the oestrogen component of combined oral contraceptives, with a consequent loss of effect. Women taking such preparations concurrently should be advised not to rely on this method of contraception alone for 1 month after the end of the antibiotic course. In addition, antibiotics are known to potentiate the action of warfarin, which may upset the therapeutic control. The patient should therefore be advised to contact their anticoagulant centre for appropriate follow-up.

Control of Pain and Anxiety

Pain and anxiety control are central to successful endodontic treatment. Drugs available for local analgesia and for sedation are both safe and effective, but as with any potent therapeutic agents, they need to be used with skill and discretion, particularly in patients who are taking other medications regularly. A whole spectrum of techniques for controlling pain and anxiety are applicable in endodontics as in other dental treatment. These range from simple persuasion and a comforting and sympathetic manner to sedation. Local anaesthetic techniques are well established, and 2 to 4 mL of lignocaine (lidocaine) 2% with 1:80 000 adrenaline (epinephrine) is a safe and effective

TABLE 2-2   **Useful Antibacterial Drugs**
Treatment of Infections
Phenoxymethylpenicillin capsules, 250 mg
One or two 6 hourly, at least 30 minutes before food, for 4–7 days
Amoxicillin capsules, 250 mg
One or two 8 hourly for 4–7 days
Augmentin capsules, 375 mg
One or two 8 hourly for 4–7 days
Metronidazole tablets, 200 mg
One or two 8 hourly for 3–5 days

TABLE 2-3   **Useful Analgesics**
Mild to Moderate Pain
Aspirin tablets or aspirin tablets dispersible, 300 mg 　　One to three every 4–6 hours as necessary, maximum 　　　4 g/day Paracetamol tablets, 500 mg 　　One to two every 6 hours as necessary, maximum 　　　4 g/day Ibuprofen tablets, 200 mg 　　One to two every 4–6 hours as necessary, preferably 　　　after food, maximum 2.4 g/day
Moderate to Severe Pain
Dihydrocodeine tablets, 30 mg 　　30 mg every 4–6 hours as necessary after food, 　　　maximum 1.8 g/day
Severe Pain
Pethidine tablets, 50 mg 　　One to two every 4 hours, maximum 6 g/day

preparation for all patients. An aspirating syringe system should be used to avoid inadvertent intravascular injection. Only in very rare cases where true allergy to lidocaine is proven, should an alternative solution (e.g. prilocaine with felypressin) be used.

Conscious sedation using either an inhaled mixture of nitrous oxide and oxygen, or intravenous administration of midazolam, is a safe and effective way of overcoming anxiety. Such techniques are only rarely required for root canal treatment; however, sedation may more often be required for periradicular surgery.

ANALGESICS

Analgesics may be used to treat existing pain or to reduce postoperative pain (Table 2-3). Analgesics administered preoperatively, as a pre-emptive measure, are useful in reducing postoperative pain. Aspirin and paracetamol (acetaminophen) remain the most effective and widely used remedies for local pain of mild to moderate severity. Aspirin is contraindicated in patients with peptic ulcerations, bleeding diatheses or who are taking systemic corticosteroids. Its use is also not advised in children because of the risk of causing Reye's syndrome. When paracetamol is used, it is

essential to warn patients not to exceed the daily maximum dose of 4 g because of the risk of severe and sometimes fatal liver damage. Other nonsteroidal antiinflammatory drugs (NSAIDs), such as ibuprofen, may be used if preferred and may be used in combination with paracetamol if required.

Dihydrocodeine tartrate is used to relieve more severe pain but frequently causes unpleasant side effects, including dizziness and nausea, and may prove ineffective. On rare occasions when severe pain persists, pethidine 50 mg, one or two tablets every 4 hours, can be administered and the patient's condition is reviewed the next day.

Local treatment (e.g. drainage and irrigation of a root canal) rendering a tooth free of occlusal contact, replacement of a failed temporary filling after root canal cleaning or irrigation of a surgical wound are far more effective ways of dealing with pain than the indiscriminate use of analgesics.

Dental Practitioner's Formulary

The *Dental Practitioner's Formulary*, which is published together with the *British National Formulary*[28] and jointly by the British Medical Association and the Royal Pharmaceutical Society of Great Britain, is a succinct and authoritative guide to prescribing for the dentist and is regularly updated. It is an invaluable source of advice and information and should be available in every dental surgery. The sections on antibiotics and analgesics, as well as information on potential drug interactions, prescribing during pregnancy and medical emergencies in dental practice, are particularly useful. Further information on medical aspects of dentistry is available in textbooks such as *Scully's Medical Problems in Dentistry*.[53]

Learning Outcomes

After completing this chapter, the reader should be able to explain and discuss the:
- differential diagnosis of orofacial pain;
- relevance of concurrent, systemic disease, as well as medications, to treatment planning and management of endodontic patients;
- use of analgesics and antibiotics in endodontic patients.

REFERENCES

1. Hampton JR, Harrison MJ, Mitchell JR, et al. Relative contributions of history-taking, physical examination and laboratory investigations to diagnosis and management of medical outpatients. British Medical Journal 1975;2: 486–9.
2. Roshan M, Rao AP. A study on relative contributions of the history, physical examination and investigations in making medical diagnosis. Journal of the Association of Physicians of India 2000;48:771–5.
3. Department of Health. The Health and Social Care Act 2008: Code of Practice on the prevention and control of infections and related guidance, <https://www.gov.uk/government/uploads/system/uploads/attachment_data/file/449049/Code_of_practice_280715_acc.pdf>; 2010.
4. Yatani H, Komiyama O, Matsuka Y, et al. Systematic review and recommendations for nonodontogenic toothache. Journal of Oral Rehabilitation 2014;41:843–52.
5. Nixdorf DR, Moana-Filho EJ, Law AS, et al. Frequency of persistent tooth pain after root canal therapy: a systematic review and meta-analysis. Journal of Endodontics 2010;36: 224–30.
6. Zakrzewska J, Harrison SD. Assessment and management of orofacial pain. Pain research and clinical management series, vol. 14. Amsterdam: Elsevier; 2002.
7. Zakrzewska JM, editor. Orofacial pain. Oxford, UK: Oxford University Press; 2009.
8. Solomon PE, Prkahin KM, Farewell V. Enhancing sensitivity to facial expression of pain. Pain 1997;71:279–84.
9. Royal College of Surgeons of England. Temporomandibular disorders (TMDs): an update and management guidance for primary care from the UK Specialist Interest Group in Orofacial Pain and TMDs (USOT). Clinical Standards Committee, Faculty of Dental Surgery, <https://www.rcseng.ac.uk/fds/publications-clinical-guidelines/clinical_guidelines/documents/temporomandibular-disorders-guideline-2013>; 2013.
10. Whooley MA, Avins AL, Miranda J, et al. Case-finding instruments for depression. Two questions are as good as many. Journal of General Internal Medicine 1997;12:439–45.
11. Nixdorf DR, Drangsholt MT, Ettlin DA, et al. Classifying orofacial pains: a new proposal of taxonomy based on ontology. Journal of Oral Rehabilitation 2012;39:161–9.
12. Ahovuo-Saloranta A, Rautakorpi UM, Borisenko OV, et al. (2014) Antibiotics for acute maxillary sinusitis in adults. Cochrane Database of Systematic Reviews 2014;(2):Art. No.: CD000243.
13. Beck-Mannagetta J, Necek D. Radiologic findings in aspergillosis of the maxillary sinus. Oral Surgery, Oral Medicine, Oral Pathology 1986;62:345–9.
14. Segura-Egea JJ, Martín-González J, Castellanos-Cosano L. Endodontic medicine: connections between apical periodontitis and systemic diseases. International Endodontic Journal 2015;48:933–51.
15. Segura-Egea JJ, Castellanos-Cosano L, Machuca G, et al. Diabetes mellitus, periapical inflammation and endodontic treatment outcome. Medicina Oral, Patologia Oral y Cirugia Bucal 2012;17:e356–61.
16. Lima SM, Grisi DC, Kogawa EM, et al. Diabetes mellitus and inflammatory pulpal and periapical disease: a review. International Endodontic Journal 2013;46:700–9.
17. Näsström K, Forsberg B, Petersson A, et al. Narrowing of the dental pulp chamber in patients with renal diseases. Oral Surgery, Oral Medicine, Oral Pathology 1985;59:242–6.
18. Durack DT. Prevention of infective endocarditis. New England Journal of Medicine 1995;332:38–44.
19. Gould FK, Elliott TSJ, Foweraker J, et al. Guidelines for the prevention of endocarditis: report of the Working Party of the British Society for Antimicrobial Chemotherapy. The Journal of Antimicrobial Chemotherapy 2006;57:1035–42.
20. Wilson W, Taubert K, Gewitz M, et al. Prevention of infective endocarditis. Guidelines from the American Heart Association: A Guideline from the American Heart Association Rheumatic Fever, Endocarditis and Kawasaki Disease Committee, Council on Cardiovascular Disease in the Young and the Council on Clinical Cardiology, Council on Cardiovascular Surgery and Anaesthesia and the Quality of Care and Outcomes Research Interdisciplinary Working Group. Circulation 2007;116:1736–54.
21. National Institute for Health and Care Excellence. Prophylaxis against infective endocarditis: NICE guidelines (CG64), <https://www.nice.org.uk/guidance/cg64>; 2008.
22. Duval X, Delahaye F, Alla F, et al. Temporal trends in infective endocarditis in the context of prophylaxis guideline modifications: three successive population-based surveys. Journal of the American College of Cardiology 2012;59:1968–76.
23. Pasquali SK, He X, Mohamad Z, et al. Trends in endocarditis hospitalizations at US children's hospitals: impact of the 2007 American Heart Association antibiotic prophylaxis guidelines. American Heart Journal 2012;163:894–9.
24. Thornhill MH, Dayer MJ, Forde JM, et al. Impact of the NICE guideline recommending cessation of antibiotic prophylaxis for prevention of infective endocarditis: before and after study. British Medical Journal 2011;342:d2392.
25. Dayer MJ, Jones S, Prendergast B, et al. Incidence of infective endocarditis in England, 2000-13: a secular trend, interrupted time-series analysis. Lancet 2015;385:1219–28.
26. Duval X, Hoen B. Prophylaxis for infective endocarditis: let's end the debate. Lancet 2015;385:1164–5.
27. National Institute for Health and Care Excellence. Prophylaxis against infective endocarditis: NICE guidelines (CG64), <https://www.nice.org.uk/guidance/cg64/chapter/Update-information>; 2015.
28. British National Formulary. London: BMJ Publishing Group Ltd and Royal Pharmaceutical Society; 2015.
29. Rider OJ, Rider EB. The changing face of oral anticoagulants. British Dental Journal 2013;215:17–20.
30. O'Connell JE, Stassen LF. New oral anticoagulants and their implications for dental patients. Journal of the Irish Dental Association 2014;60:137–43.
31. National Patient Safety Agency. Managing patients who are taking warfarin and undergoing dental treatment. NRLS-0233G-Anticoagulants~al-poster-2009-01-v2; 2009.
32. British Committee for Standards in Haematology. Guidelines for the management of patients on oral anticoagulants requiring dental surgery, <http://www.bcshguidelines.com/documents/WarfarinandentalSurgery_bjh_264_2007.pdf>; 2011.
33. Mingarro-de-Leon A, Chavell-Lopez B, Gavalda-Esteve C. Dental Management of patients receiving anticoagulant and/or antiplatelet treatment. Journal of Clinical and Experimental Dentistry 2014;6:155–61.
34. Ardekian L, Gaspar R, Peled M, et al. Does low-dose aspirin therapy complicate oral surgical procedures? Journal of the American Dental Association 2000;131:331–5.

35. Morimoto Y, Niwa H. On the use of prothrombin complex concentrate in patients with coagulopathy requiring tooth extraction. Oral Medicine, Oral Pathology, Oral Radiology and Endodontics 2010;110:7–10.

36. Lillis T, Ziakis A, Koskinas K, et al. Safety of dental extractions during uninterrupted single or dual antiplatelet treatment. American Journal of Cardiology 2011;108:964–7.

37. Stopeck AT, Lipton A, Body JJ, et al. Denosumab compared with zoledronic acid for the treatment of bone metastases in patients with advanced breast cancer: a randomized double blind. Journal Clinical Oncology 2010;8:5132–9.

38. American Association of Oral and Maxillofacial Surgeons (2014), Ruggiero SL, Dodson TB, et al. American Association of Oral and Maxillofacial Surgeons position paper on medication-related osteonecrosis of the jaw – 2014 update. Journal of Oral Maxillofacial Surgery 2014;72:1938–56.

39. Allen MR, Kubek DJ, Burr DB. Cancer treatment dosing regimens of zoledronic acid result in near-complete suppression of mandible intracortical bone remodeling in beagle dogs. Journal of Bone and Mineral Research 2010;25:98–105.

40. Allen MR, Burr DB. Mandible matrix necrosis in beagle dogs following 3 years of daily oral bisphosphonate treatment. Journal of Oral and Maxillofacial Surgery 2008;66:987–94.

41. Edwards BJ, Hellstein JW, Jacobsen PL, et al. Updated recommendations for managing the care of patients receiving oral bisphosphonate therapy: An advisory statement from the American Dental Association Council on Scientific Affairs. Journal of the American Dental Association 2008;139:1674–7.

42. Yamazaki T, Yamori M, Ishizaki T, et al. Increased incidence of osteonecrosis of the jaw after tooth extraction in patients treated with bisphosphonates: a cohort study. International Journal of Oral and Maxillofacial Surgery 2012;41:1397–403.

43. Marx RE, Cillo JE, Ulloa JJ. Oral bisphosphonate-induced osteonecrosis: Risk factors, prediliction of risk using serum CTX testing, prevention and treatment. Journal of Oral and Maxillofacial Surgery 2007;65:2397–410.

44. Scottish Dental Clinical Effectiveness Programme. Oral Health Management of Patients Prescribed Bisphosphonates, <http://www.sdcep.org.uk/wp-content/uploads/2013/03/SDCEP+Bisphosphonates+Guidance.pdf>; 2011.

45. Hellstein JW, Adler RA, Edwards B, et al. American Dental Association Council on Scientific Affairs Expert Panel on Antiresorptive Agents. Managing the care of patients receiving antiresorptive therapy for prevention and treatment of osteoporosis: executive summary of recommendations from the American Dental Association Council on Scientific Affairs. Journal of the American Dental Association 2011;142:1243–51.

46. Nagle D, Reader A, Beck M, et al. Effect of systemic penicillin on pain in untreated irreversible pulpitis. Oral Surgery, Oral Medicine, Oral Pathology, Oral Radiology & Endodontics 2000;90:636–40.

47. Fedorowicz Z, van Zuuren EJ, Farman AG, et al. Antibiotic use for irreversible pulpitis. Cochrane Database of Systematic Reviews 2013;(12):Art. No.: CD004969.

48. Cope A, Francis N, Wood F, et al. Systemic antibiotics for symptomatic apical periodontitis and acute apical abscess in adults. Cochrane Database of Systematic Reviews 2014;(6):Art. No.: CD010136.

49. World Health Organisation. Antibiotic resistance: synthesis of recommendations by expert policy groups, <http://apps.who.int/iris/bitstream/10665/66895/1/WHO_CDS_CSR_DRS_2001.10.pdf?ua=1>; 2001.

50. Adult antimicrobial prescribing in primary dental care for general dental practitioners. 2nd ed. London: Faculty of General Dental Practice (UK), Royal College of Surgeons of England; 2012.

51. Public Health England. Start smart – then focus. Antimicrobial Stewardship Toolkit for English Hospitals, <https://www.gov.uk/government/uploads/system/uploads/attachment_data/file/417032/Start_Smart_Then_Focus_FINAL.PDF>; 2015.

52. National Institute for Health and Care Excellence. Antimicrobial stewardship: systems and processes for effective antimicrobial medicine use. NICE guidelines (NG15), <http://www.nice.org.uk/guidance/ng15>; 2015.

53. Scully C. Scully's medical problems in dentistry. 7th ed. Edinburgh: Churchill Livingstone; 2014.

CHAPTER 3

Diagnosis

N. P. Chandler and B. S. Chong

Chapter Contents

Summary

Diagnosis is the first step in the care and management of any patient. A systematic and organized approach is important to avoid misdiagnosis. Special tests and additional investigations may be necessary to help confirm a provisional diagnosis. Until and unless a clear diagnosis is possible, invasive and irreversible treatment may have to be delayed. However, once a valid diagnosis is confirmed and in conjunction with the patient, various treatment options can be considered. A plan is formulated and then carried out to resolve the patient's complaint. Referral to a specialist may be indicated to help establish a diagnosis, or if complex endodontic treatment, is required.

Introduction

Diagnosis is the process of identifying a disease or an abnormal condition by collecting and evaluating the patient's presenting signs and symptoms, as well as the results of further investigations. A clear diagnosis can only be reached when information is collected systematically and interpreted accurately. If a firm diagnosis cannot be reached, irreversible treatment may have to be delayed. The maxim 'first do no harm' is a reminder that it may be better to do nothing than risk treatment which causes more harm than good. A referral to an appropriate specialist might be appropriate if a diagnosis cannot be established.

History

Taking an accurate history from the patient is the first step in diagnosis. The clinician can then decide the direction of the diagnostic process; for example, whether additional investigations or special tests are required. Subject to confirmation, a tentative diagnosis may be possible at this stage.

As well as helping establish the reasons for the patient's attendance, the history may also reveal the patient's attitude toward and motivation for dental treatment. The clinician may be alerted to potential patient management problems, for example, difficulties in achieving adequate anaesthesia or an intolerance to the use of a dental dam or having instruments in the mouth.

PRESENTING COMPLAINT

Patients should be questioned sympathetically and asked to describe their complaint in their own words; this should then be documented. Their cooperation and ability to describe their problem accurately will greatly aid diagnosis. The questions asked should be open-ended and not leading; for example, 'What brings you to see me today?' With endodontic problems, pain and/or swelling are usually the predominant complaints. Typically with pain, a series of follow-up questions is necessary to help establish the character, duration, severity and other features of pain or discomfort (see Chapter 2, Table 2-1).

HISTORY OF PRESENTING COMPLAINT

Often the presenting complaint is not new, but previous symptoms may have been mild or temporarily abated. The patient may be unaware that treatment is still required or may have chosen to ignore the problem. However, a historical perspective and the chronology of the presenting complaint are still necessary as they will provide relevant information for arriving at a diagnosis.

DENTAL HISTORY

Some patients only visit their dentist when they are in pain, whereas others visit on a regular basis. It is also important to determine whether the patient has recently had dental treatment in the region of interest. Unless it is purely coincidental, recent treatment may be related to the presenting complaint. Other snippets of information gleaned from the dental history may provide clues to possible factors contributing to the patient's complaint. For example, a history of dental trauma may explain symptoms of irreversible pulpitis associated with an otherwise unrestored tooth.

MEDICAL HISTORY

An up-to-date medical history is required. Unless already documented, the patient is requested to complete a medical history form beforehand, which the clinician will then discuss with the patient. Some medical conditions or medications may have an impact on patient management. In addition, patients should be asked if they are allergic to latex (dental dam and glove materials), household bleach (sodium hypochlorite irrigant) and other materials they will come in contact with during endodontic treatment. The subject of the patient's general health and the potential effect on endodontic treatment is covered in Chapter 2.

Examination

EXTRAORAL

The patient's general well-being and demeanour will be noticeable during consultation. Signs of facial asymmetry, swelling and/or trismus may also be apparent (Figure 3-1). However, less obvious signs may only be revealed after closer examination. The lymph glands, temporomandibular joint and muscles of mastication are assessed. The degree of mouth opening is noted because, if limited, access for root canal treatment may be challenging.

INTRAORAL
Soft Tissues

The general state of the soft tissues should be assessed. Scalloping of the lateral borders of the tongue and/or

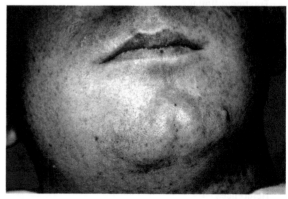

FIGURE 3-1 An extraoral swelling and associated facial asymmetry that is obvious when meeting the patient.

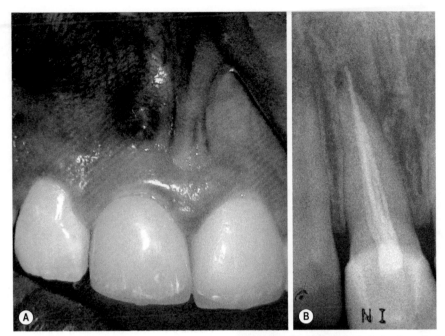

FIGURE 3-2 (A) Clinical view of the buccal sinus tract associated with a maxillary central incisor. (B) Periapical radiograph of the tooth showing an overextended and suboptimal root canal filling.

frictional keratosis of the buccal mucosa may indicate a parafunctional habit. The area of interest requires a more detailed assessment. Swelling or the presence of a sinus tract should be noted (Figure 3-2).

Hard Tissues

The dentition, including the state and quality of existing restorations, is assessed; this will provide an overall clinical view of the patient's dental history (Figure 3-3). Together with the oral hygiene status, periodontal charting and caries experience are relevant when devising a treatment plan.

If evident, the severity and distribution of tooth surface loss should be recorded. Localized wear facets and fracture lines may indicate an occlusal component to the patient's symptoms (Figure 3-4). If a cracked tooth is suspected, it may be necessary to assess individual cusps by occlusal loading. Transillumination (using a light source placed on the side of the tooth) may help reveal the otherwise hard to detect fracture lines (Figure 3-5). Special dyes, such as methylene blue (Vista-Blue, Vista Dental Products, Racine, WI, USA) may also be used to accentuate a fracture line

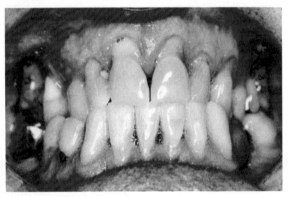

FIGURE 3-3 The state of dentition will provide an overall clinical view of the patient's past dental history.

once its approximate position is known. The use of magnification and enhanced illumination with loupes, or a dental operating microscope, greatly aid visualization (see Chapter 6). The prognosis of a cracked tooth is dependent on the direction and extent of the crack/s. A cast restoration may be placed to act as a splint to prevent further crack propagation; however, root canal

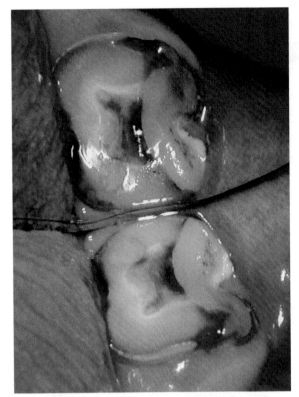

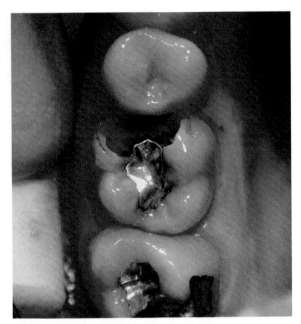

FIGURE 3-6 A large carious cavity in a maxillary right first molar. The clinical picture suggests possible pulpal involvement and the need for root canal treatment.

FIGURE 3-4 Excessive tooth surface loss in this mandibular left second molar has resulted in pulpal symptoms.

treatment may be needed beforehand if pulp vitality is compromised.

Specific Tooth/Teeth

The area of interest and the particular tooth/teeth are then considered in more detail. The occlusion and strategic nature of the tooth are assessed, for example, if a tooth is unopposed or nonfunctional. The colour of the tooth should be compared with adjacent teeth; any darkening of the clinical crown may be related to a history of trauma.[1] The possible causes of pulpal or periapical diseases are noted, for example, the presence of primary or secondary caries (Figure 3-6), fracture lines (Figure 3-7) and extensive dentine exposure due to tooth surface loss. The restorability of the tooth must be assessed. The extent of any caries, size of existing restorations and amount of remaining tooth structure will provide an indication about restorability; there is further discussion on this subject later.

Palpation. The buccal/labial and palatal/lingual mucosa are palpated. Light finger pressure is applied in a rolling motion on the soft tissues normally using

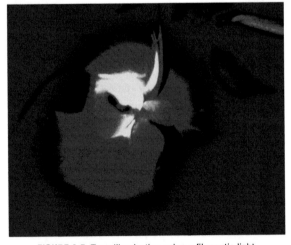

FIGURE 3-5 Transillumination using a fibreoptic light.

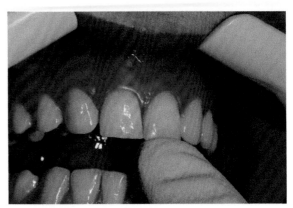
FIGURE 3-9 Tooth percussion performed using a finger.

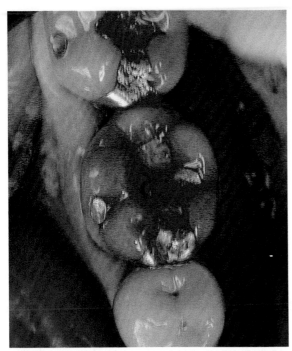
FIGURE 3-7 A mandibular right first molar with stained crack lines and an old amalgam restoration that is leaking, with evidence of secondary caries beneath.

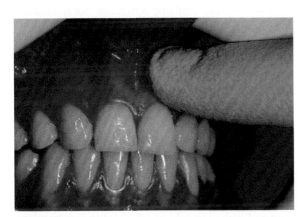
FIGURE 3-8 Light finger pressure is applied in a rolling motion to palpate the soft tissues.

an index finger (Figure 3-8). Signs of tenderness usually indicate inflammation of the underlying tissue.

Mobility. Using fingers alone or combined with a mirror handle, any abnormal tooth mobility should be noted. Common causes of increased mobility include periodontal disease, root fracture and acute apical periodontitis. The extent of any mobility is noted and scored according to the widely used system[34]:

Grade 1: just distinguishable sign of tooth movement greater than normal;

Grade 2: tooth movement of 1 mm from its normal position in any direction;

Grade 3: tooth movement of greater than 1 mm in any direction.

Percussion. Teeth are percussed in an axial and buccal direction using a forefinger (Figure 3-9) or the end of a mirror handle. Tenderness to gentle percussion indicates inflammation of the periodontal ligament surrounding the tooth; this may be pulpal or periodontal in origin.

Periodontal Probing. Probing depths should be assessed by 'walking' a periodontal probe around the entire circumference of the tooth (Figure 3-10). The probing profile for root fractures and iatrogenic perforations is characteristically an isolated localized loss of attachment. A nonmetallic periodontal probe, e.g., 'PerioWise' (Premier Dental Products, Plymouth Meeting, PA, USA), is valuable for the detection of these narrow periodontal defects. Furcation involvement may indicate advanced periodontal disease (Figure 3-11) or an iatrogenic root perforation.

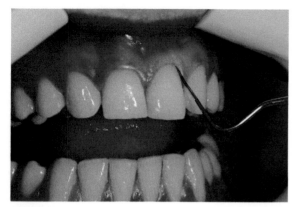

FIGURE 3-10 The periodontal probe must be 'walked' around the tooth to ensure that any isolated narrow periodontal defects are not overlooked.

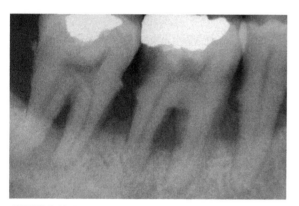

FIGURE 3-11 Advanced periodontal disease and extensive caries.

Investigations

PULP SENSITIVITY TESTS

Currently available sensitivity tests assess the neural response and not the vascular supply of the pulp, and the assumption with these tests is that the neural status reflects the blood supply status of the tooth.[2-4] With any sensitivity test, an explanation should be given to the patient about the rationale for the test. Otherwise, particularly with an anxious patient, false positive responses will result. An adjacent tooth or a similar tooth in another quadrant, considered healthy, should be tested first; this will act as the control and allow the patient to experience the likely response.

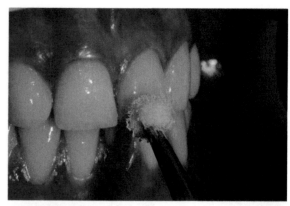

FIGURE 3-12 Cold thermal test; a refrigerant is sprayed on a small cotton pledget and applied to the tooth.

Thermal Tests

Cold Test. Cold thermal tests work by causing the contraction of the dentinal fluid within the dentine tubules; this rapid outward flow of movement results in 'hydrodynamic forces' acting on the Aδ fibres.[5,6] There is a sharp sensation lasting for up to a few seconds after the cold stimulus has been removed from the tooth.[7] Several types of cold test are available, the key difference between them being the operating temperature.

Commercially available refrigerant spray containing tetrafluoroethane (−50°C) is convenient and easy to use. It is sprayed onto a small cotton pledget and applied to the tooth (Figure 3-12). Carbon dioxide snow (−78.5°C) is also very effective in thermal testing. Carbon dioxide is expressed into a plunger mechanism from a pressurized gas cylinder and then compressed into a stick of carbon dioxide snow. This is then placed on the tooth being tested using a special applicator. Being the coldest, carbon dioxide snow is particularly useful for assessing teeth that have been restored with full coverage restorations.

Teeth may also be isolated individually with dental dam and bathed in cold water. This test is particularly useful when a patient complains of poorly localized pain provoked by cold (Figure 3-13). The colder the applied stimulus the more reliable the test as there is a greater temperature reduction within the dentine–pulp complex.[8,9] This is important in posterior teeth as the thickness of both the dentine and enamel is greater than that in anterior teeth. A negative response may result because the applied stimulus is not cold

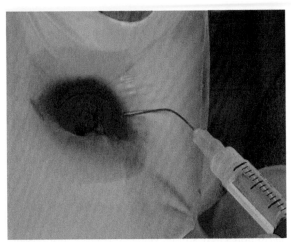

FIGURE 3-13 A tooth is isolated using a dental dam and bathed with cold water; this is repeated for each tooth in the quadrant to try to reproduce the patient's symptoms.

enough. A prolonged and lingering response usually indicates irreversible pulpitis. Cold tests appear to be more effective in assessing nerve status than heat tests.[10,11]

Heat Test. Heat may be applied to a tooth using a heat-softened gutta-percha stick (GP Temporary Stopping, DiaDent Europe, Almere, The Netherlands). A thin layer of petroleum jelly should first be applied to the test surface to prevent the material from sticking to the tooth. Another way of applying heat to a tooth is by running a rubber prophylaxis cup dry, in a slow handpiece, to generate frictional heat on the crown of the tooth.[12] However, this method is seldom used as a false positive response may be obtained because of the vibrations.

Individual teeth may also be isolated using dental dam and warm water. Furthermore, this test is particularly useful when the patient complains of poorly localized heat sensitivity. Prolonged application of heat to a tooth can result in the stimulation of C-fibres, resulting in lingering pain.[13] For testing purposes and for this reason, heat should only be applied to a tooth for a maximum of 5 seconds.

Electric Pulp Test

Electric pulp testers (EPTs) are battery-operated units (Figure 3-14A) that produce negative pulses of

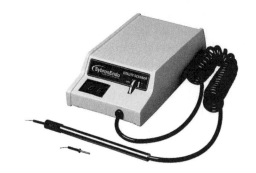

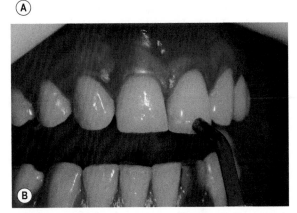

FIGURE 3-14 (A) A typical electric pulp tester. (B) The probe is placed on the incisal third of the crown of the tooth; toothpaste is used as a contact medium for improved conduction.

electricity, with a maximum current of a few milliamperes. The current can be adjusted; it is either controlled by the operator or it increases automatically when the unit is activated. The tooth to be assessed is isolated using cotton wool and dried. Depending on the type of tester, the patient is asked to hold the handle of the probe or a lip hook is placed to form one loop of the circuit. The tip of the probe is usually coated with a conducting medium (e.g., toothpaste or fluoride gel) to improve electrical transmission to the tooth. When the probe is placed onto the tooth (Figure 3-14B), the circuit is complete. If desired, the application of a dental dam, strips of dam material or Mylar may be used interproximally to reduce the likelihood of electrical conduction to the adjacent teeth.[3]

As the test proceeds, the strength of the electrical stimulus will increase, and when sensation is elicited, the patient is advised to either let go of the handle of the probe (which breaks the circuit) or signal the clinician so the probe may be removed. The reading on the EPT, either numerical or arbitrary, is then recorded. If numerical, the digital readout is relative rather than an accurate quantitative measurement of the health status of the pulp. Apart from a total lack of response suggesting a lack of vitality, EPT readings are merely an indication, a comparative measurement, as healthy teeth will respond over a range of values. The threshold for obtaining a positive response depends on the position of the probe on the tooth and the thickness of the enamel and dentine. The probe of the EPT should be placed adjacent to the pulp horn as this is where there is the highest density of nerves.[14] In the case of anterior teeth and premolars, this is at the incisal and mid-third region of the tooth, respectively[15–17] (see Figure 3-14B). The thicker the enamel and dentine, the higher the excitation threshold; for this reason, the probe should be placed where the enamel is thinnest.[18] This explains why for a given test, the excitation thresholds increase from incisor to premolar to molar teeth as the thickness of the overlying enamel and dentine increases.[19]

A tingling or warm sensation indicates a healthy, 'positive' response. This is a result of Aδ fibres being stimulated, resulting in an ionic shift in the dentinal fluid causing a localized depolarization and the generation of an action potential from the healthy nerve.[20] A lingering, dull ache after the removal of the EPT probe is a result of stimulation of the C-fibres, which is indicative of irreversible pulpal inflammation. No response from electric pulp testing indicates that the tooth is nonvital, i.e. the pulp is necrotic. Saliva conduction through the periodontal ligament may result in a false positive reading; a negative response may also be due to the failure to complete the electrical circuit. A review on EPT includes the reminder that these pulp tests can be unreliable, especially in the case of immature and concussed teeth.[21]

A study to evaluate the ability of thermal and electrical tests to register pulp vitality[2] reported that the probability of a nonsensitive reaction representing a necrotic pulp was 89% with the cold test, 88% with the electrical test and 48% with the heat test. It also indicated that the probability of a sensitive reaction

representing a vital pulp was 90% with the cold test, 84% with the electrical test, and 83% with the heat test. These results would suggest in descending order of accuracy the cold test, followed by the electrical test and heat test.

Test Cavity Preparation

Historically, test cavity preparation has been suggested as a technique to assess the pulp status when all other tests are inconclusive. Local anaesthetic is not administered, and a small bur is used with copious irrigation to prepare a small cavity into dentine. If the patient feels sensitivity, this may indicate that the tooth is vital; alternatively, it may indicate that the tooth is unhealthy as Aδ fibres may still be viable in necrotic pulp tissue. No response indicates a lack of pulpal vitality. However, if the pulp tissue has receded away from the centre of the tooth and an excessive amount of tertiary dentine has been deposited within the root canal system, the dentinal tubules being transected may not communicate with the vital odontoblastic processes, hence a negative response.

The patient's response to all sensitivity testing is subjective.[22,23] There is a poor correlation between signs and symptoms and pulpal and periapical histopathology.[11,24–26] When the results of five studies were analysed in an attempt to correlate clinical findings with the histopathological status of teeth, it was concluded that the results of these tests were more likely to be correct when teeth are healthy than diseased.[27] Sensitivity tests by themselves are of limited value; they should be used when indicated as an adjunct, as part of the diagnostic process.[28]

BITE/CUSP LOADING TESTS

Tenderness to bite is indicative of inflammation of the periodontium and a common presenting symptom. The more specific cusp loading bite test using some form of wedging device is indicated for patients with a suspected cusp, tooth or root fracture presenting with poorly localized pain on biting.[29] The patient is instructed to bite firmly on a cotton roll (Figure 3-15A) or a commercially available wedging device (Figure 3-15B) e.g. 'Tooth Slooth' (Professional Results, Inc., Laguna Niguel, CA, USA) or 'Fracfinder' (Denbur, Inc., Oak Brook, IL, USA). The biting pressure results in the temporary separation of the fractured segments,

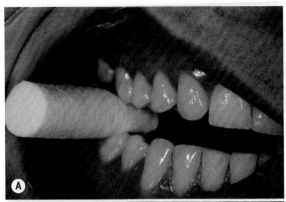

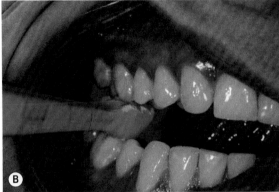

FIGURE 3-15 Bite/cusp loading test. (A) The patient is asked to bite on a cotton roll to try and reproduce symptoms of localized tenderness to chewing. (B) A wedging device is used to apply pressure to individual cusps.

thus reproducing the patient's symptoms; neighbouring teeth are used as controls.

SELECTIVE LOCAL ANAESTHESIA

If symptoms, particularly pain, are poorly localized or referred, it will be difficult to identify the source. Often, patients may be able to indicate that the pain is from the left or right side of their mouth, but they may be unsure if it originates from the mandible or maxilla. If pulp sensitivity testing is equivocal, then selective local anaesthesia may be helpful. Using the intraligamental local anaesthetic injection technique, the clinician should first selectively anaesthetize teeth in the maxillary quadrant starting from the distal sulcus of the most posterior tooth. The local anaesthetic is then administered more forward, one tooth at a time, until the pain disappears. If the pain persists

after an appropriate interval, selective local anaesthesia should similarly be performed in the mandibular quadrant. Selective local anaesthesia is usually better at pinpointing the arch or quadrant rather than a specific tooth.

BLOOD FLOW ASSESSMENT

Various 'physiometric' tests have been investigated to evaluate the blood supply within the pulp space of the tooth. They include laser Doppler flowmetry (LDF), pulse oximetry[30] and the measurement of tooth temperature using thermocouples, thermistors, infrared thermography and cholesteric liquid crystals; most of these methods are experimental.

LDF, which is noninvasive, appears to be the most promising technique.[31] A probe which emits a low-energy laser beam is placed against the surface of the tooth. This laser beam travels along the enamel prisms and dentinal tubules to reach the pulp tissue (Figure 3-16). On reaching the pulp tissue, some of the light from the laser beam is absorbed and scattered by red blood cells within the capillary plexus, resulting in a Doppler shift in the frequency of the light reflected back to the probe.[32,33] The LDF amplifies this reflected light and detects its pulsatility and signal strength. Fourier analysis, a mathematical technique, can be used to improve the diagnostic accuracy of LDF. Besides assessing the blood supply of the tooth, the other major advantages of LDF include more objective and reliable results compared with sensitivity tests.[34] LDF is particularly helpful when the results of other investigations are inconclusive[35]; it has also been used to detect the pulpal status of traumatized teeth.[34,36] Unfortunately, LDF has disadvantages, which include being more time consuming to perform, its technique-sensitive use and its cost. Nevertheless, it may be used on extensively restored or carious teeth.[37,38]

RADIOGRAPHS

Radiographs are an essential component of the diagnostic process,[39] but when used in isolation, they will not indicate the pulp condition or treatment needs.[40,41] Images from conventional radiography are captured on X-ray films or digital sensors. With the latter, the sensors are either charged-coupled devices (CCDs) or storage phosphor plates (SPPs). CCD sensors are

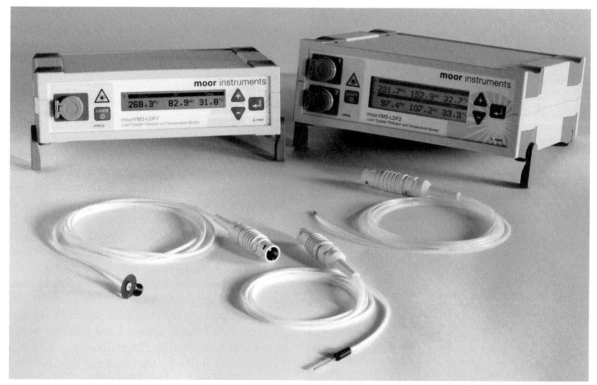

FIGURE 3-16 Moor VMS laser Doppler flowmeter (Moor Instruments Ltd, Axminster, UK.).

relatively bulky and are available in wired or wireless versions; captured images allow immediate viewing. SPP sensors are almost equivalent in thickness to conventional X-ray films and there is no wire connection, but the irradiated sensors have to be scanned in a processing unit before the images can be viewed.

Periapical radiographs may be supplemented with bitewing radiographs; this view may reveal additional information regarding the quality of any restoration present, extent of caries in relation to the pulp, calcifications in the pulp chamber and crestal bone levels (Figure 3-17).[42] Radiographs should be taken using the paralleling technique aided by a beam-aiming device rather than the bisecting angle technique. The paralleling technique reduces geometric distortions, thus resulting in more accurate images of the apical anatomy.[43] In addition, the use of a beam-aiming device allows similar positioning to be reproduced when radiographs are taken at a later date for review or comparative purposes.[44,45] Conventional radiographs condense the complex three-dimensional anatomy of the tooth and its surrounding alveolar anatomy into a two-dimensional image. The parallax technique may be used to detect, for example, additional root canals and improve the perception of the spatial relationship of the root apices to their relevant surrounding structures (Figure 3-18).

Cone beam computed tomography (CBCT) for dentistry was introduced in the late 1990s.[46,47] The X-ray beam is cone shaped and aimed through the area of interest, with the source and detector rotating about this point (fulcrum). As a cylindrical volume of data or field of view (FOV) is collected, only a single rotation is needed, in contrast to medical CT. It has been reported that a higher prevalence of apical periodontitis is revealed with CBCT compared with conventional radiographs[48]; CBCT is more accurate in diagnosing periapical pathosis compared with

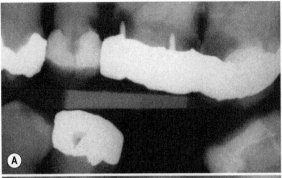

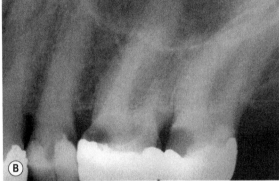

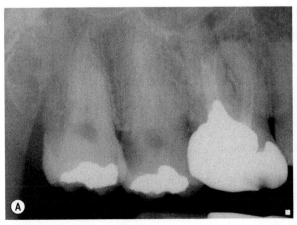

FIGURE 3-17 (A) A bitewing and (B) periapical radiograph of the maxillary left quadrant provide information about the quality of existing restorations, extent of caries, crestal bone levels, pulp calcifications, root morphology and apical condition.

conventional radiographs (Figure 3-19).[49] Although the technique may allow a more objective assessment of the healing of previously root-treated teeth, there is, however, a risk of false positive diagnoses of periapical pathosis, which may lead to unnecessary treatment.[50] The key limitation of CBCT is the greater radiation dose compared with conventional dental radiography.[51] The clinician is also responsible for interpreting the entire image volume.[52] Therefore, CBCT is not indicated as a standard assessment method and should be justified on an individual basis where the potential benefits outweigh the potential risks to a patient; the basic principles for CBCT usage should include a risk versus benefit analysis, keeping the patient's radiation exposure as low as reasonably possible as well as ensuring that the prescribing clinician has specific training in interpreting and utilizing the diagnostic information.[53–55] The smallest possible FOV, smallest voxel size, lowest mA setting and shortest exposure time in conjunction with a pulsed exposure mode of acquisition are recommended.[53,54,56,57]

Differential Diagnosis

Differential diagnosis is the process of distinguishing between diseases or conditions with similar

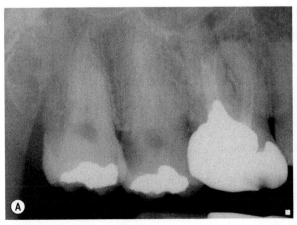
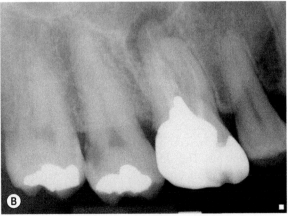

FIGURE 3-18 Additional radiographs may be helpful. The first periapical radiograph (A) reveals an inadequately treated maxillary right first molar and distal caries in the adjacent second molar; the second, parallax radiograph (B) reveals more details.

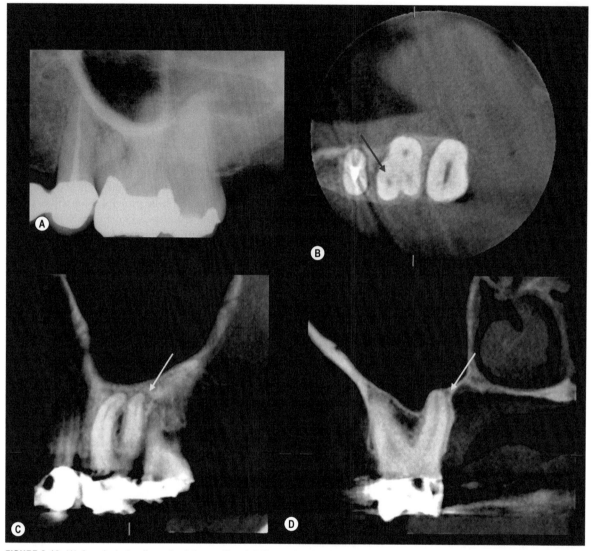

FIGURE 3-19 (A) A periapical radiograph of the maxillary left first molar showing apparently normal periapical health. (B) Axial, (C) sagittal and (D) coronal reconstructed views from cone beam computed tomography showing the presence of a periapical radiolucency associated with the distobuccal and palatal roots (*yellow arrow*) and the presence of only one mesiobuccal canal (*red arrow*).

characteristics by comparing their presenting signs and symptoms. The differential diagnosis of dental pain is covered in Chapter 2; pulpal and periapical conditions are considered in this chapter.

There is no universally agreed diagnostic terminology, classification scheme or system for pulpal and periapical diseases. The terms *symptomatic/asymptomatic* have been suggested to replace *acute/chronic*. This reflects the nature of the patient's presenting complaint instead of the histological description. The terms *apical*, *periapical* and *periradicular* are often used interchangeably. In this chapter, the more conservative terms have been retained.

PULPAL CONDITIONS

Normal Pulp

A tooth with a normal pulp will be symptom-free. The results of a clinical examination will be unremarkable, and the tooth will respond normally to sensitivity testing.

Reversible Pulpitis

A mild or transient pulpal inflammation may result in a sharp pain in the tooth lasting for up to 5 to 10 seconds, which does not linger after the applied stimulus has been removed. Common causes of reversible pulpitis include caries and coronal leakage. Radiographs may confirm the presence of caries or a defective restoration; the periapical tissues will appear normal. Removal of the causal factor/s will usually result in alleviation of pulpal inflammation and the patient's symptoms.

Irreversible Pulpitis

The pulp has suffered a more severe insult and is irreversibly inflamed; therefore, the tooth cannot be treated conservatively. Symptoms of irreversible pulpitis may range from a throbbing pain, initiated by hot or cold stimuli and lasting minutes to hours, to spontaneous intermittent bouts of aching pain lasting for hours. Symptoms may be made worse when the patient lies down or bends over, resulting in increased intrapulpal pressure. As mentioned earlier, the results of the clinical examination do not necessarily correlate with the true histopathological status of the pulp.[11,58] This is especially true with irreversible pulpitis, which may progress from relatively symptom-free or symptomless to pulp necrosis and subsequent apical periodontitis.[59]

Clinical examination may reveal caries or a defective restoration; this may be confirmed with radiographs, but the periapical tissues may appear normal. An attempt to reproduce the patient's symptoms is prudent to confirm the diagnosis. With the application of thermal stimulus, there is usually an initial sharp, shooting Aδ fibre-type pain lasting for a few seconds, and then after a few seconds of quiescence, a dull, throbbing C-fibre ache develops which may take minutes or hours to subside even after the stimulus has been removed.[60,61] Once the offending tooth has

been identified and irreversible pulpitis confirmed, preservation of the pulp is not possible and pulp removal is necessary.

Pulp Necrosis

The term *pulp necrosis* describes the partial or complete necrosis of the pulp caused by a loss of blood or inadequate blood supply. If the necrotic tissue has not become infected, the periapical tissues will appear radiographically normal. Until the periodontium is involved, the tooth is usually symptom-free. Single-rooted teeth usually do not respond to sensitivity testing. However, in multirooted teeth, parts of the pulp may still be completely or partially vital; as a result, sensitivity testing may produce a negative or positive response, depending on the status of the neural supply adjacent to the tooth surface being tested. Root canal treatment is indicated if the diagnosis of pulp necrosis is confirmed.

PERIAPICAL CONDITIONS

Normal Periapical Tissues

The tooth is symptom-free, and there is no tenderness to palpation or percussion. Radiographs show a normal periodontal ligament space and no evidence of periapical disease.

Acute Apical Periodontitis

The tooth in question will be exquisitely tender to touch, biting or percussion. Radiographs may reveal a slight widening of the periodontal ligament space. A negative response to sensitivity testing indicates an endodontic cause.

Acute Periapical Abscess

Patients suffering from acute periapical abscess will usually present complaining of an intense throbbing pain. The problem tooth will be very tender to touch with percussion and palpation. There may be discernible mobility as the tooth is elevated from its bony socket. The tooth will not respond to sensitivity tests. An intraoral or extraoral swelling may be present (Figure 3-20). In severe cases, there may be lymphadenopathy and malaise, and the patient may have an elevated temperature. On radiographs, the periapical tissues may appear normal or there may be a periapical

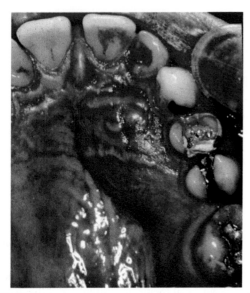

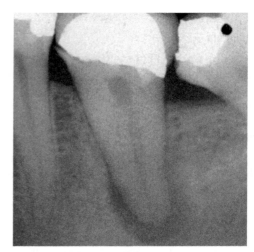

FIGURE 3-21 A mandibular left first molar with chronic apical periodontitis. The tooth has a full-coverage crown and is symptom-free, but the periapical radiograph reveals a radiolucency.

FIGURE 3-20 An acute periapical abscess related to the maxillary left first premolar. The palatal swelling will have to be incised and drained and root canal treatment commenced if the tooth is to be retained.

radiolucency. The abscess will have to be drained via the root canal by commencing root canal treatment, and incision and drainage will also be required for any fluctuant swelling (see Figure 3-20).

Chronic Apical Periodontitis

Patients may be symptom-free, or they may report that the tooth feels different, or is slightly tender to chewing. Clinically, the tooth may be tender to percussion or palpation and does not respond to sensitivity testing. On radiographs, there may be a widening of the periodontal ligament space or more often, a periapical radiolucency may be present (Figure 3-21). A 'phoenix' abscess is an acute exacerbation of chronic apical periodontitis and more commonly, arises in a tooth with a preexisting periapical radiolucency.

Chronic Periapical Abscess

The tooth is usually symptom-free and not sensitive to biting pressure, but it may 'feel different' to the patient on percussion. It will not respond to pulp sensitivity tests, and there will be a periapical radiolucency on radiographs. A chronic periapical abscess

may be distinguished from chronic apical periodontitis because the former will usually be associated with a draining sinus tract. If the sinus tract is sited at the gingival margin, there will be a localized, narrow periodontal defect. A gutta-percha cone may be gently inserted into a sinus tract and a radiograph is taken to track the source and confirm the location of the problem tooth (Figure 3-22).

Restorability

If a tooth is to be retained as a functional unit in the dental arch after root canal treatment, it has to be restored to both form and function. The restorability of the tooth must be considered before providing treatment. If there are any doubts about restorability, it may be necessary to remove the entire existing restoration to check.[62] Only after it has been established that there is sufficient sound coronal tooth structure, remaining should treatment proceed. This approach has the added benefit of allowing the clinician to visualize and consider the eventual postendodontic restoration required.

Systems have been devised to assist the clinician in deciding the prognosis of teeth and how to restore the root-treated tooth.[63,64] With one of these, the 'Tooth Restorability Index',[63] the tooth is divided into

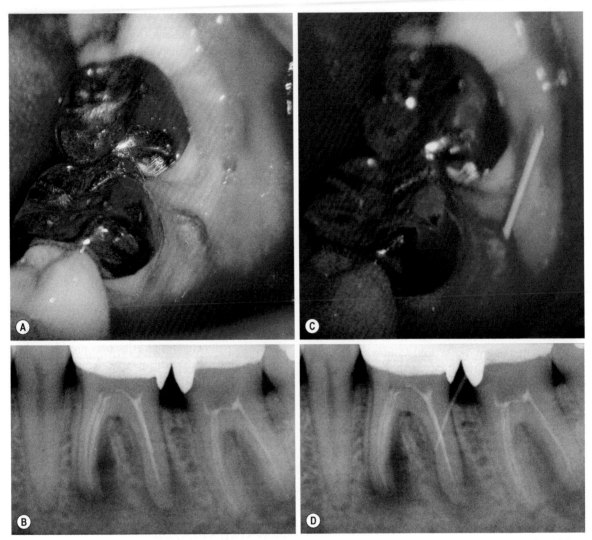

FIGURE 3-22 (A) A buccal sinus tract situated between two mandibular left molars. (B) A periapical radiograph shows that both teeth have suboptimal root fillings. (C) A gutta-percha cone is inserted into the sinus tract to trace the source, and (D) a second radiograph confirms the culprit is the mandibular left first molar. (From Chong 2004,[63] with permission of Quintessence Publishing Co. Ltd.)

sextants before restoration. The amount of remaining sound coronal tooth structure in each sextant is given a grade ranging from 0 to 3 depending on its quantity, height and width. The scores from each sextant are then combined, and the final score will help guide the clinician in planning which type of postendodontic restoration is suitable for the tooth. The restoration of endodontically treated teeth is covered in Chapter 15.

Treatment Options

On reaching a diagnosis, the patient should be advised of the different treatment options available. As part of the decision-making process, the advantages, disadvantages and the prognosis for each treatment option should be discussed. The treatment plan should be tailored to the patient's specific problem, considering the patient's preference. In

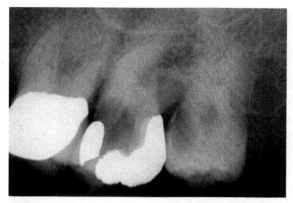

FIGURE 3-23 A complex endodontic case that may be best referred to a specialist for management. Apart from extensive caries, especially in the second molar, both teeth have complicated root morphology and significant canal sclerosis. Access to these teeth will also be challenging.

addition, the clinician should be competent and confident in carrying out the treatment plan. If not, the case may be best referred to a specialist for management (Figure 3-23). Endodontic case assessment forms[65,66] have been devised to help clinicians evaluate the potential complexity of endodontic treatment. Similar forms have been found to be useful for assessing the potential complexity of endodontic treatment; thereby, helping the general practitioner decide whether to refer the patient to a specialist.[67]

WATCH AND REVIEW

If there is no clear diagnosis or the patient is undecided on treatment, then a more cautious approach may be adopted. The tooth is monitored until a definitive diagnosis or decision on treatment is reached. If appropriate and necessary, only symptomatic treatment is provided, for example, analgesics for pain for a short period.

SAVE THE TOOTH

If a tooth is potentially saveable and the patient preference is for its retention, then treatment should be provided in the effort to save the tooth.

LOSE THE TOOTH

If the prognosis is likely to be poor despite intervention or the patient does not want to retain a potentially salvageable tooth, then extraction may be necessary after appropriate consent. Consideration may then be needed for the provision of a replacement after a tooth is lost.

Specific Endodontic Treatment Options

PULP MONITORING

If there is insufficient and inconclusive evidence that endodontic intervention is required, periodic reviews may be necessary to monitor the pulpal status. A common example is with cases of trauma, where teeth have to be reassessed and special tests may need to be repeated to monitor and evaluate pulpal health. The rationale for such an approach must be carefully explained to the patient; if there are any new developments, the need for treatment should be reconsidered.

PULP PRESERVATION

The aim of this treatment option is to maintain pulpal vitality by removing irritants that may provoke pulpal inflammation. The treatments commonly used to preserve pulp vitality include indirect pulp capping, direct pulp capping and pulpotomy; this subject is covered in Chapter 5.

PULP EXTIRPATION

When the vital pulp is irreversibly damaged, its removal is inevitable. Pulp extirpation is often the first stage in root canal treatment and a necessary emergency procedure to render the patient pain-free.

ROOT CANAL TREATMENT

Root canal treatment is needed for teeth with irreversible pulpitis or apical periodontitis. Treatment may be completed in a single visit if the tooth is not infected, if the patient prefers and if there is sufficient time available for this approach. Otherwise, the pulp may first have to be extirpated and futher appointments scheduled for completion of the root canal treatment. If the tooth is infected or there is concern about achieving predictable disinfection of the root canal system, more than one visit may be necessary. A successful treatment outcome should never be sacrificed for the sake of procedural expediency; this is discussed in Chapter 7.

ROOT CANAL RETREATMENT

Although a tooth has already been root treated, if there are signs and symptoms indicative of treatment failure and the tooth is to be retained, then root canal retreatment is required.[68] Retreatment may be via a nonsurgical or a surgical approach. There is coverage on nonsurgical and surgical retreatment in Chapters 14 and 10, respectively.

Learning Outcomes

At completion of this chapter, the reader should be able to recognize and discuss the:

- systematic approach needed to achieve a diagnosis;
- importance of deferring irreversible, invasive treatment until there is a clear diagnosis;
- special tests or additional investigations required to confirm the provisional diagnosis;
- conditions associated with pulp or periapical diseases and their differential diagnoses;
- general and specific endodontic treatment options;
- process of formulating a treatment plan based on the diagnosis;
- appropriate referral to a specialist if a diagnosis cannot be established or complex endodontic treatment is required.

REFERENCES

1. Roy R, Chandler NP. Tooth discolouration following dental trauma. ENDO (Lond Engl) 2007;1:181–7.
2. Petersson K, Söderström C, Kiani-Anaraki M, et al. Evaluation of the ability of thermal and electrical tests to register pulp vitality. Endodontics and Dental Traumatology 1999;15:127–31.
3. Pitt Ford TR, Patel S. Technical equipment for assessment of dental pulp status. Endodontic Topics 2004;7:2–13.
4. Mejàre IA, Axelsson S, Davidson T, et al. Diagnosis of the condition of the dental pulp: a systematic review. International Endodontic Journal 2012;45:597–613.
5. Brännström M. A Hydrodynamic Mechanism in the Transmission of Pain-producing Stimuli in Dentine. In: Anderson DJ, editor. Sensory Mechanisms in Dentine. Oxford, UK: Pergamon Press; 1963. p. 73–9.
6. Brännström M. Hydrodynamic theory of dental pain: sensation in preparations, caries and dentinal crack syndromes. Journal of Endodontics 1986;12:453–7.
7. Trowbridge HO, Franks M, Korostoff E, et al. Sensory response to thermal stimulation in human teeth. Journal of Endodontics 1980;6:405–12.
8. Augsburger RA, Peters DD. In vitro effects of ice, skin refrigerant, and CO_2 snow on intrapulpal temperature. Journal of Endodontics 1981;7:110–16.
9. Ingram TA, Peters DD. Evaluation of the effects of carbon dioxide used as a pulpal test. Part 2. In vivo effect on canine enamel and pulpal tissue. Journal of Endodontics 1983;9:296–303.
10. Ehrmann EH. Pulp testers and pulp testing with particular reference to the use of dry ice. Australian Dental Journal 1977;22:272–9.
11. Seltzer S, Bender IB, Ziontz M. The dynamics of pulpal inflammation: correlation between diagnostic data and actual histological findings in the pulp. Oral Surgery, Oral Medicine, Oral Pathology 1963;16:973–7.
12. Rickoff B, Trowbridge H, Baker J, et al. Effects of thermal vitality tests on human dental pulp. Journal of Endodontics 1988;14:482–5.
13. Närhi MVO. The characteristics of intradental sensory units and their responses to stimulation. Journal of Dental Research 1985;64:564–71.
14. Lin J, Chandler NP, Purton D, et al. Appropriate electrode placement site for electric pulp testing first molar teeth. Journal of Endodontics 2007;33:1296–8.
15. Byers MR, Dong WK. Autoradiographic location of sensory nerve endings in dentin of monkey teeth. Anatomical Records 1983;205:441–54.
16. Byers MR. Dental sensory receptors. International Review of Neurobiology 1984;25:39–94.
17. Lilja J. Innervation of different parts of the predentine and dentine in young human premolars. Acta Odontologica Scandinavica 1979;37:339–46.
18. Bender IB, Landau MA, Fonsecca S, et al. The optimum placement-site of the electrode in electric pulp testing of the 12 anterior teeth. Journal of the American Dental Association 1989;118:305–10.
19. Rubach WC, Mitchell DF. Periodontal disease, age, and pulp status. Oral Surgery, Oral Medicine, Oral Pathology 1965;19:482–93.
20. Pantera EA, Anderson RW, Pantera CT. Reliability of electric pulp testing after pulpal testing with dichlorodifluoromethane. Journal of Endodontics 1993;19:312–14.
21. Lin J, Chandler NP. Electric pulp testing: a review. International Endodontic Journal 2008;41:365–74.
22. Eli I. Dental anxiety: a cause for possible misdiagnosis of tooth vitality. International Endodontic Journal 1993;26:251–3.
23. Klepac RK, Dowling J, Hauge G, et al. Reports of pain after dental treatment, electrical tooth stimulation and cutaneous shock. Journal of the American Dental Association 1980;100:692–5.
24. Baume LJ. Diagnosis of diseases of the pulp. Oral Surgery, Oral Medicine, Oral Pathology 1970;29:102–16.
25. Dummer PMH, Hicks R, Huws D. Clinical signs and symptoms in pulp disease. International Endodontic Journal 1980;13:27–35.
26. Garfunkel A, Sela J, Almansky M. Dental pulp pathosis: clinicopathological correlation based on 109 cases. Oral Surgery, Oral Medicine, Oral Pathology 1973;35:110–17.
27. Hyman JJ, Cohen ME. The predictive value of endodontic diagnostic tests. Oral Surgery, Oral Medicine, Oral Pathology 1984;58:343–6.

28. Chambers IG. The role and methods of pulp testing in oral diagnosis: a review. International Endodontic Journal 1982;15: 1–5.

29. Cameron CE. The cracked-tooth syndrome: additional findings. Journal of the American Dental Association 1976;93: 971–5.

30. Calil E, Caldeira CL, Gavini G, et al. Determination of pulp vitality in vivo with pulse oximetry. International Endodontic Journal 2008;41:741–6.

31. Gazelius B, Olgart L, Edwall B, et al. Non-invasive recording of blood flow in human dental pulp. Endodontics and Dental Traumatology 1986;2:219–21.

32. Odor TM, Watson TF, Pitt-Ford TR, et al. Pattern of transmission of laser light in teeth. International Endodontic Journal 1996;29:228–34.

33. Chandler NP, Pitt Ford TR, Watson TF. Pattern of transmission of laser light through carious molar teeth. International Endodontic Journal 2001;34:526–32.

34. Olgart L, Gazelius B, Lindh-Strömberg U. Laser Doppler flowmetry in assessing vitality in luxated permanent teeth. International Endodontic Journal 1988;21:300–6.

35. Roy E, Alliot-Licht B, Dajean-Trutaud S, et al. Evaluation of the ability of laser Doppler flowmetry for the assessment of pulp vitality in general dental practice. Oral Surgery, Oral Medicine, Oral Pathology, Oral Radiology and Endodontology 2008;106:615–20.

36. Emshoff R, Moschen I, Strobl H. Use of laser Doppler flowmetry to predict vitality of luxated or avulsed permanent teeth. Oral Surgery, Oral Medicine, Oral Pathology, Oral Radiology, and Endodontics 2004;98:750–5.

37. Chandler NP, Pitt Ford TR, Monteith BD. Effect of restorations on pulpal blood flow in molars measured by laser Doppler flowmetry. International Endodontic Journal 2010;43:41–6.

38. Chandler NP, Pitt Ford TR, Monteith BD. Laser light passage through restored and carious posterior teeth. Journal of Oral Rehabilitation 2014;41:630–4.

39. Patel S, Dawood A, Whaites E, et al. New dimensions in endodontic imaging: Part 1. Conventional and alternative radiographic systems. International Endodontic Journal 2009; 42:447–62.

40. Tidmarsh BG. Radiographic interpretation of endodontic lesions- a shadow of reality. International Dental Journal 1987;37:10–15.

41. Petersson K, Wennberg A, Olsson B. Radiographic and clinical estimation of endodontic treatment need. Endodontics and Dental Traumatology 1986;2:62–4.

42. Chandler NP, Pitt Ford TR, Monteith BD. Coronal pulp size in molars: a study of bitewing radiographs. International Endodontic Journal 2003;36:757–63.

43. Forsberg J, Halse A. Radiographic simulation of a periapical lesion comparing the paralleling and the bisecting-angle techniques. International Endodontic Journal 1994;27: 133–8.

44. Forsberg J. Radiographic reproduction of endodontic 'working length' comparing the paralleling and the bisecting-angle techniques. Oral Surgery, Oral Medicine, Oral Pathology, Oral Radiology, and Endodontics 1987;64:353–60.

45. Forsberg J. A comparison of the paralleling and bisecting-angle radiographic techniques in endodontics. International Endodontic Journal 1987;20:177–82.

46. De Vos W, Casselman J, Swennen GR. Cone-beam computerized tomography (CBCT) imaging of the oral and maxillofacial region: a systematic review of the literature. International Journal of Oral and Maxillofacial Surgery 2009;38:609–25.

47. Scarfe WC, Levin MD, Gane D, et al. Use of cone beam computed tomography in endodontics. International Journal of Dentistry 2009;2009:634567. doi:10.1155/2009/634567.

48. de Paula-Silva FW, Wu MK, Leonardo MR, et al. Accuracy of periapical radiography and cone-beam computed tomography scans in diagnosing apical periodontitis using histopathological findings as a gold standard. Journal of Endodontics 2009;35:1009–12.

49. Low KM, Dula K, Burgin W, et al. Comparison of periapical radiography and limited cone-beam tomography in posterior maxillary teeth referred for apical surgery. Journal of Endodontics 2008;34:557–62.

50. Pope O, Sathorn C, Parashos P. A comparative investigation of cone-beam computed tomography and periapical radiography in the diagnosis of a healthy periapex. Journal of Endodontics 2014;40:360–5.

51. Pauwels R, Beinsberger J, Collaert B, et al. Effective dose range for dental cone beam computed tomography scanners. European Journal of Radiology 2012;81:267–71.

52. Patel S, Durack C, Abella F, et al. European Society of Endodontology position statement: the use of CBCT in endodontics. International Endodontic Journal 2014;47: 502–4.

53. SEDENTEXCT. European Commission. Radiation protection No 172 cone beam CT for dental and maxillofacial radiology (evidence-based guidelines), <http://www.sedentexct.eu/files/radiation_protection_172.pdf>; 2012.

54. Patel S, Saunders WP. Radiographs in endodontics. In: Horner K, Eaton KA, editors. Selection criteria for dental radiography. 3rd ed. London: Faculty of General Dental Practice (UK); 2013. p. 83–96.

55. Patel S, Durack C, Abella F, et al. Cone beam computed tomography in Endodontics – a review. International Endodontic Journal 2015;48:3–15.

56. AAE & AAOMR. Use of cone beam computed tomography in endodontics, 2015 update. Joint position statement of the American Association of Endodontists and the American Academy of Oral and Maxillofacial Radiology, <http://www.aae.org/uploadedfiles/clinical_resources/guidelines_and_position_statements/cbctstatement_2015update.pdf>; 2015.

57. European Society of Endodontology developed by: Patel S, Durack C, Abella F, et al. European Society of Endodontology position statement: The use of CBCT in endodontics. International Endodontic Journal 2014;47:502–4.

58. Lundy T, Stanley HR. Correlation of pulpal histopathology and clinical symptoms in human teeth subjected to experimental irritation. Oral Surgery, Oral Medicine, Oral Pathology 1969;27:187–201.

59. Michaelson PL, Holland GR. Is pulpitis painful? International Endodontic Journal 2002;35:829–32.

60. Jyvasjarvi E, Kniffki DK. Cold stimulation of teeth: a comparison between the responses of cat intradental A- and C-fibers and human sensations. Journal of Physiology 1987;391: 193–207.

61. Mengel MK, Stiefenhofer AE, Jyvasjarvi E, et al. Pain sensation during cold stimulation of the teeth: differential reflection of A delta and C fibre activity? Pain 1993;55:159–69.

62. Abbott PV. Assessing restored teeth with pulp and periapical diseases for the presence of cracks, caries and marginal breakdown. Australian Dental Journal 2004;49:33–9.

63. McDonald A, Setchell D. Developing a tooth restorability index. Dental Update 2005;32:343–8.

64. Samet N, Jotkowitz A. Classification and prognosis evaluation of individual teeth. A comprehensive approach. Quintessence International 2009;40:377–87.

65. American Association of Endodontists. Endodontic case difficulty assessment and referral, <http://www.aae.org/NR/rdonlyres/CD6A4FE5-EEAC-47AE-8B53–6DF01D324E31/0/casedifficultarticle.pdf>; 2005.

66. Canadian Academy of Endodontics. Case classification according to degrees of difficulty and risk. In: Standards of Practice, <http://www.caendo.ca/about_cae/standards/standards_english.pdf>; 2006.

67. Ree MH, Timmerman MF, Wesselink PR. An evaluation of the usefulness of two endodontic case assessment forms by general dentists. International Endodontic Journal 2003;36:545–55.

68. Chong BS. Managing endodontic failure in practice. London: Quintessence Publishing Co. Ltd; 2004.

CHAPTER 4

Pulp Space Anatomy and Access Cavities

J. Camilleri

Chapter Contents

Summary

Knowledge of pulp space anatomy is essential to achieving the objectives of endodontic treatment. The use of three-dimensional tomography has revealed and confirmed the complex and divergent anatomy of the pulp space. Classical, preconceptualized access cavity designs are informative in the understanding of pulp space anatomy. However, they have been replaced by emergent and customized access cavity designs, which are prepared according to treatment requirements. Unnecessary and excessive destruction of tooth tissue during access cavity preparation remains unwarranted. The wider adoption of magnification and enhanced illumination, especially the clinical use of an operating microscope, is invaluable as it greatly aids access cavity preparation and allows the detailed examination of the pulp space.

Introduction

Root canal treatment is carried out to treat or prevent apical periodontitis. Current practice involves chemo-mechanical cleaning followed by the complete sealing of the pulp space. In addition, the need for a good coronal restoration is integral to ensuring a favourable treatment outcome.

A clear understanding of the anatomy of human teeth is an essential prerequisite for achieving the objectives of adequate access, thorough cleaning, effective disinfection and complete obturation of the pulp space. Most procedural errors occur due to inadequate understanding of the pulp space anatomy. Both students and clinicians need to familiarize themselves with the intricacies, complexities and aberrations that are likely to occur within the pulp space. The importance of developing a visual picture of the expected locations and numbers of canals in a particular tooth cannot be overemphasized.

The internal anatomy of human teeth has been studied by many investigators, providing a valuable insight into the size, shape and form of the pulp space. Root canal anatomy has been studied using various techniques; filling the root canal space with injected silicone and tooth dissolution by concentrated acid provided visualization of the intricate root canal anatomy.[1] Another frequent method has been the use of dyes to fill and define the root canal space followed by tooth clearing.[2,3] Clearing renders the tooth rubbery; thus, recently a newer method of preparation, which preserves the natural tooth hardness, has been reported.[4] Root canal morphology can also be assessed using the Bramante muffle technique[5] and also by sectioning and visualization of ground sections using light microscopy and scanning electron microscopy. Clinical dental radiography shows the roots and pulp canal space in two dimensions only; microradiography enhances the radiographic technique.[6] The limitations of the bucccal to palatal/lingual view have been highlighted by taking radiographs in two planes.[7] The pulp space volume is invariably much greater than the clinical radiograph would suggest. Microcomputed tomography has allowed the appreciation of pulp space anatomy in three dimensions (Figure 4-1).[8,9] More recently, cone beam computed tomography (CBCT) has increased our knowledge of the pulp space[10] and allowed the identification of missed anatomy[11,12]; see Chapter 3, on the use of CBCT.

Pulp Space Anatomy

Anatomically, the dental pulp space is surrounded by dentine to form the pulp–dentine complex. Dentine forms the bulk of the mineralized tissue of the tooth. The dentinal tubules, which are interconnected, make up 20% to 30% of the total volume of dentine.[13] The number of tubules per square millimetre more than doubles, and the area occupied by tubules increases threefold from the dentine near the amelodentinal junction to that near the pulp.[14] These differences have a significant clinical effect on the permeability of dentine.[15] Dentinal tubules are an important reservoir

of microorganisms when pulpal necrosis occurs.[16] Bacteria may remain in the dentinal tubules, leading to persistent infection of the root canal system even after the completion of root canal treatment.

The pulp space is divided into two parts: the pulp chamber, which is usually described as that portion within the crown, and the pulp canal or root canal, which lies within the confines of the root. The pulp chamber is a single cavity, the dimensions of which vary according to the outline of the crown and the structure of the roots. Thus, if the crown has well-developed cusps, the pulp chamber projects into well-developed pulp horns. In multirooted teeth, the depth of the pulp chamber depends on the position of the root furcation and may extend beyond the anatomical crown. In young teeth, the outline of the pulp chamber resembles the shape of the exterior of the dentine. With age, the dentinal tubules and pulp chamber reduce in size by the laying down of intratubular dentine, secondary dentine and tertiary dentine, particularly in areas where there have been caries, tooth wear and exposure to operative treatment (Figure 4-2). The pulp chamber may then become irregular in outline. With age, there is also a gradual decrease in pulp space volume, number of nerves, blood vessels and cells within, but there is also an increase in the fibrous and mineral components. The rate at which the pulps age varies from one tooth to another and from one patient to another. Calcific changes can lead to the pulp space appearing entirely obliterated radiologically. Although radiologically unidentifiable, a residual canal almost certainly remains within the root as a pathway for microbes to reach the apex and cause periapical changes.

The pulp of root canals is continuous with the pulp chamber, and normally, the greatest diameter is at the pulp chamber level. Since the roots tend to taper toward their apices, the canals also have a tapering form which is constricted at the end, also called the apical constriction, before emerging at the apical foramina, near the root end; rarely do the foramina open at the exact anatomical apex of the tooth. During root development, the pulp and periodontal tissues separate, maintaining neural and vascular connections through the apical foramina.

The pulp space is complex, and root canals may divide and rejoin and possess forms that are

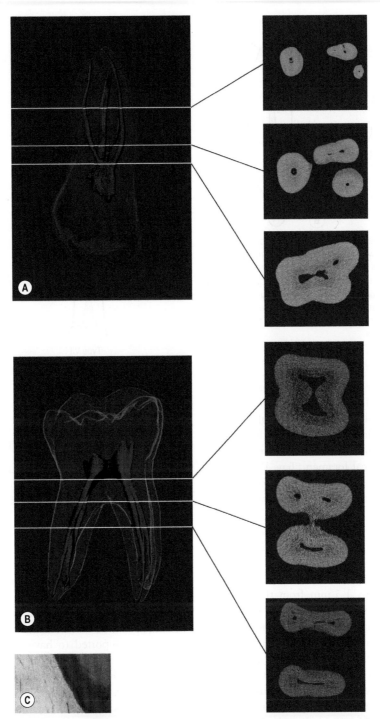

FIGURE 4-1 Three-dimensional images reconstructed from microcomputed tomography data; cross-sections at various levels indicated by corresponding lines. (A) Maxillary molar. (B) Mandibular molar. (C) Cellular arrangement of the odontoblast layer. (From Peters 2008, with permission of Quintessence Publishing Co. Ltd.)

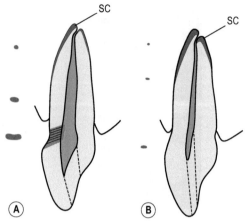

FIGURE 4-2 Alteration of the pulp size with age. (A) Tooth of a young adult; large pulp chamber with tertiary dentine under tubules affected by cervical abrasion; small amount of secondary cementum (SC) at apex. (B) Tooth of an older patient showing smaller pulp space and greater amounts of secondary cementum that have altered the relationship of the apical constriction to the foramen. Access cavities are indicated by dotted lines. To the left: cross-sections of the root canals are shown at selected levels.

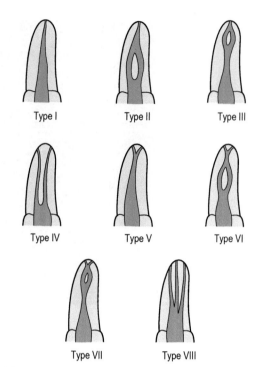

FIGURE 4-3 Types of canal configuration, classification according to Vertucci (1984).

considerably more involved than many anatomy textbooks have implied. Many roots have additional canals and a variety of canal configurations. Eight separate pulp space configurations have been identified (Figure 4-3).[17] In the simplest form, each root has a single canal and a single apical foramen (Type I). However, other canal complexities are commonly present and exit the root as one, two or more apical canals (Types II–VIII).

Since roots tend to be broader buccolingually than they are mesiodistally, the pulp space is similarly oval in cross-section. The diameter of the root canal decreases toward the apical foramen and reaches its narrowest point 1.0 to 1.5 mm from the foramen. This point, the apical constriction lies within the dentine just before the first layers of cementum and is the narrowest point to which the canal tapers. During root development, the apical part of the pulp is described as being 'open'. As the tooth matures, the funnel-shaped foramen closes and constricts to a normal root shape with a small apical foramen. The position of the apical foramen may also be altered, relative to the root apex, with the deposition of secondary cementum.

Accessory and Lateral Canals

The pulpal and periodontal tissues not only maintain connection through the apical foramina but also through accessory and lateral canals. A lateral canal can be found anywhere along the length of a root and tends to be at right angles to the main root canal. Accessory canals usually branch off the main root canal somewhere in the apical region. The presence of lateral canals in the furcation areas of molar teeth is well documented, and their incidence is relatively high. Patent lateral canals are present in the coronal or middle third of 59% of molars.[18] A total of 76% of molars are reported to have openings in the furcation.[19] It has been shown, using a vascular injection technique, that these accessory canals often had a greater diameter than the apical foramina, and the blood vessels passing through them often had a greater diameter than those in the apical foramina.[20] The accessory and lateral canals may be demonstrated histologically by clearing techniques or clinically on

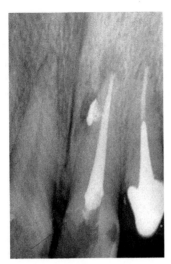

FIGURE 4-4 Radiograph of a maxillary central incisor. A lateral canal is revealed after placement of the root filling. (Reproduced courtesy of I. Khalil.)

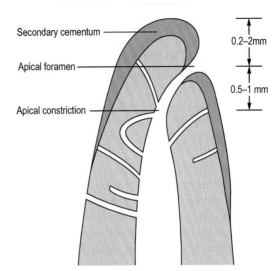

FIGURE 4-5 Diagrammatic section through apical third of root. The position of the apical foramen varies with age and may be 0.2 to 2.0 mm from the anatomical apex. The apical constriction may be 0.5 to 1.0 mm from the foramen.

radiographs (Figure 4-4). The presence of these canals in teeth with necrotic pulps allows microbial toxins to stimulate inflammatory responses in the periapical tissues.

Location of Apical Foramina

The majority of endodontists consider that the apical extent of canal preparation should be determined by the position of the apical constriction in the region of the dentine-cementum junction (Figure 4-5). Provided that this constriction is not destroyed, the periapical tissues are not damaged during root canal preparation and obturation.

Studies indicated that the apical foramen rarely coincides in position with the anatomical apex. According to various radiological and morphological studies of different teeth,[21-26] the mean distance between the apical foramen and the most apical end of the root is between 0.2 and 2.0 mm. Furthermore, the apical constriction tends to occur about 0.5 to 1.0 mm from the apical foramen.[22] Ideally, the apical constriction should be used as a natural 'stop' or 'end point' in root canal treatment, and the integrity of the constriction should be maintained during treatment if complications are to be avoided. This position can usually be located accurately with an apex locator.[27-29]

Variations in Pulp Space Anatomy

Variations in tooth form have interested scientists and anthropologists as well as dentists. These studies of variations have primarily been concentrated on the systematic description of dental crown morphology rather than root form. Variations in root form and number are likely to have a direct influence on the configuration of the root canals in affected teeth. One variation which has received some attention is the three-rooted mandibular first molar; surveys of Mongoloid populations indicate a high prevalence.[30-32] The prevalence of other Mongoloid root traits has been less studied.[33-36] In clinical practice it is not always possible to observe these variations from radiographs.

In the condition *dens invaginatus*, the surface of the tooth formed with a deep pit into the pulp space during tooth development, which subsequently becomes a route for infection into the pulp. Depending on the severity of the condition, commonly classified based on Oehler's system,[37] endodontic treatment will be difficult or very challenging[38]; nowadays, the management of such cases may be facilitated by CBCT.[39] The most commonly affected tooth is the maxillary lateral incisor.[37,40,41]

In the opposite condition, *dens evaginatus,* the surface of the tooth formed into a very protuberant cusp during tooth development. There is a high risk of this cusp fracturing during function, creating a route for infection of the pulp space. The mandibular premolar, the condition known as Leong's premolar,[42] is most frequently affected and is more often found in Mongoloid people.[43] It is best managed by prophylactic treatment.[44]

The descriptions of the frequently occurring root and canal forms of permanent teeth are based largely on studies conducted in Europe and North America and relate to teeth of predominantly Caucasoid origin. The descriptions may not be wholly applicable to teeth of non-Caucasoid origin. For example, the average lengths of teeth, around which there is wide variation, apply to Caucasoid populations. Practitioners who regularly treat Mongoloid populations are aware that roots are usually shorter. Racial differences and its influence on pulp space anatomy should always be kept in mind.

Effects of Tertiary Dentine on Pulp Space

Tertiary dentine is formed by odontoblasts in response to irritation from caries, restorative dentistry or tooth wear. The amount formed is dependent on the degree and duration of irritation. The function of this dentine is to wall off the pulp from the irritants; this is, generally, of great benefit. However, when root canal treatment is indicated, the coronal pulp is then exceedingly small and therefore difficult to locate. In addition, canal orifices become narrowed by deposition of tertiary dentine, making their identification difficult.

There is no substitute for good knowledge of pulpal anatomy; however, the clinician should be aided by a good quality preoperative radiograph from which the depth and direction of the root canals can be gauged. When inside the centre of the tooth and attempting to locate the pulp space, illumination and magnification are major assets. While this can be provided by a headlamp and loupes, it is best achieved using an operating microscope. The increased illumination reveals the different colours of circumpulpal and tertiary dentine, so that the access to the root canals can be correctly orientated.

Pulp Space Anatomy and Access Cavities

Each line drawing accompanying the description of pulp space anatomy represents, from left to right:
- longitudinal mesiodistal section, viewed from the lingual in anterior teeth and from the buccal in posterior teeth;
- longitudinal buccolingual section viewed from the mesial, and also the axial angulation of the tooth relative to the horizontal occlusal plane;
- horizontal sections through the root(s): (above) 3 mm from apex; (below) at the cervical level;
- incisal or occlusal view.

The classical outline of the access cavity is shown as a dotted line. The size of the pulp cavity shortly after completion of root formation is shown in pink, and in the aging population in brown. Line drawings are accompanied, where appropriate, by photographs of cleared specimens to give an insight into the variations of canal form that exist in the adult dentition.

Access cavity design should not be thought of as a one size fits all. Rather designs should be developed to suit the specific pulpal anatomy of individual teeth.[45] The classical outline of access cavities is helpful in the appreciation of pulp space anatomy. However, it must be emphasized that rather than preconceptualized designs, access cavities should be prepared according to access requirements. While unnecessary and excessive destruction of tooth tissue must be avoided, it is important to remember that all caries and the roof of the pulp chamber must be completely removed. After caries removal, a good temporary restoration should be placed to prevent coronal leakage.

Several authors[46,47] have recognized the importance of the systematic development of the pulp space during tooth formation to the understanding of access cavity preparation. This recognition has led to a number of 'laws' being postulated to serve as a guide to clinicians in developing the access cavity and locating accurately root canal orifices (Table 4-1).

MAXILLARY CENTRAL AND LATERAL INCISORS

The outlines and pulp cavities of maxillary central and lateral incisors are similar (Figures 4-6 and 4-7). Central incisors are larger with a mean length of 23 mm. Lateral incisors are smaller with a mean

TABLE 4-1 Laws Relating To Pulp Chamber Anatomy

Law of centrality	The floor of the pulp chamber is always located in the centre of the tooth at the level of the cemento-enamel junction (CEJ).
Law of concentricity	At the level of the CEJ, the shape of the pulp chamber mimics the external anatomy of the tooth.
Law of the CEJ	The distance from the external surface of the tooth to the wall of the pulp chamber is the same throughout the circumference of the tooth at the level of the CEJ. The CEJ is the most reliable and consistent feature for ascertaining the position of the pulp chamber.
First law of symmetry	With the exception of the maxillary molars, the orifices of the canals are equidistant either side of a line drawn mesial to distal through the floor of the pulp chamber.
Second law of symmetry	With the exception of the maxillary molars, the orifices of the canals lie on a line perpendicular to the line drawn mesial to distal through the floor of the pulp chamber.
The law of colour change	The dentine of the floor of the pulp chamber is, invariably, a darker colour than the roof and walls. With good magnification and illumination this allows the clinician to differentiate and selectively remove tissue.
First law of orifice location	The orifices of the root canals are located where the walls and the floor meet.
Second law of orifice location	The orifices of the root canals are located at the angles in the floor/wall junctions.
Third law of orifice location	The orifices of the root canals are located at the ends of the root developmental fusion lines.

(Adapted from Krasner & Rankow 2004 and Peters 2008.)

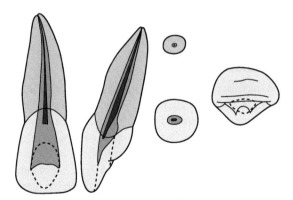

FIGURE 4-6 Maxillary central incisor with a Type I configuration.

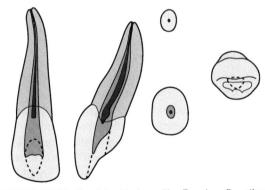

FIGURE 4-7 Maxillary lateral incisor with a Type I configuration.

length of 21 to 22 mm. The canal form is usually Type I, and it is extremely rare for these teeth to have more than one root or more than one root canal. Where abnormalities do occur they seem to affect the maxillary lateral incisor, which may present with an extra root, second root canal, *dens invaginatus,* gemination or fusion.[48,49] The pulp chamber, when viewed labiopalatally, is pointed toward the

incisal and widest at the cervical level. Mesiodistally both pulp chambers follow the general outline of their crowns and are thus widest at their incisal levels. The central incisors of young patients normally have three pulp horns. Lateral incisors usually have two pulp horns, and the incisal outline of the pulp chamber tends to be more rounded than that of central incisors.

The root canal differs greatly in outline when viewed mesiodistally and labiopalatally. The former view generally shows a fine straight canal that is seen on a radiograph. Labiopalatally the canal is much wider and often shows a constriction just apical to the cervix; this view is rarely seen on radiographs and it is important to remember that during treatment all canals have this third dimension. The canal is tapered with an oval or irregular cross-section cervically that becomes round only very near the apex. There is generally very little apical curvature in central incisors. The apex of lateral incisors is often curved in a distal/palatal direction. Sometimes the plane in which it lies means that the apex is not easily discernible during radiographic canal length determination.

As the teeth age, the anatomy of the pulp space alters with the deposition of secondary dentine. The roof of the pulp chamber recedes, in some cases to the cervical level, and the canal appears very narrow mesiodistally on a radiograph. It is often possible to negotiate a canal that appears very fine or nonexistent on a preoperative radiograph. When some incisors are traumatized, their pulps may mineralize, that is, the pulp canal becomes obliterated; subsequent root canal treatment can be extremely difficult as the mineralization frequently occurs throughout the length of the pulp space.

Access Cavities to Maxillary Incisors

Access cavities in anterior teeth will vary in size and shape according to the dimension of the pulp. They should be designed so that a straight line approach is possible to the apical third of the root without the instruments bending or binding against the walls of the access cavity or root canal. As the pulp is broader incisally than it is cervically, the outline should be triangular and must extend far enough mesially and distally to include the pulp horns. An access cavity that is too small and close to the cingulum leads to severe stresses on the instrument with binding against the access cavity walls and risks ledge formation apically (Figure 4-8). The access cavity should extend far enough incisally to allow the instrument to reach the apical part of the canal. Sometimes, the incisal edge may be involved if access is to be adequate.

Once adequate access has been made into the pulp chamber, the cervical constriction should be removed

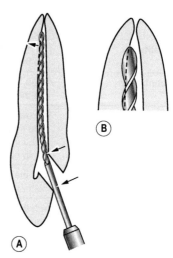

FIGURE 4-8 (A) The access cavity is too small and close to the cingulum, impeding passage of instruments, and therefore a ledge may be created apically. The incorrect access also hinders cleaning of the pulp chamber and near the apex. (B) Enlargement of the apex showing labial ledge and uninstrumented palatal side.

to facilitate instrumentation of the apical part. The accuracy of initial access is particularly important in the older patient because the pulp space is more difficult to find. It is prudent to begin the access cavity close to the incisal edge so that the pulp space can be approached in a straight line.

MAXILLARY CANINE

The maxillary canine is the longest tooth, with a mean length of 26.5 mm; therefore, longer root canal instruments are often required. It seldom has more than one root canal; the pulp chamber is quite narrow and there is only one pulp horn. The general shape of the pulp space is similar to the incisors. The Type I root canal form is oval and does not begin to become circular in a cross-section until the apical third (Figure 4-9). The canal is usually straight but may show a distal apical curvature; the direction of the curvature depends on the direction of movement of the tooth during eruption.

Access Cavity to Maxillary Canine

The access cavity for a maxillary canine should be prepared on the palatal aspect of the tooth. Oval-shaped, the access cavity should extend from the cingulum toward the canine edge; extension

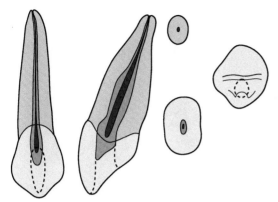

FIGURE 4-9 Maxillary canine with a Type I configuration.

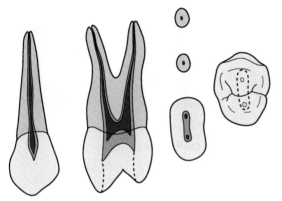

FIGURE 4-10 Maxillary first premolar with two roots.

mediodistally is, normally, not necessary as there is only one pulp horn.

MAXILLARY FIRST PREMOLAR

This tooth generally has two roots with two canals. The frequency of single-rooted maxillary first premolars ranges from 31% to 39% in Caucasians.[50,51] In people of Mongoloid origin, the frequency of maxillary first premolars with one root is in excess of 60%.[52–54] Three roots have been reported in 6% of cases.[50] A typical Caucasoid specimen has two well-developed fully formed roots that normally begin in the middle third of the roots (Figure 4-10). The single-rooted condition prevalent in Mongoloid people represents a fusion of two separate roots.

Irrespective of origin, this tooth normally has two canals, and in the case of single-rooted specimens,

these canals may open through a common apical foramen. Many types of canal configurations can be found in this tooth (Figure 4-11), and the presence of lateral canals, particularly in the apical region, can be as high as 49%.[51] The three-rooted form tends to have three canals: two located buccally and one palatally. Careful study of a preoperative radiograph should help reveal the root canal morphology. However, this morphology may be difficult to visualize radiologically, particularly when the apex is very fine.

The mean length of first premolars is 21 mm. The pulp chamber is wide buccopalatally with two distinct pulp horns, but it is narrow mesiodistally. The floor is rounded with the highest point in the centre and generally just apical to the level of the cervix. The orifices into the root canals are funnel shaped and lie buccally and palatally under the cusp tips. As the tooth ages, secondary dentine is deposited on the roof of the pulp chamber, and this has the effect of bringing the roof very much closer to the floor. The floor level remains apical to the cervix, and the thickened roof may reach apical to the cervix. The root canals are normally separate and very rarely blend into the ribbon-like type of canal frequently seen in the second premolar. They are usually straight with a round cross-section.

MAXILLARY SECOND PREMOLAR

The maxillary second premolar tends to be single rooted. The Type I canal form is prevalent; however, over 25% of these teeth may present as Types II and III, and a further 25% may have Types IV to VII forms with two canals at the apex.[53,55] Thus, the typical maxillary second premolar may be envisaged as having one root with a single canal (Figure 4-12). Less frequently two roots may be present, and while the outward appearance may be similar to the first premolar, the floor of the pulp chamber is well apical to the cervix. The mean length of the second premolar is slightly longer than the first premolar at 21.5 mm.

The pulp chamber is wide buccopalatally and has two well-defined pulp horns. The root canal is also wide buccopalatally but narrow mesiodistally. It tapers apically but rarely develops a circular cross-section except in the apical 2 to 3 mm. Often, the root of this single-rooted tooth branches into two sections in the middle third of the root. These branches almost

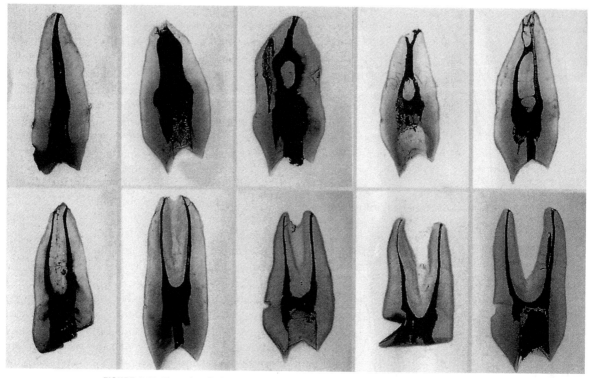

FIGURE 4-11 Cleared teeth showing various canal configurations in maxillary first premolars.

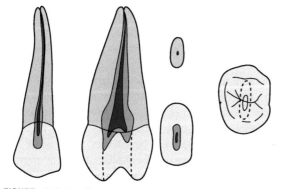

FIGURE 4-12 Maxillary second premolar with a Type I canal configuration.

invariably join to form a common canal, which has a relatively large foramen. The canal is usually straight, but the apex may curve to the distal. As the tooth matures, the roof of the pulp chamber recedes away from the crown.

Access Cavities to Maxillary Premolars

This access should be through the occlusal surface. The access cavity is a narrow slot in a buccolingual direction. In the case of the first premolar, the orifices of the root canal are readily visible as they lie just apical to the cervix; however, pulp calcifications may make canal identification challenging, and vertical misalignment, directed too mesially, is a not uncommon error. The second premolar root canal is ribbon-shaped and, because it lies well apical to the cervix, may not be readily visible. In preparing an access cavity, an inexperienced operator without magnification may easily mistake the pulp horns for the canal orifices.

MAXILLARY FIRST MOLAR

Maxillary first molars are generally three-rooted with four root canals (Figure 4-13). The additional canal is located in the mesiobuccal root.[12] The canal form of the mesiobuccal root has been extensively investigated. Studies *in vitro* indicate that a second canal is

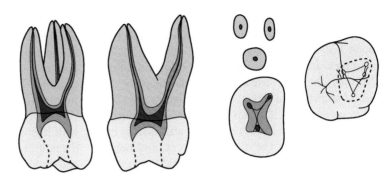

FIGURE 4-13 Maxillary first molar.

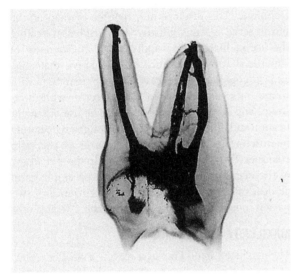

FIGURE 4-14 Cleared maxillary first molar with a Type II canal configuration in the mesiobuccal root.

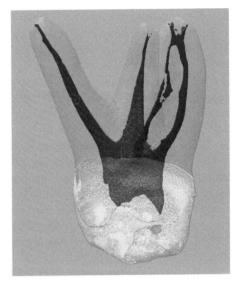

FIGURE 4-15 Computer-generated reconstructed image, from microcomputed tomography, of a maxillary first molar with a Type VI canal configuration in the mesiobuccal root. (Reproduced courtesy of Bauru Dental School, Sao Paolo State University, Brazil.)

present in up to 90% of teeth.[56–60] The canal configuration is usually Type II (Figure 4-14); however, the presence of a Type IV form with two separate apical foramina has been reported to be as high as 48%.[57] Studies *in vivo*[56,61–63] have, historically, reported a lower prevalence of the second mesiobuccal canal; however, as an operating microscope is used more routinely nowadays, unless otherwise proven, a second canal is assumed to be present. Three-dimensional tomographic radiography continues to reveal the complexity of root canal systems within the mesiobuccal root (Figure 4-15). The palatal and distobuccal roots usually present a Type I configuration.

In Caucasians, the mean length of this tooth is 22 mm, as the palatal root is slightly longer than the buccal roots. In Mongoloid teeth, there is a tendency for the roots to be closer together and the average length to be slightly shorter. The pulp chamber is quadrilateral in shape and wider buccopalatally than mesiodistally. It has four pulp horns, of which the mesiobuccal is the longest and sharpest in outline. The distobuccal pulp horn is smaller than the mesiobuccal but larger than the two palatal pulp horns. The floor of the pulp chamber is normally just apical to the cervix and is rounded and dome-shaped. The orifices of the main pulp canals are funnel-shaped and lie symmetrically in the middle of the appropriate root. The second mesiobuccal canal, if present, lies mesial to a line joining the main mesiobuccal and palatal canal orifices. It can be located anywhere between the two canals but is most frequently found adjacent to the main mesiobuccal canal under a lip of dentine. Furthermore, the transverse cross-sectional shape of the pulp chamber 1 mm above the pulpal floor is trapezoidal in most teeth.[59] For this reason, the mesiobuccal canal opening is closer to the buccal wall than is the distobuccal orifice. The distobuccal root, and hence the opening into the root canal, is closer to the middle of the tooth than to the distal wall. The palatal root canal orifice lies in the middle of the palatal root and is normally easy to identify.

The cross-section of the root canals varies considerably. The mesiobuccal canals are usually the most challenging to instrument as they leave the pulp chamber in a mesial direction before curving distopalatally. The second mesiobuccal canal is generally very fine and may join the main canal. The orifice of this canal may be concealed by a dentine lip, which needs to be removed to detect the orifice. As both mesiobuccal canals lie in a buccopalatal plane, they are often superimposed on radiographs. The distobuccal canal leaves the pulp chamber in a distal direction. It is ovoid in shape and again narrower mesiodistally. It tapers toward the apex and becomes circular in cross-section. The canal normally curves mesially in the apical half of the root. The palatal canal is the largest and longest of the three canals and leaves the pulp chamber as a round canal, which gradually tapers apically. In 50% of roots, it is not straight but curves buccally in the apical 3 to 4 mm. This curvature may not be apparent on a clinical radiograph and unless appreciated, it may lead to incorrect length measurement and canal transportation after instrumentation.

As the tooth ages, secondary dentine is deposited chiefly on the roof of the pulp chamber; thus reducing the depth of the pulp chamber. The presence of tertiary dentine further complicates canal location. As the pulp chamber becomes progressively obliterated, access preparation becomes more challenging. It is relatively easy for the inexperienced operator, and particularly with high-speed handpieces, to perforate the floor of the pulp chamber. Access should be achieved patiently and with precision. The distance from the cusp tips to the roof of the pulp chamber should be measured on a preoperative radiograph, taken using the paralleling technique. This distance may then be marked on the bur to serve as a depth gauge. It is prudent to restrict the use of high-speed handpieces to the removal of superficial tooth substance or restorative materials, and to complete the access cavity preparation with round burs with low-speed handpieces or with ultrasound and special endodontic tips. The use of magnification and illumination, usually through an operating microscope, allows better visualization of the pulp chamber. The variable nature of the pulp space anatomy of the maxillary first molar has received emphasis in clinical case reports including the occurrence of two palatal roots and multiple palatal canals.[65–68]

MAXILLARY SECOND MOLAR

The maxillary second molar is usually a smaller replica of the first molar (Figure 4-16). The roots are less divergent, and fusion between two roots is much more frequent than in the maxillary first molar. Teeth with three canals and three apical foramina are prevalent, but studies have also reported a high incidence of second mesiobuccal canals[12,69]; the mean length is 21 mm. Root fusion has been demonstrated in up to

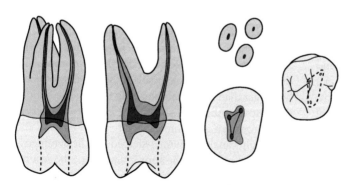

FIGURE 4-16 Maxillary second molar.

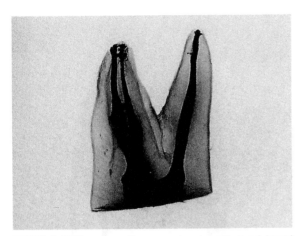

FIGURE 4-17 Cleared maxillary second molar with fused buccal roots.

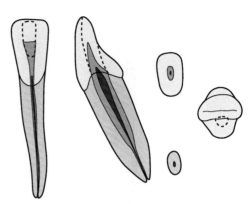

FIGURE 4-19 Mandibular central incisor with a Type I canal configuration.

MAXILLARY THIRD MOLAR

The maxillary third molar displays a great deal of variability in terms of morphology. It may possess three separate roots, but more often partial or complete fusion occurs.[69] The pulp space anatomy is less predictable, and these teeth may have a reduced number of canals.

Access Cavities to Maxillary Molars

The traditional access cavity outline for maxillary teeth is normally in the mesial two-thirds of the occlusal surface leaving the oblique ridge intact, and is triangular with the base of the triangle toward the buccal, and the apex palatally. It has been suggested that this traditional shape should be modified in the case of the first molar to a trapezoid shape.[64] As the distobuccal canal is not as close to the buccal surface as the mesiobuccal canal, less tooth tissue removal is needed from this area.

MANDIBULAR CENTRAL AND LATERAL INCISORS

Both types of teeth have a mean length of 21 mm, although the central incisor may be a little shorter than the lateral incisor. The root canal morphology may be placed into one of three configurations[70]:

- Type I – a single main canal extending from the pulp chamber to the apical foramen (Figure 4-19);
- Type II/III – two main root canals that merge in the middle or apical third of the root into a single canal with one apical foramen (Figure 4-20);

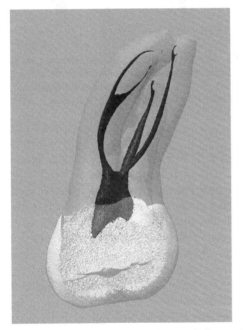

FIGURE 4-18 Computer-generated reconstructed image, from microcomputed tomography, of a maxillary second molar with a Type V canal configuration in the mesiobuccal root. (Reproduced courtesy of Bauru Dental School, Sao Paolo State University, Brazil.)

55% of Caucasoid maxillary second molars, whereas in Mongoloid groups this figure may be up to 85%.[31,53] Where root fusion does occur, the canals and their orifices are much closer together (Figures 4-17 and 4-18).

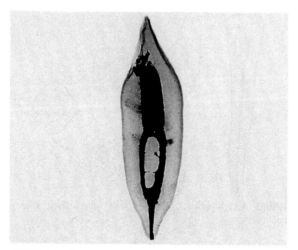

FIGURE 4-20 Cleared mandibular central incisor with a Type II canal configuration.

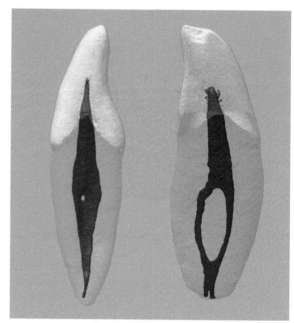

FIGURE 4-22 Computer-generated reconstructed image, from microcomputed tomography, of mandibular incisors showing a Type I (left) and a Type II (right) canal configuration. (Reproduced courtesy of Bauru Dental School, Sao Paolo State University, Brazil.)

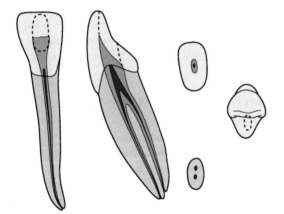

FIGURE 4-21 Mandibular lateral incisor with a Type IV canal configuration.

- Type IV – two main canals that remain distinct throughout the length of the tooth and exit through two major apical foramina (Figure 4-21).

The Type I and Type II morphologies are shown in Figure 4-22. Studies indicate that the Type I canal form is most prevalent, Types II and III less prevalent, and Type IV is the least prevalent. The presence of two canals has been recorded to be as high as 41%[70]; however, the highest recorded figure for two separate apical foramina (Type IV) has been 5%.[71] There is some evidence to suggest that there is a lower frequency of two canals in mandibular central and lateral incisors in Mongoloid people.[72]

The pulp chamber is a smaller replica of that in the maxillary incisors. It is pointed incisally with three pulp horns that are not well developed, is oval in cross-section and wider labiolingually than it is mesiodistally. When the tooth has a single root canal, it is normally straight but may curve to the distal and less often to the labial. The tooth ages in a similar way to the maxillary incisors, and the incisal part of the pulp chamber may recede to a level apical to the cervix. The pulps of these teeth may mineralize in response to traumatic injury.

Access Cavities to Mandibular Incisors

Essentially these cavities are similar to those in maxillary incisors. However, because of the more pronounced labial curvature of the crown and because the canals, particularly in older patients, are so fine, it is sometimes necessary to involve the incisal edge of the tooth. It is important to be as conservative as possible

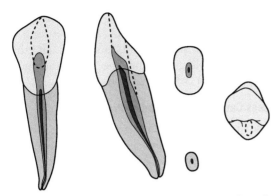

FIGURE 4-23 Mandibular canine with a Type I canal configuration.

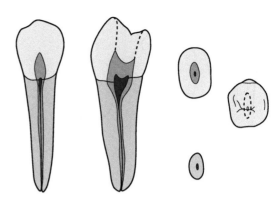

FIGURE 4-24 Mandibular second premolar with a Type I canal configuration.

and not remove more tooth tissue than necessary. Moreover, the bulk of the cingulum should be retained.

MANDIBULAR CANINE

This tooth resembles the maxillary canine, although its dimensions are smaller. It rarely has two roots, and the mean length is 22.5 mm. The Type I canal form is most prevalent (Figure 4-23); the frequency of two canals is 14%.[73] However, less than 6% of mandibular canines display the Type IV canal form with two separate apical foramina.[57,74]

Access Cavities to Mandibular Canines

The access cavity to a mandibular canine is similar to that of the maxillary tooth and should be prepared on the lingual aspect of the tooth. The shape should be oval and extend from the cingulum incisally. However, because of the more pronounced labial curvature of the crown, like in the lower incisors, it is sometimes necessary to involve the incisal edge of the tooth.

MANDIBULAR PREMOLARS

These teeth are usually single-rooted; however, the mandibular first premolar may present with a division of roots in the apical half. The Type I canal configuration is the most prevalent. Where two canals are present, they are more likely in the first premolar (Figure 4-24) and may involve up to one-third of teeth.[53,57,75–77] Additional canals may be suspected if a root canal that is visible radiologically in the coronal part of the root appears to stop abruptly as it is traced apically. Where division of canals occurs, the tendency is for them to remain separate, to produce a Type IV/V

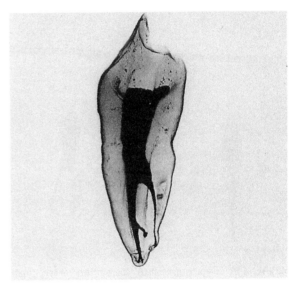

FIGURE 4-25 Cleared mandibular first premolar with a Type IV canal configuration and a lateral canal.

form (Figure 4-25). The Type II/III forms are seen in less than 5% of these teeth (Figure 4-26). The highest reported frequency of a second canal in second premolars is 11%. Less than 2% of first premolars have three canals.[53,57,77] The presence of multiple canals has been reported.[78–81] African Americans and the southern Chinese population of Hong Kong have a high prevalence of teeth with more than one canal (Figure 4-27).[57,76]

The pulp chamber is wide buccolingually, and although there are two pulp horns, only the buccal is well developed. The lingual pulp horn is very slight

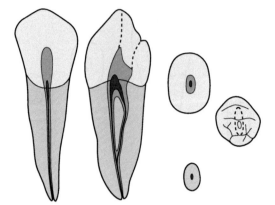

FIGURE 4-26 Mandibular first premolar with a Type II canal configuration.

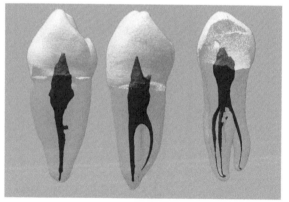

FIGURE 4-27 Computer-generated reconstructed image, from microcomputed tomography, of mandibular premolars showing different canal configurations. (Reproduced courtesy of Bauru Dental School, Sao Paolo State University, Brazil.)

in the first premolar but better developed in the second premolar. The canals of these two teeth are similar, although smaller than the canines, and thus, are wide buccolingually until they reach the middle third of the root, where they constrict.

Access Cavities to Mandibular Premolars

These should be through the occlusal surface and wide buccolingually. In the first premolar with two canals it may be necessary to extend the cavity onto the buccal surface.

MANDIBULAR FIRST MOLAR

The mandibular first molar usually has two roots, a mesial and a distal. The distal is smaller and usually rounder than the mesial. There is a variation with a supernumerary distolingual root; the reported frequency ranges from 6% to 44%.[82,83] The two-rooted molar usually has a canal configuration of three canals (Figure 4-28), and the mean length is 21 mm. Two canals are usually located in the mesial root with one in the distal. The mesial root in 40% to 45% of cases has only one apical foramen.[57,84] These canals may have a latticework arrangement of connections along their length (Figure 4-29).[85–88] Specimens with three canals in the mesial root[89] and a total of five canals have also been observed (Figure 4-30).

The single distal canal is larger, centrally placed buccolingually and more oval in cross-section than the mesial canals, and in 60% of cases, emerges on the distal side of the root surface short of the anatomical apex.[90] The incidence of two distal canals in mandibular first molars has been reported as 38%.[84] The orifices are sited buccal and lingual and are small. The

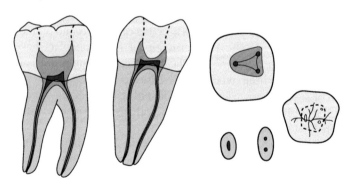

FIGURE 4-28 Mandibular first molar, with a Type IV canal configuration in the mesial root (second from left).

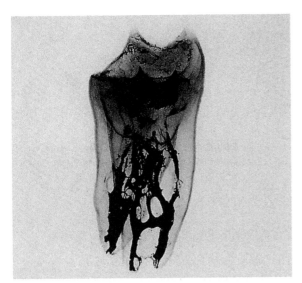

FIGURE 4-29 Cleared mandibular first molar viewed from the mesiobuccal showing connections between the mesial canals.

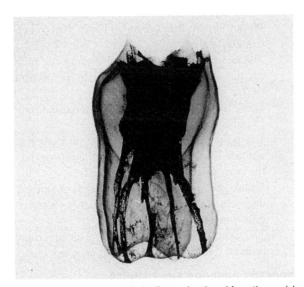

FIGURE 4-30 Cleared mandibular first molar viewed from the mesial showing five canals.

tendency for the mandibular first molar to have three roots appears to be associated with the frequency of the second distal canal, which approaches half in these teeth.[83]

The pulp chamber is wider mesially than it is distally and may have five pulp horns, the lingual pulp horns being longer and more pointed. The floor is rounded and convex toward the occlusal and lies just apical to the cervix. The root canals leave the pulp chamber through funnel-shaped openings of which the mesial tend to be much finer than the distal. Of the two mesial canals, the mesiobuccal is the more difficult canal to negotiate because of its tortuous path. It leaves the pulp chamber in a mesial direction, which alters to a distal direction in the middle third of the root. The mesiolingual canal is slightly larger in cross-section and generally follows a much straighter course, although it may curve mesially toward the apical part. When a second distal canal is present on the distolingual aspect, it tends to curve toward the buccal. With age, the pulp chamber recedes from the occlusal surface and the canals become constricted.

MANDIBULAR SECOND MOLAR

In Caucasoid populations the mandibular second molar presents as a smaller version of the mandibular first molar with a mean length of 20 mm. The mesial root has two canals and, unlike the first molar, there is usually only one distal canal. The mesial canals tend to fuse in the apical third to give rise to one main apical foramen (Figure 4-31). Studies[91–94] highlight the tendency for mandibular second molars to have fused roots in up to 52% of the Chinese population. The fusion gives rise to a horseshoe shape when the roots are viewed in cross-section. Where there is incomplete separation of roots, there may also be incomplete division of canals, giving rise to the C-shaped canal,[34,36,95–97] which increases the likelihood of canal interconnections and unpredictably placed canal orifices. One such orifice has now been termed the *median buccal canal orifice*,[98] which leads to the median buccal canal (Figure 4-32). Numerous classifications of C-shaped root canal configurations have been proposed[99] including that by Manning,[91] Melton et al[100] and Fan et al.[101,102]

MANDIBULAR THIRD MOLAR

The form of the mandibular third molar is often very varied. It generally has as many root canals as there are cusps. The roots are normally shorter than other molars. Root canal treatment on mandibular third molars may be relatively straightforward because access is facilitated by the mesial inclination of many

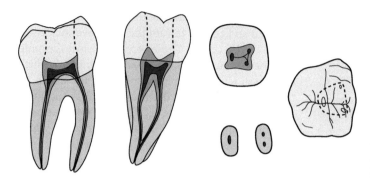

FIGURE 4-31 Mandibular second molar, with a Type II canal configuration in the mesial root (second from left).

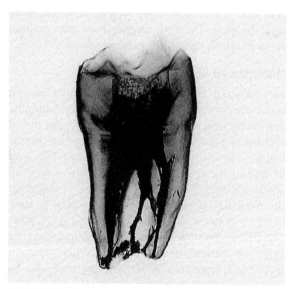

FIGURE 4-32 Cleared mandibular second molar with fused roots viewed from the buccal showing the median buccal canal.

of these teeth; however, aberrant forms of the pulp space do exist. Careful preoperative assessment is essential.

Access Cavities to Mandibular Molars

The prevalence of the second distal canal in mandibular first molars may necessitate a rectangular outline. The access cavity should be placed in the mesial three-quarters of the occlusal surface. Care should always be taken to remove the roof of the pulp chamber completely without causing damage to the floor of the pulp chamber.

Pulp Space Anatomy of Primary Teeth

The objective of endodontic treatment in primary teeth is to preserve the tooth in form and function (see Chapter 11); the endodontic techniques are modified from those for the management of permanent teeth.

The pulp cavities in primary teeth have certain common characteristics:

- Proportionally, they are much larger than in permanent teeth.
- The enamel and dentine surrounding the pulp cavities are much thinner than in permanent teeth.
- There is no clear demarcation between the pulp chamber and root canals.
- The pulp canals are more slender and tapering and are longer in proportion to the crown than the corresponding permanent teeth.
- Multirooted primary teeth show a greater degree of interconnecting branches between pulp canals.
- The pulp horns of primary molars are more pointed than suggested by cusp anatomy.

PRIMARY INCISORS AND CANINES

The pulp chambers of both maxillary and mandibular incisors and canines closely follow their crown outlines. However, the pulp tissue is much closer to the surface of the tooth, and the pulp horns are not as sharp and pronounced as in permanent teeth (Figure 4-33). The pulp canals are wide coronally and taper apically, and there is no clear demarcation between pulp chamber and root canal. Occasionally, the canals of the mandibular incisors may be divided into two

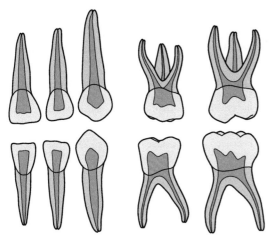

FIGURE 4-33 Pulpal space anatomy of the primary teeth.

TABLE 4-2 **Ages When Root Apices Are Considered Fully Formed**

Tooth Type	Age (Years)
Primary incisor	2
Primary canine and molar	3
Permanent first molar	9
Permanent central incisor	10
Permanent lateral incisor	11
Permanent premolar	15
Permanent second molar	17
Permanent third molar	21

branches by a mesiodistal wall of dentine. Maxillary primary central incisors have a mean length of 16 mm, whereas the lateral incisors are slightly shorter. Mandibular central incisors are 14 mm, and mandibular lateral incisors are 15 mm. The canines are the longest primary teeth, the maxillary canines being 19 mm and the mandibular 17 mm.

PRIMARY MOLARS

As in the permanent dentition the maxillary molars are three rooted (two buccal and one palatal), whereas the mandibular molars only have two roots (mesial and distal; see Figure 4-33). The pulp chambers are large in relation to tooth size, and the pulp horns are well developed, particularly in the second molars. From a restorative point of view, it is important to remember that the tip of the pulp horns may be as close as 2 mm from the enamel surface, and thus, great care must be taken in preparing cavities in these teeth if pulpal exposure is to be avoided. Due to the relatively large size of the pulp chamber, there is less hard tissue protecting the pulp.

The furcation of the roots is also very much closer to the cervical area of the crown, and thus, damage to the floor of the pulp chamber may lead to perforation. Mandibular molars normally have two root canals in each root, and the mesiobuccal root canal of the maxillary molars may divide in two. Thus, both maxillary and mandibular primary molars frequently have four canals.

Apical Closure

While calcification and cementum deposition at the apex continue throughout life, apices can be considered as fully formed several years after eruption, and approximate ages are shown in Table 4-2.

Learning Outcomes

After reading this chapter, the reader should be able to recognize and describe the:

- complex and divergent anatomy of the pulp space;
- relationship between tooth development and pulp space anatomy;
- design of access cavities for individual teeth and according to treatment requirements;
- advantages of magnification and illumination in access cavity preparation and pulp space examination.

REFERENCES

1. Davis SR, Brayton SM, Goldman M. The morphology of the prepared root canal: a study utilizing injectable silicone. Oral Surgery, Oral Medicine, Oral Pathology 1972;34:642–8.
2. Eguren AO. An endodontic technic of diaphanisation of teeth. Odontologia (Lima) 1973;17:9–11.
3. Tagger M. Clearing of teeth for study and demonstration of pulp. Journal of Dental Education 1976;40:172–4.
4. Malentacca A, Lajolo C. A new technique to make transparent teeth without decalcifying: Description of the methodology and micro-hardness assessment. Annals of Anatomy 2015; 197:11–5.

5. Bramante CM, Berbert A, Borges RP. A methodology for evaluation of root canal instrumentation. Journal of Endodontics 1987;13:243–5.

6. Thompson SA, al-Omari AO, Dummer PM. Assessing the shape of root canals: an in vitro method using microradiography. International Endodontic Journal 1995;28:61–7.

7. Dummer PM, Kelly T, Meghji A, et al. An in vitro study of the quality of root fillings in teeth obturated by lateral condensation of gutta-percha or Thermafil obturators. International Endodontic Journal 1993;26:99–105.

8. Blaskovic-Subat V, Smojver B, Maricic B, et al. A computerized method for the evaluation of root canal morphology. International Endodontic Journal 1995;28:290–6.

9. Nielsen RB, Alyassin AM, Peters DD. Microcomputed tomography: An advanced system for detailed endodontic research. Journal of Endodontics 1995;21:561–7.

10. Patel S, Dawood A, Pitt Ford T, et al. The potential application of cone beam computed tomography in the management of endodontic problems. International Endodontic Journal 2007;40:818–30.

11. Domark JD, Hatton JF, Benison RP, et al. An ex vivo comparison of digital radiography and cone-beam and micro computed tomography in the detection of the number of canals in the mesiobuccal roots of maxillary molars. Journal of Endodontics 2013;39:901–5.

12. Billis G, Pawar RR, Makdissi J, et al. A cone beam computed tomography study on the incidence and configuration of the second mesiobuccal canal in maxillary first and second molars in an adult sub-population in London. ENDO (Lond Engl) 2014;8:179–86.

13. Garberoglio R, Brännström M. Scanning electron microscopic investigation of human dentinal tubules. Archives of Oral Biology 1976;21:355–62.

14. Dourda AO, Moule AJ, Young WG. A morphometric analysis of the cross-sectional area of dentine occupied by dentinal tubules in human third molar teeth. International Endodontic Journal 1994;27:184–9.

15. Pashley DH. Mechanistic analysis of fluid distribution across the pulpodentin complex. Journal of Endodontics 1992;18:72–5.

16. Oguntebi BR. Dentine tubule infection and endodontic therapy implications. International Endodontic Journal 1994;27:218–22.

17. Vertucci FJ. Root canal anatomy of the human permanent teeth. Oral Surgery, Oral Medicine, Oral Pathology 1984;58:589–99.

18. Lowman JV, Burke RS, Pelleu GB. Patent accessory canals: incidence in molar furcation region. Oral Surgery, Oral Medicine, Oral Pathology 1973;36:580–4.

19. Burch JG, Hulen S. A study of the presence of accessory foramina and topography of molar furcations. Oral Surgery, Oral Medicine, Oral Pathology 1974;38:451–5.

20. Kramer IRH. The vascular architecture of the human dental pulp. Archives of Oral Biology 1960;2:177–89.

21. Burch JG, Hulen S. The relationship of the apical foramen to the anatomic apex of the tooth root. Oral Surgery, Oral Medicine, Oral Pathology 1972;34:262–8.

22. Chapman CE. A microscopic study of the apical region of human anterior teeth. Journal of the British Endodontic Society 1969;3:52–8.

23. Dummer PMH, McGinn JH, Rees DG. The position and topography of the apical canal constriction and apical foramen. International Endodontic Journal 1984;17:192–8.

24. Kerekes K, Tronstad L. Morphometric observations on root canals of human anterior teeth. Journal of Endodontics 1977;3:24–9.

25. Levy AB, Glatt L. Deviation of the apical foramen from the radiographic apex. Journal of the New Jersey State Dental Society 1970;41:12–3.

26. Martos J, Ferrer-Luque CM, Gonzalez-Rodriguez MP, et al. Topographical evaluation of the major apical foramen in permanent human teeth. International Endodontic Journal 2009;42:329–34.

27. Jenkins JA, Walker WA, Schindler WG, et al. An in vitro evaluation of the accuracy of the Root ZX in the presence of various irrigants. Journal of Endodontics 2001;27:209–11.

28. Shabahang S, Goon WW, Gluskin AH. An in vivo evaluation of Root ZX electronic apex locator. Journal of Endodontics 1996;22:616–18.

29. Wrbas KT, Ziegler AA, Altenburger MJ, et al. In vivo comparison of working length determination with two electronic apex locators. International Endodontic Journal 2007;40:133–8.

30. Tratman EK. Three rooted lower molars in man and their racial distribution. British Dental Journal 1938;64:264–74.

31. Turner CG. The dentition of the Arctic peoples. PhD thesis. Madison: University of Wisconsin; 1967.

32. Turner CG. Three rooted mandibular first permanent molars and the question of American Indian origins. American Journal of Physical Anthropology 1971;34:229–41.

33. Chen G, Yao H, Tong C. Investigation of the root canal configuration of mandibular first molars in a Taiwan Chinese population. International Endodontic Journal 2009;42:1044–9.

34. Seo MS, Park DS. C-shaped root canals of mandibular second molars in a Korean population: clinical observation and in vitro analysis. International Endodontic Journal 2004;37:139–44.

35. Zhang R, Wang H, Tian YY, et al. Use of cone-beam computed tomography to evaluate root and canal morphology of mandibular molars in Chinese individuals. International Endodontic Journal 2011;44:990–9.

36. Zheng Q, Zhang L, Zhou X, et al. C-shaped root canal system in mandibular second molars in a Chinese population evaluated by cone-beam computed tomography. International Endodontic Journal 2011;44:857–62.

37. Alani A, Bishop K. Dens invaginatus. Part 1: classification, prevalence and aetiology. International Endodontic Journal 2008;41:1123–36.

38. Bishop K, Alani A. Dens invaginatus. Part 2: clinical, radiographic features and management options. International Endodontic Journal 2008;41:1137–54.

39. Vier-Pelisser FV, Pelisser A, Recuero LC, et al. Use of cone beam computed tomography in the diagnosis, planning and follow up of a type III dens invaginatus case. International Endodontic Journal 2012;45:198–208.

40. De Sousa SM, Bramante CM. Dens invaginatus: treatment choices. Endodontics and Dental Traumatology 1998;14:152–8.

41. Hülsmann M. Dens invaginatus: aetiology, classification, prevalence, diagnosis, and treatment considerations. International Endodontic Journal 1997;30:79–90.

42. Ngeow WC, Chai WL. Dens evaginatus on a wisdom tooth: a diagnostic dilemma. Case report. Australian Dental Journal 1998;43:328–30.

43. Uyeno DS, Lugo A. Dens evaginatus: a review. ASDC Journal of Dentistry for Children 1996;63:328–32.

44. Koh ET, Pitt Ford TR, Kariyawasam SP, et al. Prophylactic treatment of dens evaginatus using mineral trioxide aggregate. Journal of Endodontics 2001;27:540–2.
45. Patel S, Rhodes J. A practical guide to endodontic access cavity preparation in molar teeth. British Dental Journal 2007;203: 133–40.
46. Krasner P, Rankow HJ. Anatomy of the pulp chamber floor. Journal of Endodontics 2004;30:5–16.
47. Peters OA. Accessing root canal systems: knowledge base and clinical techniques. ENDO (Lond, Engl) 2008;2:87–104.
48. Reid JS, Saunders WP, MacDonald DG. Maxillary permanent incisors with two root canals: a report of two cases. International Endodontic Journal 1993;26:246–50.
49. Thompson BH, Portell FR, Hartwell GR. Two root canals in a maxillary lateral incisor. Journal of Endodontics 1985;11: 353–5.
50. Carns EJ, Skidmore AE. Configurations and deviations of root canals of maxillary first premolars. Oral Surgery, Oral Medicine, Oral Pathology 1973;36:880–6.
51. Vertucci FJ, Gegauff A. Root canal morphology of the maxillary first premolar. Journal of the American Dental Association 1979;99:194–8.
52. Nelson CT. The teeth of the Indians of Pecos Pueblo. American Journal of Physical Anthropology 1938;23:261–93.
53. Walker RT. A comparative investigation of the root number and canal anatomy of permanent teeth in a southern Chinese population. PhD thesis. Hong Kong: University of Hong Kong; 1987.
54. Walker RT. Root form and canal anatomy of maxillary first premolars in a southern Chinese population. Endodontics and Dental Traumatology 1987;3:130–4.
55. Vertucci F, Seelig A, Gillis R. Root canal morphology of the human maxillary second premolar. Oral Surgery, Oral Medicine, Oral Pathology 1974;38:456–64.
56. Seidberg BH, Altman M, Guttuso J, et al. Frequency of two mesiobuccal root canals in maxillary permanent first molars. Journal of the American Dental Association 1973;87:852–6.
57. Pineda F, Kuttler Y. Mesiodistal and buccolingual roentgenographic investigation of 7,275 root canals. Oral Surgery, Oral Medicine, Oral Pathology 1972;33:101–10.
58. Imura N, Hata GI, Toda T, et al. Two canals in mesiobuccal roots of maxillary molars. International Endodontic Journal 1998;31:410–14.
59. Thomas RP, Moule AJ, Bryant R. Root canal morphology of maxillary permanent first molar teeth at various ages. International Endodontic Journal 1993;26:257–67.
60. Stropko J. Canal morphology of maxillary molars: clinical observations on canal configurations. Journal of Endodontics 1999;25:446–50.
61. Altman M, Guttuso J, Seidberg BH, et al. Apical root canal anatomy of human maxillary central incisors. Oral Surgery, Oral Medicine, Oral Pathology 1970;30:694–9.
62. Slowey RR. Radiographic aids in the detection of extra root canals. Oral Surgery, Oral Medicine, Oral Pathology 1974;37: 762–72.
63. Weller RN, Hartwell GR. The impact of improved access and searching techniques on detection of the mesio-lingual canal in maxillary molars. Journal of Endodontics 1989;15:82–3.
64. Ting PCS, Nga L. Clinical detection of minor mesiobuccal canal of maxillary first molars. International Endodontic Journal 1992;25:304–6.
65. Beatty RG. A five-canal maxillary first molar. Journal of Endodontics 1984;10:156–7.
66. Harris WE. Unusual root canal anatomy in a maxillary molar. Journal of Endodontics 1980;6:573–5.
67. Stone LH, Stroner WF. Maxillary molars demonstrating more than one palatal root canal. Oral Surgery, Oral Medicine, Oral Pathology 1981;51:649–52.
68. Wong M. Maxillary first molar with three palatal canals. Journal of Endodontics 1991;17:298–9.
69. Ng YL, Aung TH, Alavi A, et al. Root and canal morphology of Burmese maxillary molars. International Endodontic Journal 2001;34:620–30.
70. Benjamin KA, Dowson J. Incidence of two root canals in human mandibular incisor teeth. Oral Surgery, Oral Medicine, Oral Pathology 1974;38:122–6.
71. Rankine-Wilson RW, Henry P. The bifurcated root canal in lower anterior teeth. Journal of the American Dental Association 1965;70:1162–5.
72. Walker RT. The root canal anatomy of mandibular incisors in a southern Chinese population. International Endodontic Journal 1988;21:218–23.
73. Kaffe I, Kaufman A, Littner M, et al. Radiographic study of the root canal system of mandibular anterior teeth. International Endodontic Journal 1985;18:253–9.
74. Vertucci FJ. Root canal anatomy of the mandibular anterior teeth. Journal of the American Dental Association 1974;89: 369–71.
75. Cleghorn BM, Christie WH, Dong CCS. The root and root canal morphology of the human mandibular second premolar: A literature review. Journal of Endodontics 2007;33:1031–7.
76. Trope M, Elfenbein L, Tronstad L. Mandibular premolars with more than one root canal in different race groups. Journal of Endodontics 1986;12:343–5.
77. Vertucci FJ. Root canal morphology of mandibular premolars. Journal of the American Dental Association 1978;97:47–50.
78. Chan K, Yew SC, Chao SY. Mandibular premolar with three root canals – two case reports. International Endodontic Journal 1992;25:261–4.
79. Rhodes JS. A case of unusual anatomy: a mandibular second premolar with four canals. International Endodontic Journal 2001;34:645–8.
80. Serman NJ, Hasselgren G. The radiographic incidence of multiple roots and canals in human mandibular premolars. International Endodontic Journal 1992;25:234–7.
81. Wong M. Four root canals in a mandibular second premolar. Journal of Endodontics 1991;17:125–6.
82. Gulabivala K, Aung TH, Alavi A, et al. Root and canal morphology of Burmese mandibular molars. International Endodontic Journal 2001;34:359–70.
83. Walker RT. The root form and canal anatomy of mandibular first molars in a southern Chinese population. Endodontics and Dental Traumatology 1988;4:19–22.
84. Skidmore AE, Bjorndal AM. Root canal morphology of the human mandibular first molar. Oral Surgery, Oral Medicine, Oral Pathology 1971;32:778–84.
85. Jafarzadeh H, Wu Y-N. The C-shaped root canal configuration: a review. Journal of Endodontics 2007;33:517–23.
86. Mannocci F, Peru M, Sherriff M, et al. The isthmuses of the mesial root of mandibular molars: a micro-computed tomographic study. International Endodontic Journal 2005;38: 558–63.
87. Teixeira FB, Sano CL, Gomes BP, et al. A preliminary in vitro study of the incidence and position of the root canal isthmus in maxillary and mandibular first molars. International Endodontic Journal 2003;36:276–80.

88. von Arx T. Frequency and type of canal isthmuses in first molars detected by endoscopic inspection during periradicular surgery. International Endodontic Journal 2005;38: 160–8.

89. Fabra-Campos H. Three canals in the mesial root of mandibular first permanent molars: a clinical study. International Endodontic Journal 1989;22:39–43.

90. Tamse A, Littner MM, Kaffe I, et al. Morphological and radiographic study of the apical foramen in distal roots of mandibular molars. Part I. The location of the apical foramen on various root aspects. International Endodontic Journal 1988;21:205–10.

91. Cooke HG, Cox FL. C-shaped canal configurations in mandibular molars. Journal of the American Dental Association 1979;99:836–9.

92. Manning SA. Root canal anatomy of mandibular second molars. Part I. International Endodontic Journal 1990;23: 34–9.

93. Manning SA. Root canal anatomy of mandibular second molars. Part II. C-shaped canals. International Endodontic Journal 1990;23:40–5.

94. Yang ZP, Yang SF, Lin YC, et al. C-shaped root canals in mandibular second molars in a Chinese population. Endodontics and Dental Traumatology 1988;4:160–3.

95. Fan W, Fan B, Gutmann JL, et al. Identification of C-shaped canal systems in mandibular second molars. Part I. Radio-graphic and anatomic features revealed by intraradicular contrast medium. Journal of Endodontics 2007;33:806–10.

96. Fan B, Gao Y, Fan W, et al. Identification of a C-shaped canal system in mandibular second molars. Part II. The effect of bone image superimposition and intraradicular contrast medium on radiograph interpretation. Journal of Endodontics 2008;34:160–5.

97. Fan W, Fan B, Gutmann JL, et al. Identification of a C-shaped canal system in mandibular second molars. Part III: Anatomic features revealed by digital subtraction radiography. Journal of Endodontics 2008;34:1187–90.

98. Walker RT. Root form and canal anatomy of mandibular second molars in a southern Chinese population. Journal of Endodontics 1988;14:325–9.

99. Fernandes M, de Ataide I, Wagle R. C-shaped root canal configuration: A review of literature. Journal of Conservative Dentistry 2014;17:312–19.

100. Melton DC, Krell KV, Fuller MW. Anatomical and histological features of C-shaped canals in mandibular second molars. J Endodontics 1991;17:384–8.

101. Fan B, Cheung GS, Fan M, et al. C-shaped canal system in mandibular second molars: Part I. Anatomical features. Journal of Endodontics 2004;30:899–903.

102. Fan B, Cheung GS, Fan M, et al. C-shaped canal system in mandibular second molars: Part II. Radiographic features. Journal of Endodontics 2004;30:904–8.

CHAPTER 5

Maintaining Dental Pulp Vitality

H. F. Duncan, A. J. Smith and P. R. Cooper

Chapter Contents

Summary

The maintenance of pulp vitality and the prevention of apical periodontitis are fundamental principles of operative dentistry and endodontics. The pulp is naturally protected by dentine and exhibits an array of defensive strategies to protect itself against irritation. A comprehensive understanding of the nature of these irritants and the pulpal response is essential to prevent damage and to harness natural defenses. Recent advances in material technology, molecular biology and regenerative medicine have led to a greater predictability in managing deep caries and the development of novel cell-free homing and cell-based regenerative strategies to reconstitute vital tissue in the root canal space.

Introduction

It is imperative for clinicians to accept that the best root canal filling is healthy pulp tissue. Therefore, every inflamed pulp should not be removed, and pulp conservation should not be viewed as an old-fashioned or unsuccessful procedure. Recent rapid advances in stem cell biology and regenerative medicine have heralded a new wave of experimental and clinical treatment modalities aimed at maintaining or reestablishing pulp vitality. Consequently, regenerative or reparative techniques should be encouraged within the discipline of modern endodontics; they are comparatively more conservative, more biologically acceptable and less technically demanding than conventional root canal treatment.

Pulp and Dentine Function

The pulp occupies the core of the tooth and is the tissue from which dentine is formed. Odontoblasts line the interface between the dentine and pulp forming an interconnected tissue, often known as the pulp–dentine complex, which is normally protected from irritation by an intact layer of enamel. When the enamel is breached by caries, erosion, attrition or operative procedures, the pulp is at risk. In young patients the dentinal tubules are wider and the pulp closer to the surface, so a similarly sized breach of enamel will have a greater effect on the pulp than that in an older patient. The greater the area of exposed dentine, the greater the effect on the pulp. Therefore, the potential damage from crown preparations, extensive tooth surface loss and larger cavities is comparatively greater. Odontoblast processes project from the odontoblasts into the dentine in tubules, which are generally patent and filled with tissue fluid.[1] Irritation to the distal extremities of the tubules stimulates pulp inflammation and the formation of tertiary dentine and tubular sclerosis; these hard tissues aim to wall off the irritants from the pulp, which should then become less inflamed. It has been demonstrated that if buccal cavities are prepared in otherwise sound teeth and are left open to microbial contamination, the pulp underneath the exposed tubules becomes inflamed[2]; however, if the irritant is removed and a suitable restoration is placed, the inflammation subsides and tertiary dentine is formed.[3] There are two types of tertiary dentine formation, which include (1) reactionary dentine, which is formed by existing odontoblasts in response to mild irritation, and (2) reparative tertiary dentine, which is formed by newly recruited and differentiated odontoblast-like cells in response to severe irritation after the death of the original odontoblasts.[4,5] If tertiary dentine is formed quickly in response to a more severe stimuli, the tubular pattern is less regular and can sometimes even be more atubular than when it is formed slowly in response to mild stimuli.

Pulp Irritants

The dental pulp may be challenged by a variety of stimuli, broadly classified as being of microbial, chemical or mechanical origin. These irritants often act in synchrony; for example, mechanical and microbial stimuli may combine to provoke pulpal inflammation.

MICROBIAL

Dental Caries

This has traditionally been regarded as the main cause of pulpal damage as it has been seminally demonstrated that in the absence of bacteria, pulpal inflammation does not occur[6]; however, a decline in the incidence of caries in recent years has increased the role of other aetiologies. As a carious lesion progresses, the enamel surface breaks down and the dentine is exposed to bacteria; the pulp responds by localized inflammation and hard tissue deposition.[7] Intratubular dentine deposition leads to tubular sclerosis; tertiary dentine deposition 'walls off' the irritation and, after a short interval, the pulp is likely to recover.[8] As the early carious dentine lesion progresses toward the pulp, the sclerotic zone of dentine becomes demineralized and the lesion subsequently advances into the tertiary dentine. When bacteria invade this dentine, severe inflammatory pulp changes occur, which will lead to localized abscess formation if allowed to progress[9]; however, significant levels of inflammatory cells are not observed in the pulp until the caries has penetrated to within ≈0.5 mm.[10] Therefore, until the caries is very deep, the pulp is not likely to be irreversibly damaged. As a result, recovery of the pulp should occur after removal of carious dentine and insertion of an effective sealing restoration.[3] Since it is difficult to assess the actual state of the pulp accurately from clinical signs and symptoms, it is important to monitor teeth with deep caries.[11]

Advancing carious lesions are classically divided into zones: an outer zone of destruction, a central zone of bacterial penetration and an inner zone of demineralization reflecting the time course of the pathogenesis of caries. The zone of destruction contains dentine traditionally regarded as being destroyed by the microbiota; however, recent data have suggested that evidence of bacterial input to the degradation of the organic matrix of carious dentine is limited and may be mediated by host-derived matrix metalloproteinases (MMPs).[12,13] The soft carious dentine of this zone can be readily removed with hand excavators in active lesions and often has a lighter colour. In slowly progressing or arrested lesions, this dentine is darker and has a harder consistency. The next zone, the zone of bacterial penetration, contains microorganisms within the dentinal tubules. The structure of the dentine, when examined in a demineralized histological section, is otherwise normal. Some tubules are deeply infected while others contain no microorganisms. A variety of microorganisms from this zone have been identified by culturing techniques – *Lactobacilli, Streptococci* and *Actinomyces* species.[14,15] More recently, molecular and pyrosequencing techniques have suggested that the microbiota is more complex than previously thought with many uncultivable species.[16,17] Deep carious dentine has been shown to contain, predominantly, anaerobic bacteria, including *Propionibacteria, Prevotella, Eubacteria, Arachnia* and *Lactobacilli*.[18,19] Ahead of the zone of microorganism penetration is a zone of demineralization, frequently considered to be devoid of bacteria because the conditions for bacterial survival are too unfavourable; however, small numbers of anaerobic bacteria have been demonstrated to be present in this zone.[20]

Bacterial Microleakage

Bacterial microleakage occurs around all restorations as microorganisms from the oral cavity colonize the 'gap' around the restoration.[9] The lack of importance of bacterial contamination or rigorous disinfection at the time of cavity preparation has been shown in studies of pulpal exposures,[21,22] and a correlation between bacterial leakage around restorations and pulpal inflammation has been demonstrated.[23] The pulpal responses to irritation from bacterial microleakage are identical to caries – inflammation, tubular sclerosis and formation of tertiary dentine.[24] Nevertheless, measures should be taken to prevent pulp damage during the first few months after restoration placement by placing a cavity liner/base, a dentine-bonding agent or glass ionomer cement. In operative dentistry, the main reason for placing a cavity liner/base is to prevent damage to the pulp from bacterial leakage around restorations as former reasons, such as material irritancy or thermal protection, have been severely criticized.[25]

In many instances, the choice of lining/base material in deep cavities without pulpal exposures would appear to be a matter of operator preference. Cements based on calcium hydroxide, glass ionomer or calcium silicate all appear to be satisfactory under amalgam and are widely used. Under resin-based restorative materials, a liner/base is rarely placed as dentine-bonding agents are often adequate. The durability of some calcium hydroxide cements has been questioned, particularly if the overlying restoration has an imperfect seal.[26,27]

CHEMICAL

Dental Materials

Dental materials were historically considered to exert an irritant effect on the pulp[28,29]; however, over the last 30 years, the pulpal toxicity of various materials has been questioned.[9,23,30,31] Resin-based composites (RBCs) have long been regarded as an irritant to the pulp, but the relative blandness of this material has now been demonstrated together with the important contribution of bacterial leakage to the pulp's reaction.[32] The RBCs contract when polymerized, causing a microscopic gap to occur between the resin and the tooth, into which bacteria penetrate (bacterial microleakage); inflamed pulps have been found in teeth with bacteria in the gap.[9] From a clinical standpoint, both etching and dentine bonding are considered necessary to prevent a pulpal inflammatory reaction. RBCs are continually evolving and appear to prevent microleakage if carefully placed, demonstrating good clinical success[33]; however, some concern remains regarding the effectiveness of their long-term bond to tooth substances.[34] Generally, it is accepted that most restorations 'leak' to varying degrees, so the prevention of microleakage is generally more important than the chemical irritancy of the material itself. Clinically, a restoration should be placed which either bonds to tooth tissue or if not, a lining/base material should be placed under the restoration, which reduces leakage.

Pulp damage may occur in relation to temporary crown materials or cements, again not because of their inherent toxicity but more as a result of marginal leakage and bacterial invasion over the large area of recently exposed dentinal tubules. Temporary crowns should not be left for long periods and must always be adequately cemented,[35] or the tubules 'blocked' by placing a bonding agent before cementing the temporary crown. Although there is now considerable evidence to show the toxic 'blandness' of restorative materials, many, particularly when freshly mixed, have been shown to be toxic to cell cultures, although dentine can moderate this effect.[36]

Bleaching

Vital bleaching procedures are an increasingly popular aspect of modern dentistry, and tooth sensitivity is a common side effect of such procedures. Sensitivity was experienced in 15% to 65% of patients undergoing bleaching,[37,38] but only a small number of patients experienced severe symptoms.[39] Chairside 'power' bleaching procedures are often associated with a rise in pulpal temperature and a higher incidence of sensitivity than home bleaching techniques.[40] The symptoms are usually reversible and generally resolve 1 to 2 weeks after the end of the procedure[41]; however, symptoms may be more severe if the patient has a history of sensitivity.[39] The symptoms can be reduced by pretreatment of the teeth with a desensitizing agent such as potassium nitrate.[42] The mechanism behind the sensitivity appears to be that the peroxide bleaching agent diffuses through the enamel and down the dentinal tubules into the pulp, triggering inflammation; however, irreversible pulp damage has not been observed even when heat-assisted bleaching techniques have been used.[43]

MECHANICAL

Operative Dentistry

Dentine preparation with rotary burs can have a damaging effect on the pulp unless measures are taken to minimize injury. High-speed cavity preparation without a water spray causes significantly more pulp damage than when a water spray is used,[44,45] and it is imperative that the operator ensures the water spray is correctly and continuously directed at the head of the bur. If the spray is obstructed by a tooth structure or excess pressure is applied to the bur during use, pulp damage may occur.[46]

The area of dentine prepared can have a profound effect on the pulp response. The more tubules exposed, the more routes there are for irritants to reach the pulp. Therefore, pulpal damage results not because of the operative procedure *per se* but because the preparation exposes avenues for microbial penetration. Logically, in a small cavity prepared to treat a carious lesion, most of the exposed dentinal tubules would have been blocked by tubular sclerosis as a result of the caries, thus providing pulp protection not evident in a noncarious tooth. The deeper the cavity, the greater the potential for damage; the pulp is closer,

odontoblast processes may have been cut, more tubules will have been exposed and the deeper dentinal tubules may have a larger diameter.[47] Only when cavities are very deep, with remaining dentine less than 0.3 mm thick, does some pulp damage occur.[45] Prolonged drying of cavities causes odontoblast aspiration, i.e., their cell bodies move into the dentinal tubules, but there is no permanent damage to the pulp.[48] Crown preparations, particularly in young patients, or with previously unrestored teeth, are potentially the most damaging to the pulp that occasionally result in irreversible damage; 10% to 15% of crowned teeth have been shown to lose vitality over a 10-year period.[49,50] When local anaesthetics containing adrenaline (epinephrine) are used for crown preparation, the pulp is at particular risk of damage because of vasoconstriction and reduced blood flow,[51,52] which renders the pulp unable to regulate its temperature and other physiological defenses.

The use of lasers for cavity preparation has been reported to have no long-term adverse pulpal effects.[53–55] However, many of the beneficial properties of a laser are due to its thermal properties, so unless rigorous safety parameters are established for every type of laser equipment, there is a substantial risk of pulpal damage when lasers are used to treat the exposed pulp. Damage has been reported when lasers were used directly on the pulp,[56] whereas other studies have suggested that lasers have no detrimental effects.[57,58]

Trauma

The extent of the traumatic damage may vary from a simple enamel craze to a split tooth that cannot be restored. Direct trauma to the incisor teeth often results in fractures that are horizontal or oblique,[59] whereas with an indirect trauma, the fractures are often longitudinal. Trauma to anterior teeth most commonly affects children, whose teeth have larger pulps and wider dentinal tubules; any injury which exposes dentine can potentially damage the pulp. Traumatic injuries may also damage the blood supply to the pulp, which may lead to calcifications or necrosis.

Exposure of Dentine

Exposure of dentine may occur as a result of a cusp fracture, by a defective restoration which fails to cover the entire area of the prepared cavity or by attrition, abrasion or erosion of the covering cementum or enamel. In the early period after exposure of dentine by trauma, parafunction or cavity preparation, the pulp is sensitive to stimuli and may become inflamed, particularly if bacteria colonize the exposed dentine and enter the tubules. The pulp responds to the low-grade irritation, as previously described, with hard tissue formation, thereby protecting itself over time and making it less sensitive to stimuli.[60] Sensitivity will only persist if the cause of the dentine exposure is exacerbated and not controlled.

Cervical sensitivity can occur in undamaged or nonrestored teeth, where the gingival tissues have receded and the root dentine is exposed; this is often a result of vigorous tooth brushing. Without protection, the exposed tubules are open and communicate with the pulp. Sensitivity may be reduced by the application of potassium oxalate or bonding resins, which not only occlude the tubules but also reduce nerve activity.[61] The repair process can be undermined by further assault either by parafunction, further abrasion or erosion. This is particularly problematic in patients who continue to expose their teeth to acid from drinks, foods, gastric reflux or regurgitation.[25,62]

Function/Parafunction

The effects of occlusion on the pulp are negligible as long as a protective covering of enamel remains intact. When the enamel is breached, the dentine is exposed and irritants have a direct pathway to the pulp via the dentinal tubules. As before, the pulp will protect itself from the damage by tubular sclerosis and tertiary dentine deposition. Loss of enamel and exposure of dentine is unlikely during normal function but can occur by attrition after extended periods of parafunction. If the parafunction is particularly severe, continued sensitivity may result because of continual wear of the dentine, rather than any direct irritation by occlusal forces. Parafunction can also result in cuspal flexure, which stimulates the pulp by an outward movement of dentinal fluid; this is exaggerated considerably if a 'crack' in the tooth develops.[63]

Management of Deep Caries

As with the treatment of any carious cavity in dentine, it is generally accepted that the margins, particularly the amelodentinal junction, should be free of caries.

However, there has been less agreement over whether all carious dentine overlying the pulp should be removed.[64,65] In a tooth with a deep carious lesion, which is considered to have a healthy pulp, partial caries removal appears to be preferable to complete caries removal and the risk of pulp exposure.[66]

A traditional view prevails that if any carious dentine remains, the carious process will continue. An opposite view, supported by clinical evidence, is that if a small amount of caries is left on the pulpal aspect of the cavity and the margins are clear, the lesion can be arrested. It appears that the change in environmental conditions and a reduction in bacterial load render the remaining carious lesion inactive. Visually, the yellow carious dentine will darken and dry over time.[67] Partial caries removal, however, is subjective as the definition of a small amount of caries will vary from one operator to another. This leads to the question: when does a little become an unacceptably large amount?

In general, there are two recognized approaches to partial caries removal in adult teeth – indirect pulp therapy and stepwise excavation. The former is a one-stage procedure in which most, but not all of the caries, is removed before the placement of a permanent restoration. This technique is gaining momentum as the treatment of choice for advanced caries in deciduous teeth.[68,69] In comparison, stepwise excavation is a two-step approach in which a small amount of carious dentine is left at the first visit and the tooth dressed, before being reentered after a period of several months. This technique has also been shown to be successful in reducing the frequency of pulpal exposure.[66,70] The principle of a two-stage approach is that the reaction to the treatment can be visually assessed and the remaining decay removed later, with a decreased risk of pulp exposure. This is dependent on tertiary dentine deposition over the intervening period, but this may be difficult to assess as the volume of tertiary dentine deposited will vary from patient to patient. These differing approaches raise the question, which has not yet been fully clarified, as to whether a second intervention is really necessary. Unfortunately, although indirect pulp therapy can be carried out on permanent teeth, most of the research to date has been on deciduous teeth; therefore, data comparing the two techniques are not available.

Notably, clinical opinion often conflicts with scientific evidence when deciding if a cavity is caries free.

In one classic study, only 64% of clinically hard dentine was bacteria-free[71]; therefore, in a third of the teeth, in which the clinician considers the cavity floor to be clean, it was incorrect. Dyes which stain the superficial infected dentine, but not the deeper demineralized dentine have been advocated to address this problem[72]; however, the use of dye may lead to excessive removal of carious dentine.[73]

Light-coloured dentine is usually indicative of more active caries and darker-coloured dentine of less active or arrested caries. In addition, a deep lesion may extend into dentine modified by tubular sclerosis, dead tracts or into tertiary dentine, which can result in a darker appearance than normal but is not carious dentine. If carious dentine is left in a deep cavity, it is impossible for the clinician to ascertain whether the bacteria have invaded the pulp. The pulp may already be inflamed but free of symptoms, so placing a crown or other restoration can be an expensive mistake as the crown may need to be modified or destroyed when subsequently, root canal treatment is required. If removal of all the carious-infected dentine leads to pulp exposure, then root canal treatment is appropriate and should not be deferred, except when circumstances dictate that vital pulp treatment is preferable (see Management of Pulp Exposure).

After removal of the deep carious dentine, a protective lining/base may be placed in a very deep cavity; hard-setting calcium hydroxide materials, which stimulate pulp repair, have traditionally been used. The use of a liner/base is dependent on the proposed restorative material and the thickness of dentine remaining over the pulp. Linings/bases are rarely placed under resin restorations as the entire cavity can be etched and a dentine-bonding agent placed to seal the cavity; however, doubts remain as to whether resins provide an adequate seal in deep cavities over the long term.[74] Due to their biological properties as pulp-capping agents, calcium hydroxide and calcium silicate cements, e.g. Mineral Trioxide Aggregate (MTA) and Biodentine (Septodont, Saint-Maur-des-fossés Cedex, France), are considered the material of choice if the thickness of dentine remaining over the pulp is judged to be less than 0.5 mm. However, it should be noted that substantial washout of calcium hydroxide linings/bases under amalgam restorations occurs[26,27]; for this reason, a layer of glass ionomer can be placed over the calcium hydroxide as a secondary lining/base.

Management of Pulp Exposure

Exposure of the dental pulp can occur as a result of caries, trauma or by accident during cavity preparation. In traumatic and accidental exposures, the pulp can be regarded as being effectively noninflamed before the injury. Treatment is usually by pulp capping or partial pulpotomy, and provided that treatment is not unnecessarily delayed, a good outcome can be achieved.[75] With a carious exposure caused by sustained bacterial infection, there will be varying degrees of pulpal inflammation. Inflammation of the pulp has a significant effect on the outcome of vital pulp therapy.[66,76,77]

PULP CAPPING

Direct pulp capping is a procedure in which the pulp is covered with a protective material directly over the site of the exposure. The pulp wound should be cleansed of debris and the haemorrhage arrested by applying pressure using sterile paper points, cotton wool or, preferably, sponges (to avoid remnants of cellulose fibres of cotton); saline and sodium hypochlorite solution can also be useful. When the wound is dry, the pulp-capping agent should be gently placed over the exposure, followed, if necessary, by a glass ionomer liner/base and then a permanent restoration. Delay in placing the permanent restoration reduces the prognosis of the procedure[78] due to the likelihood of microleakage.[9]

PARTIAL PULPOTOMY

The traditional pulpotomy method involves removing the coronal pulp and placing a pulp dressing on the radicular pulp. This remains a common procedure within paediatric dentistry and has been recently proposed as a treatment option for carious-exposed pulps in permanent teeth.[79] A variation of pulpotomy was developed for the treatment of traumatized anterior teeth,[21] which is more conservative and involves removal of the superficial layer of damaged and/or inflamed pulp tissue before application of the capping material. This is advantageous as the superficial, damaged tissue is removed, which should encourage healing, and also, space is created which allows the pulp dressing to be retained within the dentine. Although similar to pulp capping, this procedure involves cutting a small 2-mm-deep cavity into the pulp with an air turbine under water spray, placing the pulp dressing and covering it with a liner/base and then a coronal restoration (Figure 5-1). In recent years, partial pulpotomy has been practised in carious, as well as traumatic, exposures with favourable outcomes, indicating that at least for practical reasons, partial pulpotomy may be the technique of choice over pulp capping if the pulp is exposed.[66,80,81]

CHOICE OF MATERIAL

Calcium hydroxide has been established as the gold standard as a pulp-capping/partial pulpotomy material over the last 50 years.[82–86] RBCs have been investigated as alternatives, but they have generally not matched the performance of calcium hydroxide in controlling pulpal inflammation or dentinal bridge formation.[87,88] Over the last 15 years, bioceramics such as MTA and more recently, Biodentine (Septodont), have emerged as the materials of choice for vital pulp therapy.[89,90]

Although the reparative mechanism of both calcium hydroxide and MTA is essentially nonspecific,[91] it appears to involve dampening pulpal inflammation, which provides an environment conducive to repair. Thereafter, bioactive molecules are liberated from the dentine[92,93] and generated by pulp cells, which stimulate the differentiation of pulpal stem cells and also further control the inflammatory response; this allows the pulp to repair.[85,94,95] Pulp progenitor cells have the ability to differentiate into odontoblast-like cells, which allows the pulp to regenerate and form dentine bridges across the exposure. The dentine bridge is not formed by calcium from the material but instead from the underlying tissues.[96] With RBCs, MTA and hard-setting calcium hydroxide, the bridge forms in relative close proximity to the material; however, with nonsetting calcium hydroxide paste, the barrier is formed with an intervening zone of necrosis.[97] The reparative dentine bridges formed under calcium hydroxide are often imperfect with tunnel defects connecting to the pulp[98,99]; this is in contrast to MTA where tunnel defects are rarely seen (Figures 5-2 and 5-3).[89] Although it appears that MTA may be the current material of choice, its nonspecific action and concerns

about tooth discolouration[100] have prompted research into targeted regenerative biomaterials aimed at stimulating biological processes.[101,102] Although the choice of material may favour the outcome of treatment, healing of pulpal exposures is predominantly dependent on the capacity of the material or surface restoration to prevent microleakage.[24,31] Therefore, regardless of the capping agent used, the prevention of microleakage is critical.

Regenerative Developments

The goal of regenerating dental tissues to their predisease state has recently gained momentum under the banner of 'Regenerative Endodontics'[103]; this encompasses a broad range of procedures ranging from simple pulp capping and pulpotomy, through non–cell-based and cell-based pulp regeneration techniques, to whole tooth generation. Many of these techniques remain experimental, but there is considerable opportunity in the future for the establishment of an array of regenerative biological solutions in endodontics. This idea is not new as the aim of pulp capping is to reconstitute a normal tissue at the pulp–dentine border that is capable of regulating tertiary dentinogenesis and has been investigated for many years.[82,104,105] These traditional regenerative techniques exploited the ability of the pulp to recover via the liberation of bioactive molecules from the damaged dentine matrix, which in turn stimulated dental pulp stem cells to differentiate into odontoblast-like cells generating dentine bridges at the site of exposure. The exact mechanism of differentiation of new odontoblast-like cells has not been fully elucidated; however, cell signalling triggered by TGF-β family members[106–108] and bone morphogenetic proteins (BMPs),[109,110] which are incorporated into the dentine matrix during formation, is thought to be key. The understanding of these mechanistic developments has not only aided future treatment techniques but has also revealed possible mechanisms for defensive dentinogenesis during pulpal irritation.

Therapeutic regenerative strategies have introduced growth factors, within a suitable carrier, directly onto the pulpal interface.[108,110] A possible benefit of bioactive pulp-capping agents is that they may be an improvement over conventional materials such as

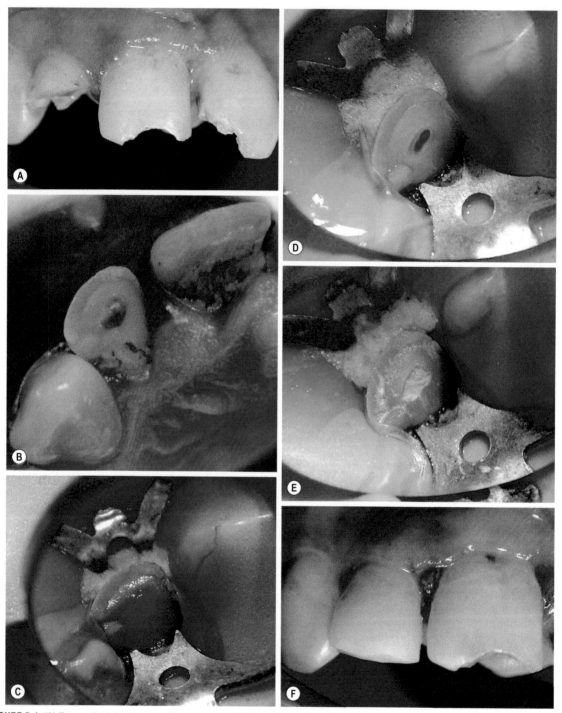

FIGURE 5-1 (A) Traumatized, fractured maxillary incisors. (B) The pulp of the maxillary right lateral incisor is exposed. (C) Dental dam placed to isolate the maxillary right lateral incisor. (D) Partial pulpotomy in which 2 mm of pulp tissue was removed with a diamond bur in a high-speed handpiece. (E) MTA placed into the partial pulpotomy 'cavity'. (F) Immediately after placement of a permanent restoration. (From Duncan *et al.* 2008 with permission of Quintessence Publishing Co Ltd.)

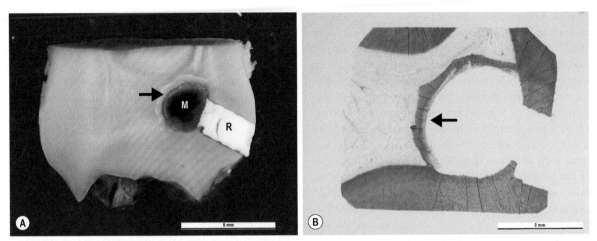

FIGURE 5-2 MTA pulp cap 3 months after placement (A) Macrophotograph showing remnants of the restorative material (*R*) and MTA capping material (*M*). A distinct hard tissue bridge (*arrowed*) can be seen (original magnifications ×6). (B) Microphotograph of part of the same histological section. Note again the thick mineralized barrier (*arrowed*) stretched across the entire length of the exposed pulp (original magnification ×8). (From Nair *et al.* 2008, with permission of Wiley-Blackwell.)

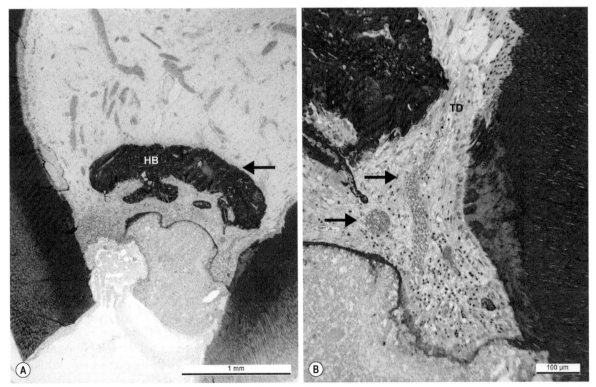

FIGURE 5-3 Calcium hydroxide pulp cap. (A) Hard tissue formation on the pulpal aspect of hard-setting calcium hydroxide capping material (*arrowed*) and a thick, calcified hard tissue barrier (*HB*) at a distance from the capping material with gaps at the periphery (original magnification ×25). (B) Higher magnification. A 'tunnel' defect (*TD*) is evident peripherally, associated with engorged blood vessels (*arrowed*) and surrounded by acute and chronic inflammatory cells (original magnification ×100).

calcium hydroxide or even MTA, which only produce a small amount of reparative dentine at the exposure site.[109] It can be postulated that a greater quantity of dentine would offer better pulp protection; however, overproduction of dentine leading to pulp space sclerosis could result in future problems during endodontic treatment.[111] These techniques, although promising, are expensive, require a suitable carrier and may have damaging side effects,[105] whereas other critical questions such as dose-response effects and the limitations of the growth factors' short biological half-life remain unanswered. Current therapeutic approaches should perhaps concentrate on the release of dormant bioactive molecules already present within the dentine and develop ways of liberating them in a controlled manner. The use of etchants[106,112] or dental materials such as MTA appears to be effective in harnessing these cytokines.[93] More traditional materials such as calcium hydroxide may not be as effective in this role, or in providing the necessary environment for repair to occur.

Future vital pulp approaches designed to address the nonspecific actions of current materials[91] could target pulpal repair mechanisms directly by using pharmacological inhibitors, such as histone deacetylase inhibitors, to reduce inflammation and increase mineralization.[101,102] Although at present, these techniques are only experimental, they potentially offer the opportunity to epigenetically induce reparative gene transcription events in pulp cells during vital pulp treatment; this provides an attractive approach as these inhibitors are relatively inexpensive compared with other specific or cell-based regenerative solutions.[113]

INFLAMMATION AND PULPITIS

The dental pulp exhibits similarities to many other connective tissues of the body; however, the rigid outer covering of hard mineralized tissue makes this a particularly challenging environment. The constraints on the pulp tissue as it swells during the inflammatory response causes significant pain to the patient, and the tissue architecture results in clinical limitations in terms of treatment options aimed at removing the causes of the injury and tooth repair. Bacterial infection is the most common injurious challenge to the pulp and results from dental caries,

clinical operative procedures and trauma. A complex and mixed microbiota, especially including gram-negative anaerobic bacteria, can subsequently flourish within a diseased pulp.[114]

Both innate and adaptive immune responses have been reported within the dental pulp tissue as it attempts to defend itself, and these inflammatory processes involve a broad array of tissue, cellular and molecular events. These events include the recruitment of immunocompetent cells from the blood, as well as the maturation and differentiation of defense cells within the pulp tissue itself. These processes aim to facilitate the removal of invading bacteria and associated host tissue debris that subsequently occurs.[115] Clearly underpinning this inflammatory response is an increased requirement for blood flow and vasodilation, necessary not only to deliver defense cells but also to provide the nourishment necessary for the host tissue to combat the infection. This fluid exudation or oedema, which occurs during the inflammatory phase, gives rise to the swelling of the pulp tissue and contributes to the significant discomfort experienced by the patient.[116-118] Some studies suggest that this is complemented by an increased involvement of the lymphatic system within the pulp, which is the case in other tissues and may be important for both immune barrier function and tissue fluid balance.[119,120] Although there have been only a limited number of investigations on pulpal lymph vasculature, studies have indicated that during inflammation, lymph vessel formation occurs.[121] During the immune response, the lymph system aims to drain filtered fluid and proteins and return them to the blood as well as remove the invading bacteria and their byproducts. The lymphatic vasculature plays an important role in the immune response due to the presence of tissue-resident dendritic cells (DCs), which transport captured antigens to the lymph nodes for presentation to lymphocytes.[122]

Notably, a plethora of molecules are involved in coordinating the complex inflammatory response, and their elaboration is mediated following environmental sensing by cells of the dentine and pulp. While the main role of odontoblasts has long been considered to be that of dentine matrix secretion, it is now apparent that these cells play a broader role in tooth defense. Indeed their role is supported by the histological structure of dentine–pulp and the intimate and intricate association of the odontoblast process and its lateral branches,[123] which ensures communication with its extracellular environment. Thus, odontoblasts are well positioned to initially detect invading bacteria as well as the dentine matrix components that are liberated during carious demineralization. However, while odontoblasts represent this first line of defense, cells deeper within the pulp core, including pulp fibroblasts, dental pulp stem cells, neurons, tissue resident immune cells and endothelial cells have all been implicated in the detection of invading cariogenic bacteria. Consequently, all these cell types should be regarded as being immunocompetent and a constitutive part of the pulp's bacterial defense response.[124]

Similar to many other structural tissue cells within the body, once odontoblasts have detected the infection they initiate host tissue immune defense. Initially, this may manifest in the release of antimicrobial peptides aimed at destroying the invading bacteria; subsequently, they will release potent signalling molecules including cytokines and chemokines, which activate the immune response. The bacterial biofilm will also adapt as the carious infection progresses deeper into the tissue, and this is due to changes in the environment in terms of nutrient and oxygen availability and interactions with the other colonizing bacteria.[125–127] The progressing and evolving bacterial biofilm will further modulate the defense reaction as the host cells differentially respond to different bacteria.[115] Notably, if the carious infection is rapidly progressing and unchecked, it may overwhelm the host tissue defense and result in the death of odontoblasts located in direct contact with the lesion. Subsequently, the infection may progress deeper into the pulp core, resulting in significant tissue damage.

In recent years, our understanding of how bacteria and their components are detected by our host cells has significantly increased. Host cellular receptors recognize pathogens or microbes, with Toll-Like Receptors (TLRs) being the major and the best characterized subset in the pulp tissue's innate immune response. Eleven members of the TLR family have now been described and the expressions of TLRs-1 to TLRs-6 and TLRs-9 have been demonstrated in odontoblasts and pulp-derived cells.[128] Ligands and activators of TLRs include surface components of bacteria, including lipopolysaccharides (LPS), lipoteichoic acids (LTS), flagellin, peptidoglycans and lipoproteins as well as microbial nucleic acids. The activation of TLRs initiates an acute inflammatory response, leading to the release of proinflammatory mediators, which activate the immune and vascular systems. The archetypal proinflammatory cytokines/chemokines include interleukin-1α (IL-1α), interleukin-1β (IL-1β) and tumour necrosis factor-α (TNF-α), and these have been shown to be important in the pulp's response to bacteria.[129–133] Once activated, these molecules act in paracrine and autocrine signalling and are regarded as being central to coordinating the inflammatory response.

The chemokine and cytokine messenger proteins released, along with those liberated by carious acid demineralization of the dentine, are relatively small but highly potent molecules. Subsequently, they generate intense signalling gradients, which lead to immune cell recruitment at sites of infection. Although a relatively small number of immune cells are already resident within the healthy pulp where they play a sentinel role, after infection there is a significant increase in the number of different cell types, including T- and B-lymphocytes, plasma cells, neutrophils and macrophages.[134–136] These cells are the effectors of the innate and adaptive immune responses, with the latter process becoming increasingly prominent as the caries extends more extensively into the pulp and the inflammation becomes more chronic in nature. The prime role for the recruited neutrophils and macrophages is the killing and phagocytosis of the invading bacteria, especially during the early and acute phase of inflammation. As the disease progresses clinically and the adaptive immune response develops, defense cells, such as natural killer (NK), T and B cells and immature DCs, will become more involved, leading to increased proinflammatory signalling and cell activation.[137,138] Although these immune cells aim to clear the infection, their deployed armament frequently leads to exacerbation of inflammation and associated tissue damage. Indeed, to combat the bacteria and traverse the pulp tissue, the immune cells release degradative enzymes and molecules, such as MMPs and reactive oxygen species (ROS). These molecules subsequently result in collateral host tissue damage due to their destruction of extracellular molecules and their deleterious effects on cells.[115]

Currently, it is apparent that although many observational studies have reported the presence of a range of immune cells and inflammatory mediators in carious pulpal tissue, there still remains a lack of functional understanding of their complex interrelationships. Indeed, a better appreciation of the cellular responses initiated during the innate response associated with acute inflammation, and the increasing complexity as adaptive immune responses come into play during chronic inflammation, is required to aid development of novel and targeted treatment approaches.

REPAIR AND REGENERATION

As has previously been highlighted, tertiary dentinogenesis is the focal secretion of dentine matrix at sites of injury in the mature dentine–pulp complex. It can be considered a defense response, in that it generates a barrier to further injurious challenge and bacterial ingress, as well as being a reparative and regenerative response for restoration of the tissue architecture and function. The extent of dental tissue injury is dependent on disease progression and intensity.[4,139,140] During milder tooth injury, such as in slowly progressing disease, the primary odontoblasts beneath the lesion survive and up regulate their

activity to secrete 'reactionary' tertiary dentine focally at the site of injury. However, when the intensity of the injury compromises odontoblast vitality and leads to cell death, dental tissue fate will be determined by the interplay between the injurious challenge, inflammatory and immune responses and the regenerative response. If the tissue environment is, subsequently, conducive for wound healing, stem/progenitor cells may be recruited to the injury site and differentiate to form a new generation of odontoblast-like cells secreting 'reparative' tertiary dentine (Figure 5-4). Thus, reparative dentinogenesis can occur after pulp exposure, where a dentine bridge can be generated after direct pulp capping. Clearly, the sequence of cellular and tissue events necessary for reactionary and reparative dentinogenesis differs appreciably in complexity between the two processes. Indeed, reactionary dentinogenesis is relatively simple and involves the up regulation of activity of the existing primary odontoblasts, whereas reparative dentinogenesis involves recruitment, proliferation and differentiation of stem/progenitor cells derived from within the dentine–pulp complex or potentially recruited from the peripheral vasculature. The odontoblast-like cells developed at the site of injury will also require an intense period

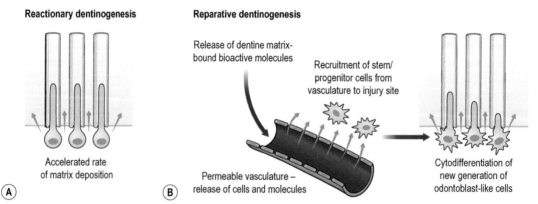

FIGURE 5-4 Characterization of reactionary and reparative tertiary dentinogenic events. (A) Reactionary dentinogenesis occurs as a result of mild injury or irritation to the tooth, such as in the case of a slowly progressing carious lesion. The existing odontoblasts survive beneath the disease lesion and up regulate their rate of dentine matrix deposition. (B) Reparative dentinogenesis occurs as a result of a more intense injury or irritation to the tooth, such as in the case of a more rapidly progressing carious lesion. Subsequently, the existing odontoblasts beneath the lesion die and are replaced by newly formed odontoblast-like cells, which are recruited and differentiated from stem/progenitor cells, e.g. dental pulp stem cells, either locally or more distantly via the vasculature. These odontoblast-like cells also deposit dentine matrix at a relatively rapid rate to provide a barrier against the tissue injury by restoring dental tissue integrity. In both cases, the dentinogenic processes may be modulated by the release of signalling molecules, such as growth factors, which are liberated due to dentine demineralization by cariogenic bacterial acids. These molecules diffuse down the dentinal tubules to trigger the cellular events described.

of up regulated secretory activity.[141] Notably, the progenitor/stem cell sources may reside in a variety of niches, which have been described within the dental pulp, and work remains ongoing to better characterize these locations, their cellular developmental origin and specific cell phenotype.[142]

The signalling of both reactionary and reparative dentinogenic events is driven by molecules present or generated at the site of injury. Interestingly, it has been known for some time that dentine fragments, generated clinically during mechanical exposure of the pulp or artificially introduced, result in the induction of mineralized tissue formation within tissue.[143,144] This observation provides clues as to the origins of the signals necessary to stimulate dental tissue wound healing and implies that dentine matrix components are able to invoke repair processes. More recent work has shown that several distinct components of the dentine and pulp matrices, including many growth factors and cytokines, can stimulate the cellular processes necessary for dental tissue wound repair.[145] These molecules can be liberated from the dentine or pulp matrix adjacent to sites of injury through carious demineralization, as well as due to tissue treatment with restorative materials and agents.

Although a complex cocktail of growth factors, cytokines, and other molecules are present, and can be released from the dentine matrix to signal tissue repair, several reports have highlighted significant roles for members of the BMP family. In particular, transforming growth factor-β1 (TGF-β1) has been shown to be sufficient and potentially central for the direct signalling of dental hard and soft tissue repair.[146–148] Furthermore, underpinning hard and soft tissue wound healing is the need for a robust and well-developed vascular system to provide the necessary cells, nutrients and oxygen supply. It is known that during tertiary dentinogenesis, local angiogenesis occurs, and this is likely driven by proangiogenic growth factors, such as vascular endothelial growth factor (VEGF) and platelet-derived growth factor (PDGF), which are released from the dentine matrix.[149,150] Also, the role of the pulp's neuronal network during tissue repair should not be underestimated, as bidirectional signalling with this system may be necessary for the complete regeneration of the dentine–pulp complex. Indeed, many neuropeptides and neurotrophic factors are expressed by neurons, odontoblasts and pulp cells, and it can also be liberated from the dentine matrix under repair-relevant conditions.[151,152]

INTERPLAY BETWEEN INFLAMMATION AND REGENERATION

Clearly, inflammation and regeneration within the tooth are temporal-spatially linked, and there is likely to be significant overlap between the signalling of the two events. Clinically, this has been suspected for some time after the use of the pulp-capping agent calcium hydroxide, which stimulates reparative dentinogenesis *in vivo*. Although its precise mechanisms of action remain controversial, it has been proposed that its hydroxyl ion release leads to a high local pH, resulting in cell necrosis beneath the restoration.[153,154] Subsequently, this cell death may lead to a 'sterile' inflammatory response driven by the release of low levels of proinflammatory mediators from the dying cells.[155] Studies on the chemically related restorative material, MTA, have indicated that this may well exert a similar mode of action to facilitate dental tissue repair. Indeed, recent *in vitro* studies have shown that relatively low levels of cytokines, including IL-1α, IL-1β, IL-2, IL-6 and IL-8, are released from mineralizing cells after exposure to MTA.[156–158] Combined, these observations support the notion that low-grade resolving inflammation, potentially combined with the liberation of molecules from the dentine matrix by calcium hydroxide and MTA, may provide conditions conducive for dental tissue repair.[92,93] Complementary to these properties may be the antimicrobial action of these two restorative materials, which may ensure that chronic bacterial-driven inflammation does not develop.

Under ideal circumstances, the immune defense response following injurious challenge to a tissue will lead to elimination of the infecting agent and, ultimately, endeavours to generate an environment conducive for wound repair. In support of this notion, studies have demonstrated that dental tissue repair occurs more successfully in germ-free and inflammation-free animals compared with infected controls.[6,159–161] There is, therefore, significant support for the premise that at relatively low concentrations, proinflammatory mediators which may be present during the early stages of disease, or following clinical intervention, may actually promote regenerative events; however, these molecules may impede repair via inhibitory signaling mechanisms if they are present at relatively high levels.

A more recent review[162] on bone regeneration provided similar conclusions to those proposed here and indicated that chronic and relatively high-grade inflammation inhibited the body's repair ability, whereas relatively low-grade inflammation was beneficial in stimulating bone metabolic activity and regeneration. Clearly, eradication of bacterial infection in the dental tissues while restoring tissue function and vitality are key goals in operative dentistry and endodontics, and this may be facilitated by the development of novel therapeutics and treatments in the area, which bridges dental tissue inflammation and regeneration. Emerging therapeutic areas, which centre on inflammation regulation via modulation of the nuclear factor-kappa B (NF-κB) pathway or immunomodulation by stem cells, may ultimately translate into clinical application; however, significant basic and clinical research is still required before this is realized.

STRATEGIES FOR REGENERATIVE ENDODONTICS

Endodontic treatment planning approaches should be based on prevention or treatment of pulpal and periapical disease, whereas subsequent operative procedures should be targeted at restoring normal tissue structure and function. Wherever possible, minimally invasive therapies which harness natural wound healing responses should be considered; however, in-depth knowledge of tissue destruction levels and the possibility of repair/regeneration are necessary in the planning stages.

Characterization of reactionary and reparative tertiary dentinogenic events (see Figure 5-4) helps to identify the key biological events in the dentine–pulp complex, which underpin regenerative endodontic procedures. It is important to recognize, however, that wound healing is a pathological process and, consequently, the regulatory control of molecular and cellular events in the pulp may differ to some extent from the physiological processes of normal tooth development and homoeostasis. By definition, the processes of reactionary and reparative dentinogenesis may affect the healing outcomes in terms of how closely newly formed tissues resemble their physiological counterparts. Thus, reactionary dentine, as simply the secretion of dentine matrix at an increased rate compared with primary/secondary dentine, will show close similarity in structure to its physiological counterparts, although pulp chamber/root canal volumes may be reduced. In contrast, reparative dentine can be heterogeneous in morphology, ranging from a normal tubular to an atubular structure.[145] Clearly, a more bone-like atubular reparative dentine will be distinctly different to more physiological dentine. Similarly, a wide spectrum of tissue architecture may be found for pulp after carious injury to the tooth and subsequent wound healing. Nevertheless, it can be seen that the structures of pulp and dentine after injury and wound healing in the tooth may well not necessarily resemble their physiological counterparts very closely. Thus, by strict definition the healing responses are perhaps more reparative than regenerative in nature.[95] Despite this, the term *regenerative endodontics* remains useful in describing treatment approaches with a biological basis aimed at restoring vital and functional tissues in the dentine–pulp complex.

Theoretically, a broad variety of strategies might be adopted for regenerative endodontics. To achieve healing, there is a requirement for cells, signalling mediator molecules to orchestrate the cellular activity and a matrix substratum (scaffold) within which the cells can operate. All of these components can be recognized within natural pulp wound healing responses and in *de novo* tissue formation and represent the elements required for tissue engineering. Although substantial progress has been made at the experimental level in terms of dental tissue engineering,[163] further work is required before this becomes a viable option for routine clinical treatment. Meanwhile, significant opportunity exists for clinical intervention to promote the events associated with natural wound healing. Such intervention may target aspects of the wound healing responses, including stem/progenitor cell recruitment, cellular signalling for cell differentiation and secretion and provision of a scaffold/matrix substratum within which healing can occur; these targets have been described as cell-free approaches (revascularization) and contrast with cell-based approaches involving the application of cells to promote the healing responses. Both approaches have been extensively discussed within the proceedings of a recent symposium.[164] At present, many of the studies of dentine–pulp regeneration have been at the experimental level and while providing exciting proof of principle, will require considerable refinement before they may be considered for routine clinical practice. This is especially true of strategies involving the application of cells, which will require focus on cellular sources, their preparation to the exacting safety standards required for good manufacturing practice and their storage, manipulation and application within the clinical endodontic setting.

CLINICAL PROCEDURES FOR REGENERATIVE ENDODONTICS

As described earlier, the concept of regenerative medicine has long been a focus for dentistry with the application of materials including calcium hydroxide,[165,166] MTA[89] and tri-calcium silicate (Biodentine, Septodont)[167] to preserve pulp vitality. These techniques have contributed significantly to the maintenance of pulp vitality and provide a valuable platform from which further therapeutic strategies may develop.

A number of single case and case series reports describing use of regenerative endodontic protocols have been published.[79,168–170] These protocols have a strong biological basis with approaches ranging from the creation of a favourable tissu e environment for the promotion of natural wound healing processes, to those based around tissue engineering principles to promote healing. The creation of an environment conducive for tissue healing will include infection and inflammation control measures to minimize pathogenic stimuli, as well as trying to optimize the recruitment of stem/progenitor cells to the injury site and facilitating signalling events for their participation in healing. In all endodontic approaches, effective control of infection and inflammation is a fundamental consideration, but regenerative procedures often require adoption of more careful control measures to minimize tissue damage and to allow preservation of tissue vitality. A more conservative approach during surgical intervention with the use of a superficial partial pulpotomy[21] may also provide more favourable outcomes for regenerative endodontics.[79] This has implications for case selection, and regenerative endodontics will more likely be used in those cases where infection and inflammation are diagnosed as being less extensive. This highlights, however, a significant constraint for endodontic patient management generally, and regenerative endodontics in particular, with the lack of robust diagnostic markers, which can underpin biological and clinical assessment of tissue injury and vitality.[171,172] To date, case selection has also provided a focus on the treatment of immature teeth in regenerative endodontics using a cell-homing method, where tissues are likely to be at an active developmental stage. The ability to stimulate completion of root formation in such cases represents a significant advantage for regenerative endodontics, but there is a need to better examine its potential for the treatment of permanent teeth.

Exciting opportunities exist for the introduction of tissue engineering approaches within regenerative endodontics with proof of principle for such approaches[173] at the experimental level. Attempts to apply tissue engineering principles at the clinical level have been attempted through what has been termed 'revascularization' procedures,[168] usually with immature necrotic teeth. The generation of a blood clot during such revascularization procedures can potentially provide a scaffold as well as perhaps targeting stem/progenitor cells and signalling mediator molecules to the site. Application of platelet-rich plasma[174] has also been attempted to encourage revascularization of the pulp. These various revascularization procedures may stimulate deposition of radicular mineralized tissue of periodontal rather than dentinogenic origin. However, if the result contributes to effective apical closure and maintenance of tissue vitality, the origin of the tissue may be of lesser importance.

FUTURE DEVELOPMENTS

The recent swathe of experimental studies involving regenerative endodontics provides much optimism for future developments in this field.[164] It is important however, to consider such developments in the context of how endodontics is practised within healthcare systems. The rapid progress in stem cell biology and translation of this into the clinical arena shows much promise for regenerative medicine generally. The setting up of stem cell banks for long-term storage of cells, often collected noninvasively from deciduous primary teeth, offers the possibility of autologous cell sources, thereby minimizing the risks of immune rejection after implantation. Nevertheless, except in specialist hospital settings, it will not be easy to provide the facilities for effective storage, handling and application of stem cells in routine endodontic practice.

There are, however, other developments that might be achieved in regenerative endodontics much more readily and which could contribute significantly to treatment outcomes. For example, there is no consensus within endodontics as to what are the optimum disinfection and irrigation protocols, which should be used during canal preparation. The agents used in these protocols can potentially impact greatly on regenerative events in the pulp, especially on the activity of signalling molecules sequestered within the dental tissues. Dentine matrix contains a rich reservoir of cytokines, growth factors and other bioactive molecules protected in a 'fossilized' state,[145] which can be exploited to stimulate regenerative events. Common irrigation agents, such as ethylenediaminetetraaecetic acid (EDTA), can release these matrix stores of signalling molecules and promote regeneration. In contrast, disinfectants like sodium hypochlorite can potentially degrade such bioactive molecules. Thus, there is scope to modify regenerative endodontic outcomes by simple manipulation and modification of disinfection and irrigation protocols. Identification of disinfectants with greater specificity toward bacteria, rather than the cells of the pulp, would also be a worthwhile development. Release of the matrix stores of signalling molecules may also be promoted by application of pulp-capping agents, including calcium hydroxide and MTA,[92,93] and optimization of protocols to favour such release may further promote pulp vitality.

It seems likely that future developments in regenerative endodontics will follow both shorter- and longer-term agendas. In the shorter term, greater attention to canal preparation and its effects on the biological status of the dentine–pulp complex, together with optimization of the use of pulp-capping agents and other materials to exploit their various properties, can be expected. In the longer term, targeted application of stem/progenitor cells and signalling molecules may allow a greater tissue engineering approach to regenerative endodontics. Together, all of these developments provide an exciting future for endodontic practice.

Maintaining Pulp Vitality during General Dental Treatment

CRACKED TEETH

A patient may complain of poorly localized pain from an unidentified posterior tooth on biting or from hot or cold drinks. Clinically and radiographically, there is often no evidence of caries, and although the offending tooth may be restored, the restoration present may not be deep. Mandibular molars are the most frequently affected.[175] The patient experiences pain due to the crack exposing multiple dentinal tubules, which bacteria and their byproducts pass down to elicit pulpal inflammation.[25] Biting on the cracked tooth creates a wedging effect, stimulating fluid movement in the crack and communicating tubules; this provokes a painful response in an already inflamed pulp. Treatment is unpredictable, but generally, cracks which are centrally placed in the axial plane are more difficult to treat than those eccentrically placed as the latter tend to exit the tooth laterally. Centrally placed cracks lead into the pulp and with time can split the tooth (Figure 5-5). The pulp can be maintained if there are only symptoms of reversible pulpitis, with

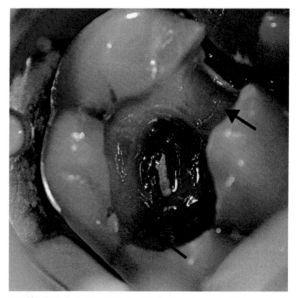

FIGURE 5-5 A maxillary molar tooth after removal of an amalgam restoration. A crack (*arrowed*) is sited centrally; the distal extension is stained.

treatments ranging from simple removal of a loose cusp and restoration placement, to placement of a temporary and then a permanent crown if no loose cusp is detected. Where there have been symptoms of irreversible pulpitis, pulpal extirpation and root canal filling or extraction may be required. During root canal treatment, it is advisable to place a band (e.g. stainless steel orthodontic band) to splint the tooth together, preventing further crack propagation. However, despite all efforts, a cracked tooth can have an unpredictable prognosis as it is impossible to know accurately the true extent of any crack/s.

ORTHODONTICS

Application of orthodontic forces will provoke a haemodynamic response in the pulp, which varies in intensity depending on several factors. Orthodontic movements, such as tipping, lead to an initial decrease in blood supply,[176] before a reactive hyperaemia increases the pulp perfusion.[177] Intrusive movements can lead to a sustained reduction in blood flow,[178] which is generally reversible but may jeopardize vitality if the tooth has been previously compromised; however, pulp necrosis is considered a rare event. Teeth with closed apices and pulps, which have been compromised particularly by previous trauma, but also by caries, restorations or periodontal disease, are more susceptible to irreversible damage and necrosis.[179,180] Although orthodontic forces have other pulpal effects, including a reduction in respiration, altered metabolism and localized cell death, these changes are probably a result of the haemodynamic alterations described and are, similarly, likely to be reversible.[181,182] In a small number of cases, orthodontic movement can stimulate an increase in calcification within the root canal, which can, in extreme cases, obstruct the entire root canal.[183] This can lead to problems of canal negotiation if the tooth requires root canal treatment at a later date.

PERIODONTAL DISEASE AND TREATMENT

Periodontal disease does not cause pulp necrosis unless the disease extends all the way to the tooth apex.[184,185] The normality of the pulp is maintained during periodontal disease because of the intact layer of cementum on the root surface. If this layer of cementum is destroyed during treatment or disease,

pulpal inflammation under the affected tubules is evident.[186] As before, the pulp responds to the stimulus by tubular sclerosis and tertiary dentine formation.[187] Therefore, even extensive periodontal disease causes little or no inflammatory changes in the pulp.[188] It has been shown that periodontal treatment, which removes cementum, may cause pulpal inflammation and the formation of tertiary dentine[186,187]; however, the response to root surface debridement is not severe and does not adversely affect pulp vitality. After root surface debridement, dentinal tubules may become opened and the teeth are hypersensitive; after several weeks the sensitivity decreases, presumably as the tubules become blocked by mineral deposits or a smear layer.[25]

INTRAALVEOLAR SURGERY AND IMPLANTS

Implants have become a popular replacement for missing teeth. Loss of vitality can occur during implant placement due to the root being damaged directly or indirectly if the neurovascular bundle apically is severed.[189] If the quantity of bone is unacceptable for a satisfactory result, bone will have to be augmented by grafts, often from the mandible or iliac crest. A common site for mandibular bone harvesting is the chin region, which due to the proximity of the incisor apices, can lead to a reduction of blood supply, reduction of pulpal sensitivity or even pulpal necrosis[189,190] The loss of pulpal sensitivity varies depending on the level of the osteotomy.[191,192] It has usually been considered that pulp necrosis and abscess formation will follow surgical cutting or severance of the root near its apex. A distance of 3 to 10 mm between the root apex and the osteotomy has been recommended to avoid pulpal degeneration or necrosis[191,193]; however, this has been disputed in an experimental study which demonstrated that no undesirable pulp sequelae occurred even when the roots were surgically cut.[194]

Learning Outcomes

At the end of this chapter the reader should be able to demonstrate knowledge of the:
- response of the pulp and dentine to irritation;
- range of pulpal irritants and their relative importance;

- ways to harness the regenerative potential of the pulp when treating deep caries lesions and pulpal exposures;
- impact of new regenerative research and how it has altered the understanding of modifying dentine–pulp structure and function, and the treatment of pulpal exposures;
- overlapping influences of inflammation, repair and regeneration on the damaged pulp;
- newer strategies in endodontics, including both cell-free and cell-based approaches;
- precautions necessary in order to maintain pulpal vitality during various dental procedures.

REFERENCES

1. Brännström M, Garberoglio R. The dentinal tubules and the odontoblast processes. A scanning electron microscopic study. Acta Odontologica Scandinavica 1972;30:291–311.
2. Mjör IA, Tronstad L. Experimentally induced pulpitis. Oral Surgery, Oral Medicine, Oral Pathology 1972;34:102–8.
3. Mjör IA, Tronstad L. The healing of experimentally induced pulpitis. Oral Surgery, Oral Medicine, Oral Pathology 1974;38:115–21.
4. Smith AJ, Cassidy N, Perry H, et al. Reactionary dentinogenesis. International Journal of Developmental Biology 1995;39:273–80.
5. Smith AJ, Lumley PJ, Tomson PL, et al. Dental regeneration and materials: a partnership. Clinical Oral Investigations 2008;12:103–8.
6. Kakehashi S, Stanley HR, Fitzgerald RJ. The effects of surgical exposures of dental pulps in germ-free and conventional laboratory rats. Oral Surgery, Oral Medicine, Oral Pathology 1965;20:340–9.
7. Smith AJ, Murray PE, Lumley PJ. Preserving the vital pulp in operative dentistry: 1. A biological approach. Dental Update 2002;29:64–9.
8. Warfvinge J, Bergenholtz G. Healing capacity of human and monkey dental pulps following experimental-induced pulpitis. Endodontics and Dental Traumatology 1986;2:256–62.
9. Bergenholtz G, Cox CF, Loesche WJ, et al. Bacterial leakage around dental restorations: its effect on the dental pulp. Journal of Oral Pathology 1982;11:439–50.
10. Reeves R, Stanley HR. The relationship of bacterial penetration and pulpal pathosis in carious teeth. Oral Surgery, Oral Medicine, Oral Pathology 1966;22:59–65.
11. Dummer PM, Hicks R, Huws D. Clinical signs and symptoms in pulp disease. International Endodontic Journal 1980;13:27–35.
12. Hannas AR, Pereira JC, Granjeiro JM, et al. The role of matrix metalloproteinases in the oral environment. Acta Odontologica Scandinavica 2007;65:1–13.
13. Mazzoni A, Tjäderhane L, Checchi V, et al. Role of dentin MMPs in caries progression and bond stability. Journal of Dental Research 2015;94:241–51.
14. Loesche WJ. Role of Streptococcus mutans in human dental decay. Microbiology Reviews 1986;50:353–80.
15. Bowden GHW. The microbial ecology of dental caries. Microbial Ecology in Health and Disease 2000;12:138–48.
16. Munson MA, Banerjee A, Watson TF, et al. Molecular analysis of the microflora associated with dental caries. Journal of Clinical Microbiology 2004;42:3023–9.
17. Kianoush N, Adler CJ, Nguyen KA, et al. Bacterial profile of dentine caries and the impact of pH on bacterial population diversity. PLoS ONE 2014;9:e92940.
18. Chhour KL, Nadkarni MA, Byun R, et al. Molecular analysis of microbial diversity in advanced caries. Journal of Clinical Microbiology 2005;43:843–9.
19. Nadkarni MA, Caldon CE, Chhour KL, et al. Carious dentine provides a habitat for a complex array of novel Prevotella-like bacteria. Journal of Clinical Microbiology 2004;42:5238–44.
20. Hoshino E, Ando N, Sato M, et al. Bacterial invasion of non-exposed dental pulp. International Endodontic Journal 1992;25:2–5.
21. Cvek M. A clinical report on partial pulpotomy and capping with calcium hydroxide in permanent incisors with complicated crown fracture. Journal of Endodontics 1978;4:232–7.
22. Cox CF, Bergenholtz G, Fitzgerald M, et al. Capping of the dental pulp mechanically exposed to the oral microflora – a 5-week observation of wound healing in the monkey. Journal of Oral Pathology 1982;11:327–39.
23. Browne RM, Tobias RS, Crombie IK, et al. Bacterial microleakage and pulpal inflammation in experimental cavities. International Endodontic Journal 1983;16:147–55.
24. Tobias RS, Plant CG, Browne RM. Reduction in pulpal inflammation beneath surface-sealed silicates. International Endodontic Journal 1982;15:173–80.
25. Brännström M. The cause of postrestorative sensitivity and its prevention. Journal of Endodontics 1986;12:475–81.
26. Novickas D, Fiocca VL, Grajower R. Linings and caries in retrieved permanent teeth with amalgam restorations. Operative Dentistry 1989;14:33–9.
27. Pereira JC, Manfio AP, Franco EB, et al. Clinical evaluation of Dycal under amalgam restorations. American Journal of Dentistry 1990;3:67–70.
28. Frank RM. Reactions of dentin and pulp to drugs and restorative materials. Journal of Dental Research 1975;54:B176–87.
29. Plant CG, Jones DW. The damaging effects of restorative materials. Part II. Pulpal effects related to physical and chemical properties. British Dental Journal 1976;140:406–12.
30. Brännström M. Communication between the oral cavity and the dental pulp associated with restorative treatment. Operative Dentistry 1984;9:57–68.
31. Cox CF, Keall CL, Keall HJ, et al. Biocompatibility of surface-sealed dental materials against exposed pulps. Journal of Prosthetic Dentistry 1987;57:1–8.
32. Cox CF, Hafez AA, Akimoto N, et al. Biocompatibility of primer, adhesive and resin composite systems on non-exposed and exposed pulps of non-human primate teeth. American Journal of Dentistry 1998;11:S55–63.
33. Opdam NJ, van de Sande FH, Bronkhorst E, et al. Longevity of posterior composite restorations: a systematic review and meta-analysis. Journal of Dental Research 2014;93:943–9.
34. Kato G, Nakabayashi N. The durability of adhesion to phosphoric acid etched, wet dentin substrates. Dental Materials 1998;14:347–52.
35. Brännström M. Reducing the risk of sensitivity and pulpal complications after the placement of crowns and fixed partial dentures. Quintessence International 1996;27:673–8.
36. Meryon SD. The model cavity method incorporating dentine. International Endodontic Journal 1988;21:79–84.

37. Haywood VB, Leonard RH, Nelson CF, et al. Effectiveness, side effects and long-term status of nightguard vital bleaching. Journal of the American Dental Association 1994;125: 1219–26.

38. Schulte JR, Morrissette DB, Gasior EJ, et al. The effects of bleaching application time on the dental pulp. Journal of the American Dental Association 1994;125:1330–5.

39. Jorgensen MG, Carroll WB. Incidence of tooth sensitivity after home whitening treatment. Journal of the American Dental Association 2002;133:1076–82.

40. Nathanson D, Parra C. Bleaching vital teeth: a review and clinical study. Compendium of Continuing Education in Dentistry 1987;8:490–7.

41. Leonard RH Jr, Smith LR, Garland GE, et al. Evaluation of side effects and patients' perceptions during tooth bleaching. Journal of Esthetic and Restorative Dentistry 2007;19:355–64.

42. Kwon SR, Swift EJ Jr. Critical appraisal. In-office tooth whitening: pulpal effects and tooth sensitivity issues. Journal of Esthetic and Restorative Dentistry 2014;26:353–8.

43. Robertson WD, Melfi RC. Pulpal response to vital bleaching procedures. Journal of Endodontics 1980;6:645–9.

44. Morrant GA. Dental instrumentation and pulpal injury. Part II. clinical considerations. Journal of the British Endodontic Society 1977;10:55–63.

45. Swerdlow H, Stanley HR. Reaction of the human dental pulp to cavity preparation. Part II at 150,000 rpm with an air-water spray. Journal of Prosthetic Dentistry 1959;9:121–31.

46. Langeland K. Prevention of pulpal damage. Dental Clinics of North America 1972;16:709–32.

47. Murray PE, About I, Lumley PJ, et al. Human cavity remaining dentin thickness and pulpal activity. American Journal of Dentistry 2002;15:41–6.

48. Brännström M. The effect of dentin desiccation and aspirated odontoblasts on the pulp. Journal of Prosthetic Dentistry 1968;20:165–71.

49. Cheung GS, Lai SC, Ng RP. Fate of vital pulps beneath a metal-ceramic crown or a bridge retainer. International Endodontic Journal 2005;38:521–30.

50. Valderhaug J, Jokstad A, Ambjørnsen E, et al. Assessment of the periapical and clinical status of crowned teeth over 25 years. Journal of Dentistry 1997;25:97–105.

51. Kim S. Ligamental injection: a physiological explanation of its efficacy. Journal of Endodontics 1986;12:486–91.

52. Pitt Ford TR, Seare MA, McDonald F. Action of adrenaline on the effect of dental local anaesthetic solutions. Endodontics and Dental Traumatology 1993;9:31–5.

53. Takamori K. A histopathological and immunohistochemical study of dental pulp and pulpal nerve fibers in rats after the cavity preparation using Er:YAG laser. Journal of Endodontics 2000;26:95–9.

54. Tanabe K, Yoshiba K, Yoshiba N, et al. Immunohistochemical study on pulpal response in rat molars after cavity preparation by Er:YAG laser. European Journal of Oral Sciences 2002;110:237–45.

55. White JM, Goodis HE, Setcos JC, et al. Effects of pulsed Nd:YAG laser energy on human teeth: a three-year follow-up study. Journal of the American Dental Association 1993;124:45–51.

56. Jukić S, Anić I, Koba K, et al. The effect of pulpotomy using CO2 and Nd:YAG lasers on dental pulp tissue. International Endodontic Journal 1997;30:175–80.

57. Moritz A, Schoop U, Goharkhay K, et al. The CO_2 laser as an aid in direct pulp capping. Journal of Endodontics 1998;24:248–51.

58. Olivi G, Genovese MD, Maturo P, et al. Pulp capping: advantages of using laser technology. European Journal of Paediatric Dentistry 2007;8:89–95.

59. Andreasen JO, Andreasen FM, Tsukiboshi M. Crown-root fractures. In: Andreasen JO, Andreasen FM, Andersson L, editors. Textbook and color atlas of traumatic injuries to the teeth. 4th ed. Copenhagen (Denmark): Munksgaard; 2007. p. 314–36.

60. Pashley DH. Dentin permeability, dentin sensitivity and treatment through tubule occlusion. Journal of Endodontics 1986;12:465–74.

61. Pollington S, van Noort R. A clinical evaluation of a resin composite and a compomer in non carious Class V lesions. A 3-year follow-up. American Journal of Dentistry 2008;21:49–52.

62. Barbour ME, Rees GD. The role of erosion, abrasion and attrition in tooth wear. Journal of Clinical Dentistry 2006;17:88–93.

63. Cameron CE. Cracked-tooth syndrome. Journal of the American Dental Association 1964;68:405–11.

64. Fisher FJ. The treatment of carious dentine. British Dental Journal 1981;150:159–62.

65. Ricketts DN, Kidd EA, Innes N, et al. Complete or ultraconservative removal of decayed tissue in unfilled teeth. Cochrane Database of Systematic Reviews 2006;3:CD003808.

66. Bjørndal L, Reit C, Bruun G, et al. Treatment of deep caries lesions in adults: randomized clinical trials comparing stepwise vs. direct complete excavation, and direct pulp capping vs. partial pulpotomy. European Journal of Oral Science 2010;118:290–7.

67. Bjørndal L, Larsen T, Thylstrup A. A clinical and microbiological study of deep carious lesions during stepwise excavation using long treatment intervals. Caries Research 1997;31:411–7.

68. Coll JA. Indirect pulp capping and primary teeth: is the primary tooth pulpotomy out of date? Journal of Endodontics 2008;34:S34–9.

69. Marchi JJ, de Araujo FB, Fröner AM, et al. Indirect pulp capping in the primary dentition: a 4-year follow-up study. Journal of Clinical Pediatric Dentistry 2006;31:68–71.

70. Magnusson BO, Sundell SO. Stepwise excavation of deep carious lesions in primary molars. Journal of the International Association of Dentistry for Children 1977;8:36–40.

71. Shovelton DS. A study of deep carious dentine. International Dental Journal 1968;18:392–405.

72. Fusayama T. Two layers of carious dentin: diagnosis and treatment. Operative Dentistry 1979;4:63–70.

73. Kidd EA, Joyston-Bechal S, Beighton D. The use of a caries detector dye during cavity preparation: a microbiological assessment. British Dental Journal 1993;174:245–8.

74. Sturdevant JR, Lundeen TF, Sluder TB, et al. Five-year study of two light-cured posterior composite resins. Dental Materials 1988;4:105–10.

75. Duncan HF, Nair PNR, Pitt Ford TR. Vital pulp treatment: clinical considerations. ENDO (London, England) 2009;3:7–17.

76. Matsuo T, Nakanishi T, Shimizu H, et al. A clinical study of direct pulp capping applied to carious-exposed pulps. Journal of Endodontics 1996;22:551–6.

77. Mejàre I, Cvek M. Partial pulpotomy in young permanent teeth with deep carious lesions. Endodontics and Dental Traumatology 1993;9:238–42.

78. Barthel CR, Rosenkranz B, Leuenberg A, et al. Pulp capping of carious exposures: treatment outcome after 5 and 10 years: a retrospective study. Journal of Endodontics 2000;26: 525–8.

79. Simon S, Perard M, Zanini M, et al. Should pulp chamber pulpotomy be seen as a permanent treatment? Some preliminary thoughts. International Endodontic Journal 2013;46: 79–87.

80. Barrieshi-Nusair KM, Qudeimat MA. A prospective clinical study of mineral trioxide aggregate for partial pulpotomy in cariously exposed permanent teeth. Journal of Endodontics 2006;32:731–5.

81. Mass E, Zilberman U. Clinical and radiographic evaluation of partial pulpotomy in carious exposure of permanent molars. Pediatric Dentistry 1993;15:257–9.

82. Glass RL, Zander HA. Pulp healing. Journal of Dental Research 1949;28:97–107.

83. Pitt Ford TR, Roberts GJ. Immediate and delayed direct pulp capping with the use of a new visible light-cured calcium hydroxide preparation. Oral Surgery, Oral Medicine, Oral Pathology 1991;71:338–42.

84. Schröder U. Evaluation of healing following experimental pulpotomy of intact human teeth and capping with calcium hydroxide. Odontologisk Revy 1972;23:329–40.

85. Schröder U. Effects of calcium hydroxide-containing pulp-capping agents on pulp cell migration, proliferation and differentiation. Journal of Dental Research 1985;64: 541–8.

86. Stanley HR, Lundy T. Dycal therapy for pulp exposures. Oral Surgery, Oral Medicine, Oral Pathology 1972;34:818–27.

87. Bergenholtz G. Evidence for bacterial causation of adverse pulpal responses in resin-based dental restorations. Critical Reviews in Oral Biology and Medicine 2000;11:467–80.

88. Fernandes AM, Silva GAB, Lopes N Jr, et al. Direct capping of human pulps with a dentin bonding system and calcium hydroxide: an immunohistochemical analysis. Oral Surgery, Oral Medicine, Oral Pathology, Oral Radiology, and Endodontics 2008;105:385–90.

89. Nair PNR, Duncan HF, Pitt Ford TR, et al. Histological, ultrastructural and quantitative investigations on the response of healthy human pulps to experimental capping with mineral trioxide aggregate: a randomised controlled trial. International Endodontic Journal 2008;41:128–50.

90. Pitt Ford TR, Torabinejad M, Abedi HR, et al. Using mineral trioxide aggregate as a pulp-capping material. Journal of the American Dental Association 1996;127:1491–4.

91. Sangwan P, Sangwan A, Duhan J, et al. Tertiary dentinogenesis with calcium hydroxide: a review of proposed mechanisms. International Endodontic Journal 2013;46:3–19.

92. Graham L, Cooper PR, Cassidy N, et al. The effect of calcium hydroxide on solubilisation of bio-active dentine matrix. Biomaterials 2006;27:2865–73.

93. Tomson PL, Grover LM, Lumley PJ, et al. Dissolution of bio-active dentine matrix components by mineral trioxide aggregate. Journal of Dentistry 2007;35:636–42.

94. Mjör IA, Dahl E, Cox CF. Healing of pulp exposures: an ultrastructural study. Journal of Oral Pathology and Medicine 1991;20:496–501.

95. Simon S, Smith AJ. Regenerative endodontics. British Dental Journal 2014;216:E13.

96. Pisanti S, Sciaky I. Origin of calcium in the repair wall after pulpal exposure in the dog. Journal of Dental Research 1964;43:641–4.

97. Tronstad L. Reaction of the exposed pulp to Dycal treatment. Oral Surgery, Oral Medicine, Oral Pathology 1974;38: 945–53.

98. Cox CF, Sübay RK, Ostro E, et al. Tunnel defects in dentin bridges: their formation following direct pulp capping. Operative Dentistry 1996;21:4–11.

99. Langeland K, Dowden WE, Tronstad L, et al. Human pulp changes of iatrogenic origin. Oral Surgery, Oral Medicine, Oral Pathology 1971;32:943–80.

100. Lenherr P, Allgayer N, Weiger R, et al. Tooth discoloration induced by endodontic materials: a laboratory study. International Endodontic Journal 2012;45:942–9.

101. Duncan HF, Smith AJ, Fleming GJ, et al. HDACi: cellular effects, opportunities for restorative dentistry. Journal of Dental Research 2011;90:1377–88.

102. Ferracane JL, Cooper PR, Smith AJ. Can interaction of materials with the dentin-pulp complex contribute to dentin regeneration? Odontology / Journal of the Society of the Nippon Dental University 2010;98:2–14.

103. Murray PE, Garcia-Godoy F, Hargreaves KM. Regenerative endodontics: a review of current status and a call for action. Journal of Endodontics 2007;33:377–90.

104. Smith AJ. Pulp responses to caries and dental repair. Caries Research 2002;36:223–32.

105. Tziafas D. The future role of a molecular approach to pulp-dentinal regeneration. Caries Research 2004;38:314–20.

106. Cassidy N, Fahey M, Prime SS, et al. Comparative analysis of transforming growth factor-β isoforms 1–3 in human and rabbit dentine matrices. Archives of Oral Biology 1997;42: 219–23.

107. Rutherford RB, Wahle J, Tucker M, et al. Induction of reparative dentine formation in monkeys by recombinant human osteogenic protein-1. Archives of Oral Biology 1993;38:571–6.

108. Tziafas D, Alvanou A, Papadimitriou S, et al. Effects of recombinant basic fibroblast growth factor, insulin-like growth factor-II and transforming growth factor-β1 on dog pulp cells in vivo. Archives of Oral Biology 1998;43:431–44.

109. Iohara K, Nakashima M, Ito M, et al. Dentin regeneration by dental pulp stem cell therapy with recombinant human bone morphogenetic protein 2. Journal of Dental Research 2004;83: 590–5.

110. Nakashima M. Induction of dentin formation on canine amputated pulp by recombinant human bone morphogenetic proteins (BMP)-2 and -4. Journal of Dental Research 1994;73:1515–22.

111. Goldberg M, Smith AJ. Cells and extracellular matrices of dentin and pulp: a biological basis for repair and tissue engineering. Critical Reviews in Oral Biology and Medicine 2004;15:13–27.

112. Zhao S, Sloan AJ, Murray PE, et al. Ultrastructural localisation of TGF-β exposure in dentine by chemical treatment. Histochemistry Journal 2000;32:489–94.

113. Duncan HF, Smith AJ, Fleming GJ, et al. Histone deacetylase inhibitors epigenetically promote reparative events in primary dental pulp cells. Experimental Cell Research 2013;319: 1534–43.

114. Siqueira JF. Pulpal infections including caries. In: Hargreaves KM, Goodis HE, Tay FR, editors. Seltzer & Bender's dental pulp. 2nd ed. Chicago: Quintessence Books; 2012. p. 205–39.

115. Cooper PR, Holder MJ, Smith AJ. Inflammation and regeneration in the dentin-pulp complex: a double-edged sword. Journal of Endodontics 2014;40:S46–51.
116. Yu CY, Boyd NM, Cringle SJ, et al. An in vivo and in vitro comparison of the effects of vasoactive mediators on pulpal blood vessels in rat incisors. Archives Oral Biology 2002; 47:723–32.
117. Edwall L, Olgart L, Haegerstam G. Influence of vasodilator substances on pulpal blood flow in the cat. Acta Odontologica Scandinavica 1973;31:289–96.
118. Kim S, Dörscher-Kim J. Hemodynamic regulation of the dental pulp in a low compliance environment. Journal of Endodontics 1989;15:404–8.
119. Oehmke MJ, Knolle E, Oehmke HJ. Lymph drainage in the human dental pulp. Microscopy Research and Technique 2003;62:187–91.
120. Marchetti C, Poggi P, Calligaro A, et al. Lymphatic vessels in the healthy human dental pulp. Acta Anatomica (Basel) 1991;140:329–34.
121. Heyeraas KJ, Berggreen E. Interstitial fluid pressure in normal and inflamed pulp. Critical Reviews in Oral Biology and Medicine 1999;10:328–36.
122. Bhingare AC, Ohno T, Tomura M, et al. Dental pulp dendritic cells migrate to regional lymph nodes. Journal of Dental Research 2014;93:288–93.
123. Lu Y, Xie Y, Zhang S, et al. DMP1-targeted Cre expression in odontoblasts and osteocytes. Journal of Dental Research 2007;86:320–5.
124. Veerayutthwilai O, Byers MR, Pham TT, et al. Differential regulation of immune responses by odontoblasts. Oral Microbiology and Immunology 2007;22:5–13.
125. Fouad AF, Verma P. Healing after regenerative procedures with and without pulpal infection. Journal of Endodontics 2014;40:S58–64.
126. Fouad AF. The microbial challenge to pulp regeneration. Advances in Dental Research 2011;23:285–9.
127. Pekovic DD, Adamkiewicz VW, Shapiro A, et al. Identification of bacteria in association with immune components in human carious dentin. Journal of Oral Pathology 1987;16:223–33.
128. Hirao K, Yumoto H, Takahashi K, et al. Roles of TLR2, TLR4, NOD2, and NOD1 in pulp fibroblasts. Journal of Dental Research 2009;88:762–7.
129. Hosoya S, Matsushima K, Ohbayashi E, et al. Stimulation of interleukin-1beta-independent interleukin-6 production in human dental pulp cells by lipopolysaccharide. Biochemical and Molecular Medicine 1996;59:138–43.
130. Matsuo T, Ebisu S, Nakanishi T, et al. Interleukin-1 alpha and interleukin-1 beta periapical exudates of infected root canals: correlations with the clinical findings of the involved teeth. Journal of Endodontics 1994;20:432–5.
131. Pezelj-Ribaric S, Anic I, Brekalo I, et al. Detection of tumor necrosis factor alpha in normal and inflamed human dental pulps. Archives of Medical Research 2002;33:482–4.
132. McLachlan JL, Smith AJ, Bujalska IJ, et al. Gene expression profiling of pulpal tissue reveals the molecular complexity of dental caries. Biochimica et Biophysica Acta 2005;1741:271–81.
133. Dinarello CA. Interleukin-1. Reviews of Infectious Diseases 1984;6:51–95.
134. Hahn CL, Falkler WA Jr, Siegel MA. A study of T and B cells in pulpal pathosis. Journal of Endodontics 1989;15:20–6.
135. Izumi T, Kobayashi I, Okamura K, et al. Immunohistochemical study on the immunocompetent cells of the pulp in human non-carious and carious teeth. Archives of Oral Biology 1995;40:609–14.
136. Iwasaki Y, Otsuka H, Yanagisawa N, et al. In situ proliferation and differentiation of macrophages in dental pulp. Cell and Tissue Research 2011;346:99–109.
137. Maghazachi AA. Compartmentalization of human natural killer cells. Molecular Immunology 2005;42:523–9.
138. Kikuchi T, Hahn CL, Tanaka S, et al. Dendritic cells stimulated with Actinobacillus actinomycetemcomitans elicit rapid gamma interferon responses by natural killer cells. Infection and Immunity 2004;72:5089–96.
139. Bjørndal L, Darvann T. A light microscopic study of odontoblastic and non-odontoblastic cells involved in tertiary dentinogenesis in well-defined cavitated carious lesions. Caries Research 1999;33:50–60.
140. Bjørndal L, Darvann T, Thylstrup A. A quantitative light microscopic study of the odontoblast and subodontoblastic reactions to active and arrested enamel caries without cavitation. Caries Research 1998;32:59–69.
141. Smith AJ, Lesot H. Induction and regulation of crown dentinogenesis: embryonic events as a template for dental tissue repair? Critical Reviews Oral Biology and Medicine 2001;12:425–37.
142. Sloan AJ, Smith AJ. Stem cells and the dental pulp: potential roles in dentine regeneration and repair. Oral Diseases 2007;13:151–7.
143. Anneroth G, Bang G. The effect of allogeneic demineralized dentin as a pulp capping agent in Java monkeys. Odontologisk Revy 1972;23:315–28.
144. Seltzer S, Bender IB. Pulp reactions to operative procedures. The dental pulp. 3rd ed. Philadelphia: Lippincott; 1984.
145. Smith AJ, Scheven BA, Takahashi Y, et al. Dentine as a bioactive extracellular matrix. Archives Oral Biology 2012;57:109–21.
146. Sloan AJ, Smith AJ. Stimulation of the dentine-pulp complex of rat incisor teeth by transforming growth factor-beta isoforms 1-3 in vitro. Archives Oral Biology 1999;44:149–56.
147. Melin M, Joffre-Romeas A, Farges JC, et al. Effects of TGFbeta1 on dental pulp cells in cultured human tooth slices. Journal of Dental Research 2000;79:1689–96.
148. Li Y, Lü X, Sun X, et al. Odontoblast-like cell differentiation and dentin formation induced with TGF-β1. Archives Oral Biology 2011;56:1221–9.
149. Roberts-Clark DJ, Smith AJ. Angiogenic growth factors in human dentine matrix. Archives Oral Biology 2000;45:1013–16.
150. Zhang R, Cooper PR, Smith G, et al. Angiogenic activity of dentin matrix components. Journal of Endodontics 2011;37:26–30.
151. Nosrat CA, Fried K, Ebendal T, et al. NGF, BDNF, NT3, NT4 and GDNF in tooth development. European Journal of Oral Science 1998;106(Suppl. 1):S94–9.
152. Nosrat I, Seiger A, Olson L, et al. Expression patterns of neurotrophic factor mRNAs in developing human teeth. Cell Tissue Research 2002;310:177–87.
153. Kardos TB, Hunter AR, Hanlin SM, et al. Odontoblast differentiation: a response to environmental calcium? Endodontics and Dental Traumatology 1998;14:105–11.
154. Schröder U, Granath LE. Early reaction of intact human teeth to calcium hydroxide following experimental pulpotomy and its significance to the development of hard tissue barrier. Odontologisk Revy 1971;22:379–95.

155. Kono H, Onda A, Yanagida T. Molecular determinants of sterile inflammation. Current Opinion in Immunology 2014;26:147–56.

156. Huang TH, Yang CC, Ding SJ, et al. Inflammatory cytokines reaction elicited by root-end filling materials. Journal of Biomedical Material Research. Part B. Applied Biomaterials 2005;73:123–8.

157. Mitchell PJ, Pitt Ford TR, Torabinejad M, et al. Osteoblast biocompatibility of mineral trioxide aggregate. Biomaterials 1999;20:167–73.

158. Koh ET, McDonald F, Pitt Ford TR, et al. Cellular response to mineral trioxide aggregate. Journal of Endodontics 1998;24:543–7.

159. Kakehashi S, Stanley HR, Fitzgerald RJ. The exposed germ-free pulp: effects of topical corticosteroid medication and restoration. Oral Surgery Oral Medicine Oral Pathology 1969;27:60–7.

160. Tsuji T, Takei K, Inoue T, et al. An experimental study on wound healing of surgically exposed dental pulp in germ-free rats. Bulletin of the Tokyo Dental College 1987;28:35–8.

161. Inoue T, Shimono M. Repair dentinogenesis following transplantation into normal and germ-free animals. Proceedings of the Finnish Dental Society 1992;88:183–94.

162. Thomas MV, Puleo DA. Infection, inflammation, and bone regeneration: a paradoxical relationship. Journal of Dental Research 2011;90:1052–61.

163. Smith AJ, Sharpe PT. Biological tooth replacement and repair. In: Lanza R, Langer R, Vacanti JP, editors. Principles of tissue engineering. 4th ed. London: Elsevier; 2014. p. 1471–85.

164. Proceedings of Pulp Regeneration – Translational Opportunities Symposium. Journal of Endodontics 2014;40:S1–90.

165. Hermann B. Ein weiterer Beitrag zur Frage der Pulpenbehandlung. Zahnärztl Rundsch 1928;37:1327–76.

166. Zander HA. Reaction of the pulp to calcium hydroxide. Journal of Dental Research 1939;18:373–9.

167. Zanini M, Sautier JM, Berdal A, et al. Biodentine induces immortalized murine pulp cell differentiation into odontoblast-like cells and stimulates biomineralization. Journal of Endodontics 2012;38:1220–6.

168. Trope J. Regenerative potential of dental pulp. Journal of Endodontics 2008;34:S13–7.

169. Diogenes A, Henry MA, Teixeira FB, et al. An update on clinical regenerative endodontics. Endodontic Topics 2013;28:2–23.

170. Shimizu E, Ricucci D, Albert J, et al. Clinical, radiographic, and histological observation of a human immature permanent tooth with chronic apical abscess after revitalization treatment. Journal of Endodontics 2013;39:1078–83.

171. Mejàre IA, Axelsson S, Davidson T, et al. Diagnosis of the condition of the dental pulp: a systematic review. International Endodontic Journal 2012;45:597–613.

172. Petersson A, Axelsson S, Davidson T, et al. Radiological diagnosis of periapical bone tissue lesions in endodontics: a systematic review. International Endodontic Journal 2012;45:783–801.

173. Cordeiro MM, Dong Z, Kaneko T, et al. Dental pulp tissue engineering with stem cells from exfoliated deciduous teeth. Journal of Endodontics 2008;34:962–9.

174. Martin G, Ricucci D, Gibbs JL, et al. Histological findings of revascularized/revitalized immature permanent molar with apical periodontitis using platelet-rich plasma. Journal of Endodontics 2013;39:138–44.

175. Cameron CE. The cracked tooth syndrome: additional findings. Journal of the American Dental Association 1976;93:971–5.

176. McDonald F, Pitt Ford TR. Blood flow changes in permanent maxillary canines during retraction. European Journal of Orthodontics 1994;16:1–9.

177. Nixon CE, Saviano JA, King GJ, et al. Histomorphometric study of dental pulp during orthodontic tooth movement. Journal of Endodontics 1993;19:13–6.

178. Sano Y, Ikawa M, Sugawara J, et al. The effect of continuous intrusive force on human pulpal blood flow. European Journal of Orthodontics 2002;24:159–66.

179. Årtun J, Urbye KS. The effect of orthodontic treatment on periodontal bone support in patients with advanced loss of marginal periodontium. American Journal of Orthodontics and Dentofacial Orthopedics 1988;93:143–8.

180. Bauss O, Röhling J, Rahman A, et al. The effect of pulpal obliteration on pulpal vitality of orthodontically intruded traumatized teeth. Journal of Endodontics 2008;34:417–20.

181. Hamersky PA, Weimer AD, Taintor JF. The effect of orthodontic force application on the pulpal tissue respiration rate in the human premolar. American Journal of Orthodontics 1980;77:368–78.

182. Hamilton RS, Gutmann JL. Endodontic-orthodontic relationships: a review of integrated treatment planning challenges. International Endodontic Journal 1999;32:343–60.

183. Delivanis HP, Sauer GJ. Incidence of canal calcification in the orthodontic patient. American Journal of Orthodontics 1982;82:58–61.

184. Langeland K, Rodrigues H, Dowden W. Periodontal disease, bacteria, and pulpal histopathology. Oral Surgery, Oral Medicine, Oral Pathology 1974;37:257–70.

185. Rotstein I, Simon JH. Diagnosis, prognosis and decision making in the treatment of combined periodontal-endodontic lesions. Periodontology 2000 2004;34:165–203.

186. Bergenholtz G, Lindhe J. Effect of experimentally induced marginal periodontitis and periodontal scaling on the dental pulp. Journal of Clinical Periodontology 1978;5:59–73.

187. Hattler AB, Listgarten MA. Pulpal response to root planing in a rat model. Journal of Endodontics 1984;10:471–6.

188. Torabinejad M, Kiger RD. A histologic evaluation of dental pulp tissue of a patient with periodontal disease. Oral Surgery, Oral Medicine, Oral Pathology 1985;59:198–200.

189. Margelos JT, Verdelis KG. Irreversible pulpal damage of teeth adjacent to recently placed osseointegrated implants. Journal of Endodontics 1995;21:479–82.

190. Davis P, Chong BS, Mannocci F. Tooth discolouration following bone harvesting for pre-implant augmentation. ENDO (Lond, Engl) 2011;5:107–11.

191. Nkenke E, Schultze-Mosgau S, Radespeil-Tröger M, et al. Morbidity of harvesting of chin grafts: a prospective study. Clinical Oral Implant Research 2001;12:495–502.

192. Raghoebar GM, Meijndert L, Kalk WW, et al. Morbidity of mandibular bone harvesting: a comparative study. International Journal of Oral and Maxillofacial Implants 2007;22:359–65.

193. Duran S, Güven O, Günhan Ö. Pulpal and apical changes secondary to segmental osteotomy in the mandible-an experimental study. Journal of Cranio-Maxillo-Facial Surgery 1995;23:256–60.

194. Hitchcock R, Ellis E, Cox CF. Intentional vital root transection: a 52-week histopathologic study in Macaca mulatta. Oral Surgery, Oral Medicine, Oral Pathology 1985;60:2–14.

CHAPTER 6

Basic Instrumentation in Endodontics

S. J. Stone and J. M. Whitworth

Chapter Contents

Summary

Endodontics is a discipline rich in technology, and it is difficult even for experienced specialists to keep track of all that is available. The principles of root canal treatment have changed little in the last 50 years, but the same cannot be said for the burgeoning array of instruments and devices that continue to flood the market, with tempting promises of safer and more efficient practice. As in all clinical disciplines, many advances have failed to meet expectations, whereas others have enjoyed a brief period of popularity before they were rendered obsolete by the next 'brightly packaged' innovation. On the other hand, some advances have stood the test of time and brought lasting benefits to clinicians and patients alike. The latest is not always the best, and favourable treatment outcomes may be achieved by a variety of means. This chapter seeks to provide an overview of instruments and devices for the safe practice of root canal treatment, including tooth isolation, access to the pulp space, the mechanical shaping of root canals, their irrigation, medication and final root canal filling. The sterilization and storage of endodontic instruments will also be considered. Inevitably, newer, improved or modified versions of existing products will continue to hit the market, making it impossible to keep totally up-to-date.

Introduction

Effective root canal treatment is accomplished by eliminating as many microorganisms from the pulp space as possible and preventing their recurrence. In practical terms, this means locating and negotiating all the root canals, before shaping, cleaning and filling them with appropriate materials. Each stage demands a particular range of instruments and devices, with high- and low-tech options available from a number of manufacturers.

Basic Instrument Pack

For convenience, a basic selection of sterile instruments should be available, packaged or set up on a tray (Figure 6-1). A front-surfaced mouth mirror produces an undistorted image for good visibility deep within the pulp chamber. The DG16 endodontic explorer is a double-ended, extra long, sharp probe designed to help in the location of root canal entrances and for the

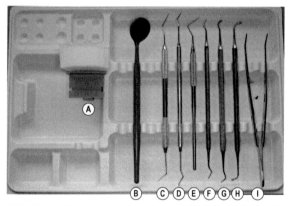

FIGURE 6-1 Basic endodontic instrument kit (left to right): (A) Endoring II (Jordco) incorporating a millimetre ruler, (B) front surface mirror, (C) DG16 explorer, (D) Briault probe, (E) periodontal probe, (F) long spoon excavator, (G) flat plastic instrument, (H) amalgam plugger, (I) endodontic locking tweezers.

detection of fractures or other features of interest. A Briault probe is helpful for exploring the integrity of restoration margins, for detecting caries and during access cavity preparation for determining whether the pulp chamber has been fully unroofed. A periodontal probe is essential for assessing bony support, for detecting the narrow, deep probing defects that are often associated with root fractures and for other measuring purposes during access cavity preparation. A long spoon excavator is helpful for removing the contents of the pulp chamber, and for the excavation of soft caries when present. Locking tweezers are ideal for handling paper points, gutta-percha cones, cotton wool pellets and root canal instruments. A millimetre ruler is essential for measurement purposes and is often combined with a sponge and holder (e.g. Endoring II, Jordco, Beaverton, OR, USA) for endodontic files during treatment (see Storage and Sterilization of Endodontic Instruments). A flat plastic instrument and an amalgam plugger are also helpful for the placement of an interappointment restoration.

Dental Dam

Root canal treatment should not be conducted on teeth unless they are properly isolated from the oral environment with a well-fitting dental dam; its many benefits include:
- protection of the patient from inhalation or ingestion of instruments, medicaments and debris;
- prevention of root canal infection by excluding saliva;
- enhanced vision and access by retracting soft tissues;
- enhanced patient comfort by excluding water-spray, endodontic materials and debris from the mouth;
- increased treatment efficiency.[1]

Sheets of dental dam are available in both latex and latex-free materials, including silicone (e.g. Flexi Dam, Roeko, Coltène/Whaledent, Cuyahoga Falls, OH, USA; Figure 6-2) and polyolefin elastomers (e.g. nonlatex dental dam, Hygenic, Coltène/Whaledent). Hypersensitivity reactions to latex[2] and to the powders with which they are often coated make latex-free and powder-free versions the options of choice in most

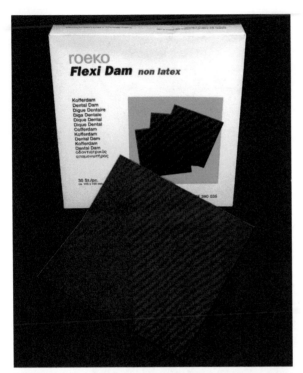

FIGURE 6-2 Flexi Dam, a nonlatex dental dam. (Coltène/Whaledent Gmbh + Co. KG)

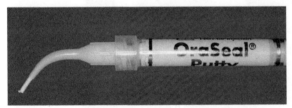

FIGURE 6-3 OraSeal caulking agent, a nonsetting dental dam sealant.

clinical settings. The dental dam is available in precut squares, measuring 15 cm^2, and in different thicknesses: thin, medium, heavy, extra heavy and special heavy; some are even scented. The heavier weight dams provide greater soft tissue retraction and protection as well as a tighter seal around the tooth. If the dam cannot be adapted perfectly and there is potential for leakage, gaps can be sealed with the application of a temporary filling material (e.g. Cavit, 3M ESPE, St Paul, MN, USA), a nonsetting caulking agent (e.g. OraSeal, Ultradent, South Jordan, UT, USA; Figure 6-3) or a light-cured silicone (e.g. Opaldam, Ultradent).

DENTAL DAM PUNCH

Holes are punched through the dental dam to accommodate the teeth to be isolated. For endodontic purposes, single tooth isolation is often sufficient, and some punches allow the size of the hole to be varied according to the size of the tooth (e.g. Ainsworth pattern, Figure 6-4A), whereas others cut a one-size hole (e.g. Ash Dam Punch, Dentsply, Weybridge, Surrey, UK, Figure 6-4B). The selection of a dental dam punch is a matter of personal preference, although holes that are too large may lead to leakage and holes that are too small may result in the dam tearing as it stretches over the tooth. The dam may also tear if the hole is not punched cleanly, and therefore punches should be kept sharp to avoid this eventuality.

DENTAL DAM CLAMPS

A dental dam is usually secured to the teeth with clamps. The majority of clamps are manufactured from stainless steel, though plastic versions are also available (e.g. SoftClamp, KerrHawe, Bioggio, Switzerland) and may be safer to use around the margins of ceramic restorations. Many designs of clamps are available from a range of manufacturers. A small selection of clamps to fit molars, premolars and incisors will suffice for most situations, with less common sizes reserved and separately packaged for special circumstances.

Aside from their size (molar, premolar and incisor), clamps may be categorized as 'active', where the beaks slope downward toward the gingival crevice (particularly helpful for engaging partially erupted teeth or teeth with little coronal bulbosity), or 'bland', where the beaks engage the tooth more horizontally, suitable for most situations where undercuts are available; clamps may also be winged or wingless (Figure 6-5), depending on the preferred method of dam application (see Methods of Application). Clamps should always be tried before application to ensure that the fit on the tooth is stable and comfortable. A stable clamp generally embraces the tooth around its margin, making a four-point contact below the point of maximum cervical bulbosity.

All clamps are at risk of fracture, especially across the bow[3], which undergoes cycles of flexion during application and removal. Therefore, it is wise to

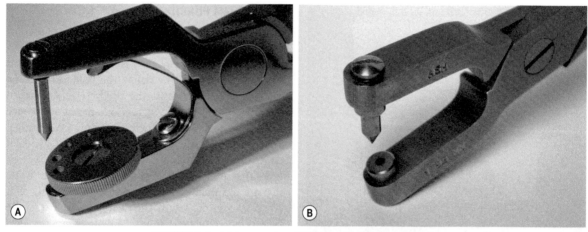

FIGURE 6-4 Dental dam punches: (A) Ainsworth; (B) Ash single hole.

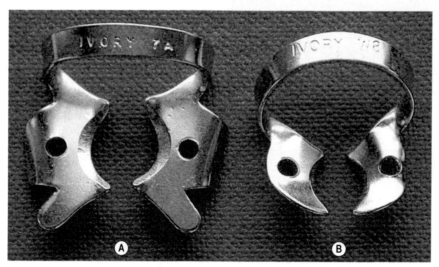

FIGURE 6-5 Dental dam clamps: (A) winged clamp with bland jaws (7A); (B) wingless clamp with retentive jaws (W8).

protect patients by attaching floss to both sides of the clamp during application. This is most simply achieved by passing a length of floss through the holes on either side of the clamp and tying it off (Figure 6-6). Once the dam has been applied, the floss can be cut and removed if so wished.

CLAMP FORCEPS

Clamps are applied, adjusted and removed with forceps. A variety of designs are available, including the Ivory (Heraeus Kulzer, Hanau, Germany) and

University of Washington (Dentsply) patterns (Figure 6-7), and selection is once again a matter of personal preference. The beaks of the clamp forceps sometimes require adjustment to ensure that they smoothly engage and disengage from the holes in the clamps; this is readily achieved by reducing the undercuts with a fine diamond bur and a high-speed handpiece.

DENTAL DAM FRAME

Once the dental dam is applied, its corners are attached to a frame, which is available in a variety of

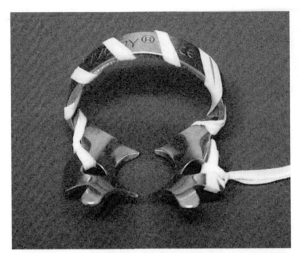

FIGURE 6-6 Dental floss tied to the dental dam clamp to aid retrieval in case of fracture or dislodgement.

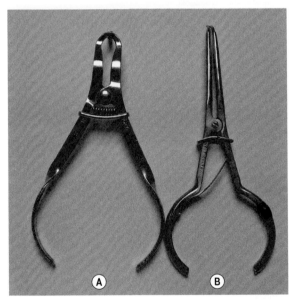

FIGURE 6-7 Dental dam clamp forceps: (A) Ivory and (B) University of Washington/Stokes.

designs (e.g. Youngs pattern, Nygaard-Ostby) and manufactured from metal (Hu-Friedy, Chicago, IL, USA; Dentsply) or plastic (Visi-Frame, Star Dental, Lancaster, PA, USA; Hygenic; Figure 6-8). Dental dams are also available with convenient, 'built-in' plastic frames (e.g. HandiDam, Dentsply; Flexi Dam,

Hygenic) and in frame-free mask form with elastics for the patient's ears (e.g. Dry Dam, Directa, Upplands, Väsby, Sweden).

METHODS OF APPLICATION

There are three main methods of dental dam application.[4] In the first method, the dental dam is attached to a winged clamp, which is gently stretched with forceps and placed below the tooth's undercuts without impinging on the gingival tissues. Once the clamp is securely attached, the dam is disengaged from the wings with a probe or plastic instrument and adapted around the cervical margin of the tooth (Figure 6-9). In the second method, a winged or wingless clamp is first attached to the tooth before stretching the punched hole in the dam over the clamp and tooth and adapting the dam around the cervical margins. In the third method, the dam is first stretched over the tooth and held in place by an assistant while the clamp (winged or wingless) is applied.

If more than one tooth is to be isolated, the dam may be stretched and 'knifed' through at each succeeding contact point. Sometimes, the application of a water-soluble lubricant, such as shaving gel or K-Y jelly (Reckitt Benckiser, Slough, Berkshire, England), or the use of floss is necessary to ensure easier passage of the dam through the contact points.

Challenging situations may call for resourcefulness; teeth that are severely broken down may be built-up with restorative material or by the placement of an orthodontic band or copper ring. Undercuts can also be created by the application of acid-etched retained composite resin, and on occasions, surgical crown-lengthening may be required beforehand. Decoronated teeth, with no undercuts, and teeth involved in bridgework may be isolated by a split-dam technique in which holes are punched for teeth at the mesial and distal limits of the planned isolation site, and then the holes are joined by cutting with scissors. The dam is applied by knifing through contact points, before securing with clamps or with latex or nonlatex stabilizing cords (e.g. Wedjets, Hygenic; Figure 6-10). On many occasions, anterior teeth can be isolated by knifing the dam through adjacent contact points and securing with Wedjets stabilizing cords. This is particularly helpful in the presence of fragile ceramic crown margins. Any leaks in the dam can, once again,

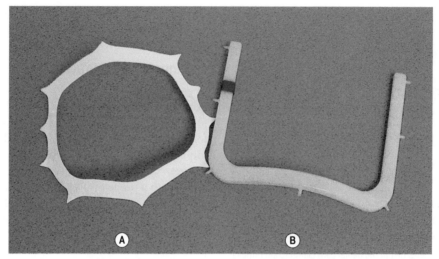

FIGURE 6-8 Dental dam frames: (A) Nygaard-Ostby; (B) Visi-Frame.

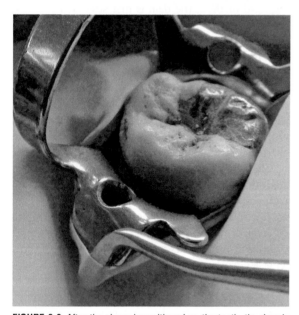

FIGURE 6-9 After the clamp is positioned on the tooth, the dam is lifted off the wings with a flat plastic instrument.

be sealed with a caulking agent such as OraSeal (Ultradent).

Instruments for Access Cavity Preparation

The first stage of root canal treatment is to gain entry to the pulp chamber. Magnification and improved illumination are always helpful.

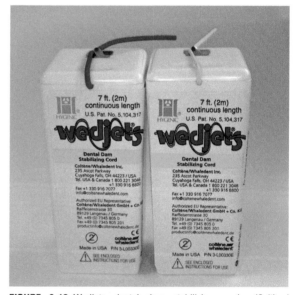

FIGURE 6-10 Wedjets dental dam stabilizing cords. (Coltène/Whaledent Inc)

MAGNIFICATION AND LIGHTING

The use of magnifying loupes, often with supplementary illumination, is well established in many branches of dentistry and brings tangible benefits to practitioners of any age (Figure 6-11). Many find loupes of a magnification level of 2.5× comfortable for endodontic and other dental applications, without becoming too heavy or cumbersome.

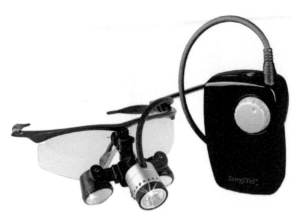

FIGURE 6-11 Magnifying loupes with supplementary light source.

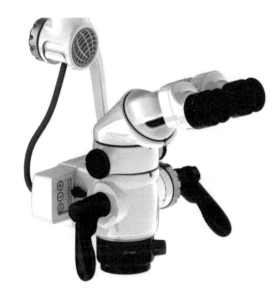

FIGURE 6-12 A dental operating microscope provides a range of magnifications and improved illumination.

Endodontics, perhaps more than any other dental discipline, has embraced the operating microscope for enhanced visualization and illumination.[5] Prominent suppliers of dental microscopes include the Global Surgical Corporation (St. Louis, MO, USA; Figure 6-12) and Carl Zeiss (Oberkochen, Germany) and offer models with a range of magnification levels from 2× to 20× or greater as well as illumination options. The operating microscope not only enhances the ability of clinicians to see and appreciate complex anatomy but it also brings the additional advantages

of improving posture, reducing fatigue, enhancing the quality of treatment and as a result, engendering renewed enthusiasm for dentistry.

BURS

Access to the pulp requires the judicious use of high-speed and slow-speed burs.

High-Speed Burs

Friction-grip diamond or tungsten carbide burs (Figure 6-13) are ideal for outlining the access cavity and gaining initial entry to the pulp. In an age of minimally invasive dentistry, pulp access may appear to require deep preparations, but in reality, the pulps of most posterior teeth are entered within a depth of 6 or 7 mm; the temptation to use long 'crown-preparation' burs that may catastrophically overcut should be avoided. Access through enamel/dentine, composite resin, amalgam and ceramic restorations is best achieved with diamond burs, whereas cast metal can often be accessed more efficiently with tungsten carbide burs. Once the pulp chamber is entered, its roof can be safely and efficiently removed with a nonend cutting, tapered, diamond (Diamendo, Dentsply) or tungsten carbide (Endo-Z, Dentsply) bur (see Figure 6-13), aligned to the long-axis to prevent over-flaring of the cavity and lightly floated around the line angles of the pulp chamber.

Slow-Speed Burs

Round burs with long, narrow shanks, such as the Goose-Neck (Hager & Meisinger, Neuss, Germany) and Long-Neck pin burs (Dentsply; Figure 6-14), are ideal for refining pulp access; the narrow shank allows the operator to observe the tip of the bur at all times. They are also helpful for 'troughing'[6] on the pulp chamber floor to detect additional anatomy, such as second mesiobuccal canals in maxillary molars, and for chasing the entrances of canals that have become obliterated by mineralized deposits.

ULTRASONICS

Piezoelectric ultrasonic units have many applications in dentistry. In endodontics, a simple, water-cooled scaler tip may be helpful to debride the pulp chamber, remove overhanging elements of the chamber roof and eliminate obstructions such as pulp stones.

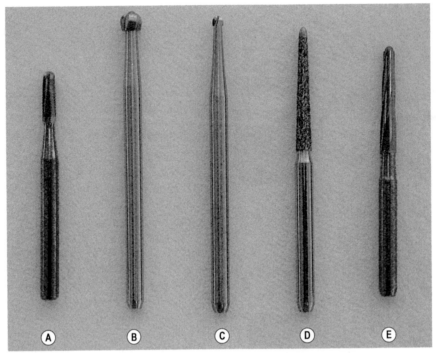

FIGURE 6-13 Access cavity burs (left to right): (A) FG 557 ISO 010 (TC); (B) FG ISO round 018 (long); (C) FG ISO round 010 (long); (D) FG safe-ended diamond 332 ISO 018 and (E) FG safe-ended TC, Endo-Z (Dentsply).

Specialized endodontic ultrasonic microtips (Figure 6-15) are also available for applications similar to those described for long-shank round burs. If used without water coolant, care should be taken to avoid overheating of the tips and burning of tissues after prolonged use.[7]

GATES-GLIDDEN BURS

Gates-Glidden burs are operated in a slow-speed handpiece and may be used to refine pulp access, particularly for enlarging canal openings and removing overhanging dentine that so often impedes the easy entry of instruments. These burs are available in six sizes, from 0.5 to 1.5 mm in diameter (Figure 6-16), and feature a noncutting pilot tip, a cutting bulb and a narrow shank, which is designed to fracture closer toward the handpiece for easier retrieval. They are available in a variety of lengths, a standard 32 mm, a shorter 24 mm and a longer 36 mm.

When using Gates-Glidden burs, care should be taken to avoid overcutting the furcal wall of curved root canals, resulting in a strip perforation.[8] For this

and other reasons, the role of the Gates-Glidden bur has diminished in recent times, with tapered nickel-titanium (NiTi) files largely taking over the role of canal orifice enlargement and creation of a 'glide path' for instrument entry. However, Gates-Glidden burs also create frictional heat and are efficient for softening and removing gutta-percha from the straight, coronal part of the root canal during endodontic retreatment.

Tools for Retrieving Posts and Fractured Files

POST REMOVAL DEVICES

Although most often only encountered during endodontic retreatment, posts constructed from metal or fibre-reinforced composites may present formidable challenges to access and require special devices for their removal.

Successful post removal is helped by first identifying the type post: is it made of metal or fibre reinforced

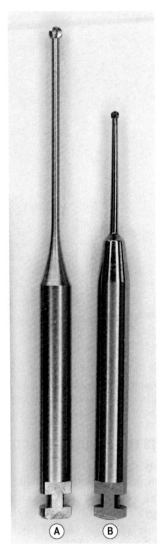

FIGURE 6-14 Goose-Neck (A) and Long-Neck pin (B) burs.

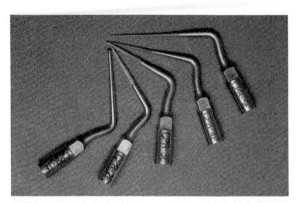

FIGURE 6-15 A set of multipurpose diamond-coated endodontic ultrasonic microtips.

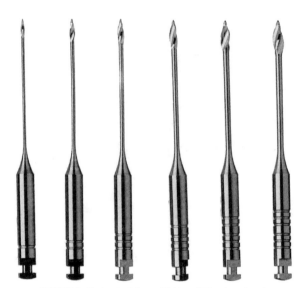

FIGURE 6-16 A set of Gates-Glidden drills, sizes 1 to 6.

composite? Is it threaded and screwed into the canal or cemented passively? Is it tapered or parallel? It is also useful to know if the post was cemented with an adhesive resin or with traditional cement such as zinc phosphate.

In most cases, the application of a water-cooled ultrasonic tip may help to disrupt the cement lute and loosen the post. Threaded posts may often be unscrewed with a dedicated screwdriver from the post kit or by working an ultrasonic tip counterclockwise around its head. Tapered and parallel-sided metal posts, particularly those cemented with traditional cements, may be first loosened using ultrasonics and then lifted from the canal with a postpulling device such as the Eggler,[9,10] Thomas/Gonon (Société FFDM-PNEUMAT, Bourges Cedex, France) or Ruddle (Sybron-nEndo, Orange, CA, USA) postpuller[11] (Figure 6-17). Both work rather like a corkscrew, applying pressure to the root as the post is extracted; however, there is a risk of root fracture. Parallel-sided metallic posts are first loosened with ultrasonics and retrieved using the

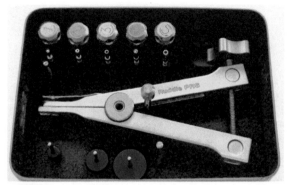

FIGURE 6-17 The Ruddle post removal kit. (Reproduced courtesy of Quality Endodontic Distributors, Peterborough, UK).

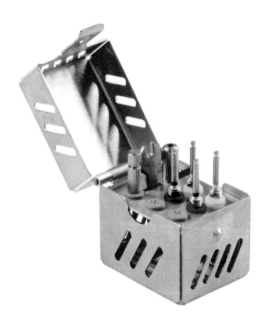

FIGURE 6-18 Masserann micro kit containing trepans, handle, extractor and spanner.

Masserann kit (Micro-Mega, Besançon, France) – a series of hollow drills (trephines) which cut through the cement lute to free the post[12] (Figure 6-18). Fibre-posts are not amenable to being pulled or loosened with ultrasonics and must be removed by working a narrow ultrasonic tip through their centre or by drilling them out with a dedicated fibre post removal bur[13] (Figure 6-19).

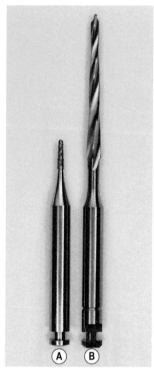

FIGURE 6-19 Fibre post removal kit (RTD, Saint Egreve, France). A small pilot bur (A) creates a pathway for an engine reamer (B) to follow.

INSTRUMENTS FOR REMOVING FRACTURED FILES

Clinicians may encounter teeth with fractured files, Gates-Glidden drills and other metallic objects such as silver points. Not all retained objects are amenable to retrieval, but a number of devices may be helpful.[11,14] The careful use of ultrasonics is often effective in vibrating and loosening metallic objects free, enabling the removal of fragments; it is prudent to ensure that the loosened fragment does not find its way into another canal opening.

Forceps

If the top end of the object is visible, it may be possible to first loosen it by ultrasonics and then extract it using fine-beaked haemostats, microsurgical needle holders or Steiglitz forceps (Hu-Friedy; Figure 6-20).

Cancellier Kit

Another way of gaining purchase to a fractured object can be facilitated with glue. The Cancellier kit

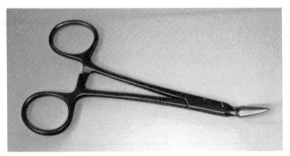

FIGURE 6-20 Steiglitz forceps, with their fine and lockable beaks, can be helpful in grasping and retrieving small metallic objects such as silver points and fractured files.

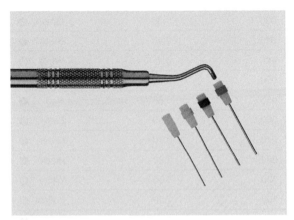

FIGURE 6-21 Cancellier kit, with tubes of different diameters and a handle.

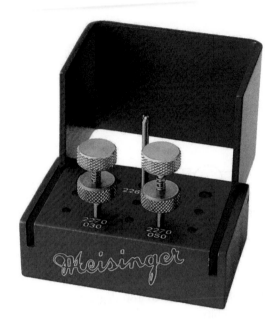

FIGURE 6-22 The Meitrac Endo safety system for retrieving small metallic objects.

(SybronEndo; Figure 6-21) provides a range of metallic tubes which may be attached to a handle. The tube that fits most closely over the object is chosen. The end of the tube is then filled with cyanoacrylate adhesive or better still, chemically curing composite resin. The tube is then inserted over the object and held while the adhesive or composite resin sets; this then engages, and when the tube is removed, pulls the object free.

Masserann Kit

In addition to its series of trephines, the Masserann kit (Micro-Mega) contains narrow tubes with internal locking features; the other hollow tube is placed over the metallic objects, the stylet inserted to engage it and then the whole assembly removed together to pull the object free.

Meitrac System

Other proprietary devices such as the Meitrac Endodontic Safety System (Hager & Meisinger; Figure 6-22) are extraction tools with smaller chucks, similar to those found on electric power drills, to engage fractured instruments, silver points or post fragments to allow them to be extracted. For more on the topic of removal of fractured instruments see Chapter 14.

Instruments for Gross Removal of Pulp Tissue

BARBED BROACHES

The insertion of a standard endodontic hand file may compact soft tissue within the canal and create an obstruction, but this can often be avoided by undertaking gross pulp tissue removal with a barbed broach first. Constructed from relatively soft stainless steel, these fine-shank instruments present a series of asymmetrically positioned barbs (Figure 6-23) created by making cuts into the surface of the instrument and elevating the cut sections outward. The barbed broach

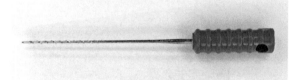

FIGURE 6-23 Barbed broach used for gross pulp tissue removal.

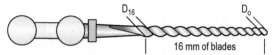

FIGURE 6-24 Illustration of an ISO hand file. ISO regulations determine the diameter of the instrument close to its tip (D_0), a taper of 0.02 mm/mm (2% taper), the diameter 16 mm from the tip (D_{16}) and the colour of the handle (See Table 6-1).

TABLE 6-1 Nominal Sizes and Colour Coding of ISO Endodontic Hand Instruments		
Size	D_0 (mm)	Colour
006	0.06	Orange ●
008	0.08	Grey ○
010	0.10	Purple ●
015	0.15	White ○
020	0.20	Yellow ○
025	0.25	Red ●
030	0.30	Blue ○
035	0.35	Green ○
040	0.40	Black ●
045	0.45	White ○
050	0.50	Yellow ○
055	0.55	Red ●
060	0.60	Blue ○
070	0.70	Green ○
080	0.80	Black ●
090	0.90	White ○
100	1.00	Yellow ○
110	1.10	Red ●
120	1.20	Blue ○
130	1.30	Green ○
140	1.40	Black ●

is inserted, rotated 90 to 180 degrees to engage the mass of pulp tissue, and then removed. Barbed broaches are also useful for removing the pledget of cotton wool that is frequently placed in pulp chambers between appointments to cover canal orifices, underneath the temporary coronal restoration. The risk of fracture of a barbed broach is minimal provided a suitable size is used, it does not engage the canal walls and it is not forcefully overrotated.

Instruments for Negotiating and Shaping Root Canals

ISO HAND INSTRUMENTS

Hand files with features defined by the International Standards Organisation (ISO) have been the mainstay of canal negotiation and shaping since the early 1960s. ISO regulations determine the diameter of the instrument where its cutting flutes end at the tip (D_0; Figure 6-24), the taper of the instrument (0.02 mm/mm, or 2%), the length of the fluted portion (always 16 mm) and the diameter of the instrument at the end of the fluted portion (D_{16}).[15] Instrument sizes are denoted by the colour of the handle (Table 6-1). ISO hand files are typically available in 21, 25 and 31 mm lengths and may be constructed from stainless steel or NiTi alloys.

The ISO does not define the specifics of cutting flute design, and two broad categories are available,

K-type and Hedstrom (H) files, each with distinct methods of application.[16]

K-Type Files

Stainless steel K-type files (Figure 6-25) remain popular for initial canal negotiation and for the development of a smoothly flowing glide-path before canal enlargement.[17] Stainless steel K-type files are produced by twisting tapered wires with a square, triangular or rhomboid cross-section to create strong instruments that can be precurved for canal negotiation. They are capable of cutting dentine with 'filing' motions (dragging or rasping instruments against canal walls as they are withdrawn) or with 'rotational' motions (twisting intermediate size 12.5 instrument so that the size increment is more gradual.

NiTi ISO hand files are generally manufactured by milling, creating cutting flutes in a NiTi wire, and overcoming many of the problems associated with instrument stiffness.[20] They are suitable for enlarging canals without deviation, but they cannot be pre-curved and are generally not suited to initial canal negotiation.[17] Popular examples include Nitiflex (Dentsply) and NiTi K-files (VDW).

H (Hedstrom) Files

Both stainless steel and NiTi H files (see Figure 6-25) are manufactured by milling and creating cutting flutes in a circular cross-section wire; the aggressive, deep-fluted blades cut in a filing (rasping) motion against the canal walls on the outward stroke.[21] The manufacturing process results in a narrow central core of metal, making H files more flexible than their K-type file equivalents but also making them more vulnerable to fracture, especially if rotated. H files are typically used for enlarging root canal entrances, with rasping strokes away from the furcation and for engaging and removing root filling materials from canals during endodontic retreatment.

NON-ISO HAND INSTRUMENTS

The development of flexible NiTi alloys, coupled with the technology to mill complex cutting flutes, has heralded a new generation of instruments of non-ISO geometries.[22] Non-ISO K-type files include GT hand files (Dentsply), ProTaper Universal hand files (Dentsply) and RaCe 123 hand files (FKG, La Chaux-de-Fonds, Switzerland). GT hand files have a uniform size 20 tip, tapers of 6% to 12% and blades milled in reverse, for single-instrument canal shaping with reverse Balanced Force motion. ProTaper Universal hand files consist of a series of eight instruments used in watch-winding or Balanced Force motion to progressively enlarge the canal and develop the desired degree of apical enlargement and taper.

MECHANICALLY DRIVEN FILES

In addition to their flexibility, NiTi alloys have greater resistance to work hardening (cyclic fatigue) and torsional failure than stainless steel alloys, making it possible to use rotating files in curved root canals with a

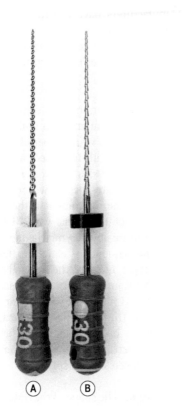

FIGURE 6-25 ISO endodontic hand files: K-type (A) and Hedstrom (B), showing differences in their cutting flutes.

instruments clockwise and counterclockwise between finger and thumb in 'watch-winding' or 'Balanced Force'[18] motions). The majority have noncutting tips to minimize the risk of instruments deviating from the long axis of curved canals during use, but as instrument sizes increase, so does instrument stiffness. Popular examples of K-type files include K Flexofiles (Dentsply), K-flex (SybronEndo), Triple-Flex files (Sybron) and Flexicut files (VDW, Munich, Germany).

Small K-type files (typically sizes 06–15) constructed from stiffer carbon steel or heat-treated stainless steel alloys are available to negotiate narrow and more challenging root canals.[19] Examples include Pathfinder CS files (SybronEndo), C-Pilot (VDW) and C+ files (Dentsply). When opening narrow canals, the 50% increase in instrument tip diameter from the size 10 to the size 15 file can be an impediment. For this reason, the C-Pilot series of files includes an greater degree of safety.[23] Since their introduction in the early 1990s, NiTi rotary files are now commonly used in both specialist and nonspecialist practices, allowing clinicians to shape canals with greater efficiency and safety.

Files Operated in Continuous (360-Degree) Clockwise Rotation

The majority of NiTi file systems introduced between 1991 and 2013 were operated in continuous clockwise motion with a dedicated motor and handpiece.[23] During this period, manufacturers sought to create instruments that operate safely with the minimum risk of fracture, while optimizing cutting efficiency and the ability to cut debris out of the canal; these instruments (Figure 6-26) often have radically different designs, all claiming to help in some unique way and address the challenges of canal shaping more effectively than others. There is consensus that NiTi rotary files are able to enlarge canals safely and effectively, though no file system can claim superior clinical outcomes in comparison with others. Instrument selection is therefore a matter of personal preference.

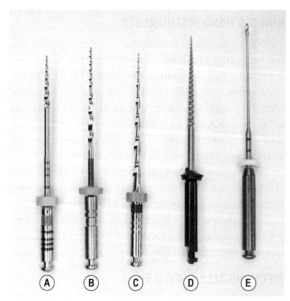

FIGURE 6-26 Examples of NiTi rotary files, each with radically different designs (from left to right): (A) GT rotary (Dentsply), (B) BioRaCe (FKG Dentaire SA), (C) Mtwo (VDW), (D) HERO (Micro-Mega), (E) Lightspeed (SybronEndo).

Manufacturers have incorporated certain features to help improve performance; these include modifications in taper, cross-section, rake angle, helical flute angle, core diameter/flute depth, tip geometry and surface treatment.

Variable Taper. Traditional step-back instrumentation at 1-mm increments with multiple ISO hand files can produce canals with a taper of approximately 5%. Rotary NiTi files with increased taper can predictably develop shapes of 5% or greater taper without the need to use as many files; however, great stresses may be placed on the instrument if they engage and cut too much of the root canal wall. Manufacturers have responded to this by varying the taper of instruments in their file sequence – e.g. Hero 642 (MicroMega) with 6% taper files for the coronal third, 4% taper for mid-third and 2% taper for apical third. Others have produced files with variable tapers, resulting in successive instruments that enlarge the coronal and middle thirds of the root canal, before moving to fixed-taper instruments for apical enlargement (e.g. ProTaper Universal, Dentsply).

Flute Design. The shape of the flutes in cross-section determines cutting efficiency and the ability of the file to remove debris. A design incorporating a reservoir for the dentine debris will help effective evacuation as the debris is transported coronally by the clockwise rotation of the instrument.

Rake Angle. The rake or cutting angle of most conventional instruments is negative so the cutting blade scrapes rather than cuts into dentine, and this is inefficient. A positive rake angle results in more effective cutting, but if the rake angle is excessively positive, the cutting blade may dig deeply into the canal walls and risk both overcutting and overstressing the file (Figure 6-27).

Helical Flute Angle. This is the angle at which the cutting flutes spiral around the shaft of the instrument (Figure 6-28). If there are too few spirals, dentine debris will accumulate quickly, the flutes will become clogged, cutting will become inefficient and the instrument may be overstressed. On the other hand, if there are too many spirals, the dentine debris has too great

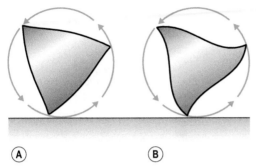

FIGURE 6-27 File rake angle – the angle at which the file blades engage dentine. Negative angles (A) are inefficient, but positive angles (B) that are too aggressive may risk dentine or instrument damage.

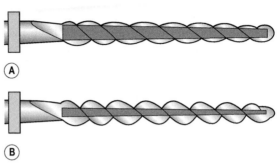

FIGURE 6-29 File core diameter/flute depth; (A) shallow flutes, with a wide core diameter, create a relatively strong but inflexible instrument, with little space for debris and the potential for inefficient cutting, (B) deep flutes, with a narrow core diameter, create a relatively flexible but less robust instrument, with increased space for debris and the potential for more efficient cutting.

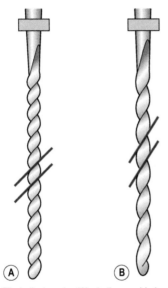

FIGURE 6-28 File helical angle; (A) shallow as blades are arranged closely together, (B) steep as blades are more widely separated; an important feature for cutting efficiency and debris removal.

a distance to travel before it is evacuated from the canal, and frictional resistance may trap and compress the debris. The ideal helical flute angle allows efficient removal of dentinal debris without clogging the instrument. Design features such as increasing the helical flute angle along the length of the file from tip to handle may assist in debris removal.

Core Diameter/Flute Depth. The core strength and flexibility of an instrument is dependent on its core cross-sectional diameter; the larger the core

diameter, the more robust and rigid the instrument but the less flexible it becomes. The core diameter is inversely related to the flute depth. The proportion of the core diameter to the outside diameter should be greatest at the tip, where strength is most important. By uniformly decreasing this proportion as the fluting moves up the taper, flute depth increases and file flexibility increases, while the strength of the instrument is maintained. An additional advantage is that dentine debris is also removed more efficiently (Figure 6-29).

Noncutting Tip. Noncutting tips are now almost universal, keeping instruments centred within the canal and serving to guide instruments as they navigate down the canal.

Surface Treatment. The majority of rotary NiTi instruments are produced by milling. As a result, defects and adherent debris are present on the surface of instruments, which may become sites of stress concentration and crack initiation. Electropolishing reduces these defects and produces a surface free of contaminants, thereby increasing the instrument's fatigue resistance.[24,25] Milling grooves, cracks, pits and areas of metal rollover are less evident on electropolished instruments. A variety of other surface treatments have also been shown to improve the hardness, wear resistance and cutting efficiency of rotary NiTi instruments. These include ionic implantation with boron,[26] the creation of a titanium nitride layer by thermal nitridation[27] and physical and chemical vapour deposition.[28,29] Other developments have allowed the manufacture of NiTi files by twisting, rather than milling, NiTi wires; for example, the Twisted File (TF; SybronEndo) has apparent improvements in instrument fracture resistance.[30]

Other Innovations. Other innovations have included the development of novel NiTi alloys, notably M-wire[31] (e.g. ProTaper Next, Dentsply) and R-phase heat-treatment technology[32] (e.g. Twisted File, SybronEndo) with their demonstrably improved resistance to fracture, and controlled memory (CM) alloys (e.g. HyFlex CM, Coltène/Whaledent) with their enhanced fracture resistance and ability to be precurved before entry to the canal. This is clearly an area of enormous technological development.[33]

Handpieces, Motors and Motions

Files in continuous clockwise rotation have the tendency to 'screw' into canals, where they may lock and fracture as it continues to be driven by the motor. Files may also be at risk of fracture if they undergo too many cycles of rotation in the canal and as they are work-hardened. Files must therefore be rotated at the speed directed by the manufacturer (typically 150–350 rpm) and inserted in and out of the canal in the recommended manner; typically, this means light up-down 'pecking' motions, or brushing against the canal walls on withdrawal.

Speed-reducing handpieces can be used with standard air-driven motors, provided the speed of the motor is known and can be reduced, or electric motors; though optimal control is achieved by the use of a dedicated electric endodontic motor (Figure 6-30), some of which are cordless (e.g. Endo-Mate TC, NSK, Kanuma, Tochigi, Japan; EndoTouch TC, SybronEndo). To improve access, some handpieces have reduced head sizes, and some manufacturers produce files with shorter handles or lengths to facilitate access to posterior teeth. Motors may also incorporate torque control settings that prevent torsional overload of the file beyond its elastic limit, or a reverse feature of backing out of the canal, reducing the risk of locking or torsional fracture.[34] Two key variables that are beyond the control of the manufacturer are the

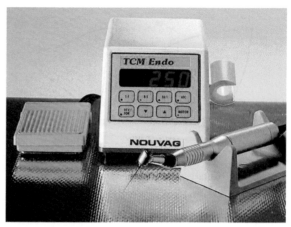

FIGURE 6-30 Speed-controllable electric motor and handpiece for rotary NiTi root canal instrumentation.

experience of the operator and the reuse of instruments[34]; the latter is not permitted in the UK.

Files Operated in Reciprocation

A newer generation of reciprocating motors, which drive files in a clockwise/counterclockwise motion as they advance into the canal, are available; examples include Reciproc (VDW; Figure 6-31) and WaveOne Gold (Dentsply), each with dedicated handpieces and motors to deliver rotations of 170 degreees counterclockwise/50 degrees clockwise at 10 cycles per second (350 rpm), and 150 degrees counterclockwise/ 30 degrees clockwise at 10 cycles per second (300 rpm), respectively. It should be noted that the cutting flutes of both instruments are milled in the opposite direction compared with conventional hand and rotary files, and that dentine is cut during the anticlockwise rotation. Other innovations include the relatively large taper of the instruments in their apical 3 mm, before reducing the taper further up the instrument to minimize excessive dentine removal. Reciproc (VDW), for example, comes in sizes R25 (tip size 25), R40 (tip size 40) and R50 (tip size 50), with the expectation that shaping will be accomplished with one instrument. The performance of these instruments has been reviewed favourably[35–37] and has enabled clinicians to shape canals with an improved degree of speed and safety. However, there are concerns about these instruments pushing debris into the periapical tissues and creating cracks in root dentine.[35] Reciprocating instruments

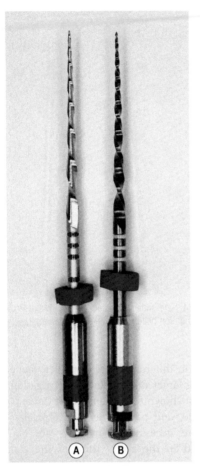

FIGURE 6-31 Examples of NiTi files driven in reciprocation: Reciproc (VDW) (A) and WaveOne Gold (Dentsply) (B).

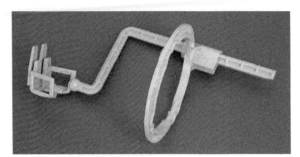

FIGURE 6-32 Endoray II beam-aiming device for periapical radiographs during root canal treatment.

have also been proven efficient in the removal of root filing materials during endodontic retreatment.[38] Recent modifications have resulted in newer versions such as WaveOne Gold (Dentsply; see Figure 6-31). Further advancement include instrument systems with motors capable of varying their motion (rotation or reciprocation) in response to canal conditions (e.g. Twisted File Adaptive, SybronEndo).[39]

Devices to Determine Working Length

Endodontic instruments and materials should be confined within the root canal. Therefore, root canal length should be determined early in treatment and checked at intervals as necessary.

MEASURING DEVICES

A key essential is a ruler or other device to measure the lengths of instruments and materials. This can be as simple as a sterilizable metal ruler, with graduations of 1 mm or 0.5 mm, a ruler incorporated into an Endoring II (Jordco; see Figure 6-1), or a measuring block with holes of predetermined depths. Rubber or silicone stops are prefitted on most endodontic files, although boxes of stops are available, often incorporating a ruler.

RADIOGRAPHIC WORKING LENGTH DETERMINATION

An instrument with its rubber or silicone stop adjusted to the estimated working length is advanced into the canal until its stop sits on a chosen coronal reference point, typically a cusp tip or incisal edge. An undistorted conventional film or digital radiograph is then exposed. Dedicated film holders and centering devices are available for paralleling views with both conventional films and digital sensors (e.g. Endoray II, Dentsply Rinn, Elgin, IL, USA; XCP-DS, Dentsply Rinn)[40] (Figure 6-32).

ELECTRONIC APEX LOCATORS

Electronic apex locators (EALs) are popular for determining working length. These devices are supplied with electrodes to contact the patient's oral mucosa, usually in the corner of the mouth, and the file; they measure the impedance to current flow between the electrodes as the instrument advances toward the apical foramen.[41] Operating with multiple current frequencies, newer EALs contain powerful microprocessors that perform mathematical quotient and algorithm

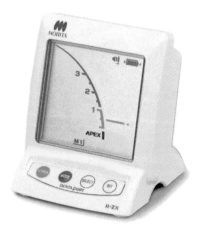

FIGURE 6-33 Root ZX electronic apex locator with digital display.

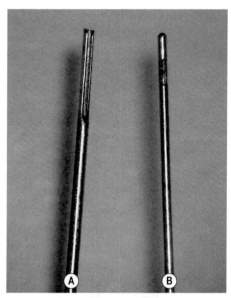

FIGURE 6-34 Safe-ended Monoject (A) and Max-i-Probe (Dentsply Rinn) (B) irrigation needles.

calculations, and provide accurate information on the point at which the instrument tip leaves the canal and contacts the periodontal ligament, even in the presence of blood and other fluids within the canal.[42] Caution is needed in the presence of metal restorations, where readings may not be accurate, and with open apices that offer little impedance to current flow. EALs available include the popular Root ZX (Morita, Suita City, Osaka, Japan; Figure 6-33), RayPex 6 (VDW) and Elements (SybronEndo) units. EALs have brought additional predictability to working length determinations and are capable of reducing, though not eliminating, the number of radiographic exposures necessary. Cordless endodontic handpieces that incorporate an electronic apex locator are also available (e.g. Tri Auto ZX, Morita).[43]

Irrigant Delivery Devices

Though essential for canal enlargement, even the best shaping instruments may leave up to 35% of canal walls untouched,[44] leaving pulp tissue and microbial biofilm in canal complexities,[45] and packed debris.[46] Irrigation therefore plays an essential role in lubricating the canal, washing out debris, dissolving pulp tissue, disturbing biofilm and dissolving smear layer from root canals and their ramifications.[45] The standard method of delivery is through an endodontic irrigating needle, attached securely via a Luer-Lok, screw-type coupling, to the syringe to prevent its dislodgement during irrigation. Irrigating needles are

available in different gauges; smaller gauge numbers indicating larger outer diameters. Irrigating solutions have been shown to exchange little beyond the tip of the needle, and narrow needles, typically 27 or 30 gauge, are necessary if irrigants are to be better exchanged in the apical third of the canal.[47] Care should be taken to avoid irrigant extrusion through the tooth apex, first by the use of dedicated irrigating needles with, for example, side vents to prevent pressure build-up (Figure 6-34) and second by ensuring that the fine needle does not extend beyond working length.[48] As the limits of instrumentation and syringe irrigation have been recognized, devices have emerged to exchange irrigant solutions more effectively, ideally creating complex patterns of turbulence to penetrate canal complexities, and remove unwanted material without increasing the risks of irrigant extrusion.[49] The best evidenced is ultrasound,[50] which can be delivered via a small file, mounted to a dedicated chuck (Figure 6-35) or less effectively by simply touching the shank of a small file that has been inserted into a canal with an ultrasonic scaler tip. Care should be taken to minimize canal wall contact with the ultrasonically energized file. Other less well-documented devices for irrigant activation include

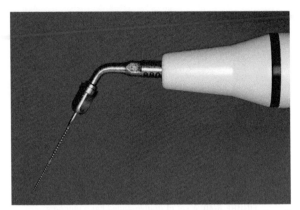

FIGURE 6-35 A small file mounted to a piezoelectric ultrasonic unit for activated irrigation.

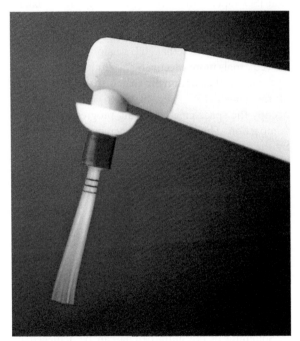

FIGURE 6-36 The EndoActivator (Dentsply), with a plastic vibrating tip available in a range of diameters, for irrigant activation.

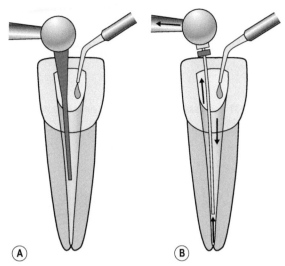

(A)   (B)

FIGURE 6-37 Illustration of the EndoVac (SybronEndo) system. Irrigant is delivered to the pulp chamber, and evacuated first by a plastic cannula placed at midroot (A), then by a metal cannula placed apically (B).

vibrating syringes (e.g. Vibringe, Cavex, Haarlem, the Netherlands),[51] a vibrating plastic filament (e.g. EndoActivator, Dentsply)[52] (Figure 6-36), and even the simple act of pumping a gutta-percha point up and down within the canal (so-called manual dynamic irrigation).[53] A more sophisticated 'hydrodynamic' approach is offered by RinnsEndo (Dürr Dental, Bietigheim-Bissingen, Germany), which rhythmically pumps and suctions irrigant to and from the canal through a narrow needle.[54] Promise is also shown by Endo-Vac (SybronEndo),[55] a negative pressure irrigating system in which irrigant is administered to the pulp chamber and drawn into the canal at high velocity by the midroot, followed by apically positioned suction cannulae, effectively eliminating the risk of apical extrusion (Figure 6-37). Irrigation systems have become a hot topic for research and development.[56]

One precaution that must not be forgotten during root canal irrigation is eye protection. Protective glasses should be worn by clinicians and patients at all times and especially when using sodium hypochlorite.[48]

Instruments for Root Canal Medication

It is often desirable to medicate root canals between appointments. Medicaments available in syringe form, with fine plastic tips for direct injection into the canal, are relatively easy to deliver. Alternatively, medicaments may be progressively fed into canals with endodontic hand files rotated counterclockwise or with a loosely fitted spiral paste filler (Figure 6-38) rotated clockwise by hand or in a slow-speed handpiece in the manner of an Archimedean screw.[57]

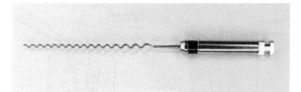

FIGURE 6-38 Spiral paste filler for the placement of intracanal medicament pastes.

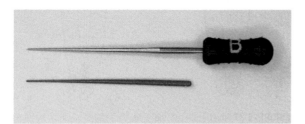

FIGURE 6-39 A stainless steel finger spreader, with a nominally size-matched gutta-percha accessory cone.

Instruments for Filling Root Canals

Root canals are generally filled by cold or warm (thermoplasticized) gutta-percha in combination with a sealer. The standard techniques of cold lateral condensation and warm vertical condensation, in addition to alternative materials and methods, are considered more fully in Chapter 9.

SEALER APPLICATION

It is customary to apply sealer to the root canal before gutta-percha is placed and compacted. Thermoplastic techniques generally demand less sealer, but cold lateral condensation requires more generous amounts; this may be achieved in the ways already described for medicating root canals. Alternatively, sonic and ultrasonic devices for activating irrigating solutions may also be used for sealer application.

LATERAL CONDENSATION

Lateral condensation of gutta-percha is achieved by the application of a spreader, which is a smooth-sided, tapered instrument with a pointed tip which is loaded vertically and encourages materials to be compressed, predominantly laterally by its wedge-like action (Figure 6-39). Spreaders are available with ISO and

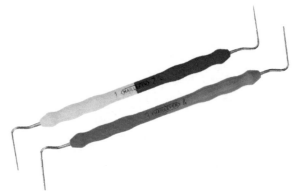

FIGURE 6-40 A set of double-ended hand pluggers.

non-ISO tapers, the latter generating higher lateral compaction forces. The majority of finger and hand spreaders are constructed from stainless steel, though it has been suggested that NiTi versions may penetrate curved canals more effectively.[58,59] Gutta-percha 'accessory points' that nominally match the size and taper of the spreader[60,61] (see Figure 6-39) are used to occupy the space created during progressive material compaction. The flow of gutta-percha can be assisted by the application of heat, or an ultrasonically energized file may be used to plasticized gutta-percha, providing a softened pathway for the deep insertion of a cold finger spreader.[62]

VERTICAL CONDENSATION

The vertical compaction of gutta-percha is achieved by the application of pluggers (Figure 6-40), smooth-sided, flat-ended instruments which are loaded vertically. Pluggers, usually double ended, are available in a range of sizes and are manufactured from stainless steel or NiTi for use in curved canals.

Softening of the gutta-percha can be achieved by the application of an instrument heated in a Bunsen burner, or ideally, the use of an electronic heat carrier (e.g. System B, SybronEndo; Elements Obturation Unit, SybronEndo; Calamus, Dentsply; Figure 6-41), which at the touch of a button heats to a chosen temperature. Each unit has a variety of tip sizes, allowing it to be fitted to different levels of the canal. When heat is used, care should be exercised to avoid overheating of the tooth and damage to the periodontal attachment apparatus.[63,64]

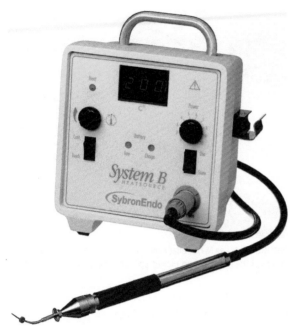

FIGURE 6-41 System B heat source for warm condensation of gutta-percha.

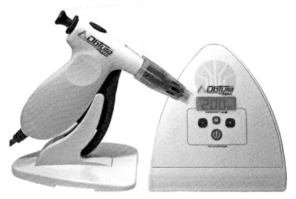

FIGURE 6-42 Obtura III Max injection-moulded thermoplastic gutta-percha system, which operates like a thermostatically controlled glue gun.

INJECTION-MOULDED THERMOPLASTIC GUTTA-PERCHA

The concept of rapidly filling root canals by the injection of molten gutta-percha is attractive, provided there is adequate resistance to prevent the extrusion of warmed material through the root apex.[65] If the apex has first been sealed with conventionally compacted gutta-percha or an alternative barrier material, such as Mineral Trioxide Aggregate (MTA), wide and irregularly shaped canals, such as those altered by internal resorption, can be safely and effectively filled this way. Working in a similar fashion to a glue gun, such devices are loaded with pellets or metal carpules containing injectable gutta-percha. Then they are heated to a chosen temperature, typically 200°C, in preparation for injection through a precurved size 20-, 23- or 25-gauge needle. Some units have manual triggers to extrude material (e.g. Obtura III Max, Obtura Spartan, Algonquin, IL, USA; Figure 6-42), whereas others have mechanical drivers, the speed of which can often be controlled (e.g. Calamus, Dentsply; BeeFill, VDW; Elements Obturation Unit, SybronEndo). The handpieces are supplied with heat guards to prevent injury to the patient's lips or skin. Injection-moulded root canal fillings are denser and well-adapted.[66] Many units including the Calamus (Dentsply) and Elements Obturation (SybronEndo) conveniently incorporate both an electronic heating device for warm vertical condensation and an injection moulding device for back-filling.

GUTTA-PERCHA CARRIER DEVICES

Another method of filling root canals rapidly is with gutta-percha coated on a carrier device. The original concept involved the application of gutta-percha to an endodontic file, which was heated, inserted to working length, and cut-off in the canal.[67] Carrier systems, subsequently, evolved through titanium to plastic carriers – the best known being Thermafil (Dentsply; Figure 6-43), with its 4% tapered plastic core and dedicated oven (Thermaprep, Dentsply). Helpful features of Thermafil carriers include their 'V' shaped cross-section, creating space for the insertion of endodontic files and facilitating their removal during retreatment. Thermafil and its numerous rival products (e.g. Soft-Core, SybronEndo) are available in a range of sizes and tapers to match different file systems. Numerous reports have highlighted the speed, simplicity and effectiveness of carrier-based root canal filling[68,69]; however, a favourable treatment outcome is dependent on the root canal system being suitably decontaminated. In many circumstances, the retrieval of gutta-percha carrier devices from root canal systems during retreatment has remained challenging.[70,71] More

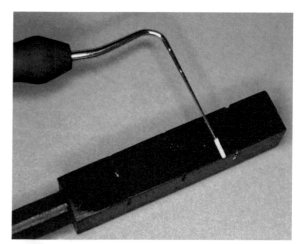

FIGURE 6-44 Lee MTA Pellet Forming Block; an MTA pellet is formed in one of the grooves and picked up with a plugger.

Teflon blocks (e.g. Lee MTA Pellet Forming Block, Hartzell, Concord, CA, USA; Figure 6-44), with channels to create moulded cylindrical pellets of differing widths, which are carried to the usage site on the tip of a plugger.

Storage and Sterilization of Endodontic Instruments

INSTRUMENT STANDS AND STORAGE SYSTEMS

Unless they have been supplied prepackaged and sterile, all endodontic instruments should be cleaned and sterilized before use. Standard instrument packs can be arranged on trays with lids or in autoclavable bags or boxes. Small instruments such as files can be autoclaved in stands (e.g. Endo-Stand, Dentsply) or in Pyrex glass test tubes with colour-coded lids to indicate their contents (Figure 6-45).

A convenient way of managing small sterile instruments such as files, Gates-Glidden burs and finger spreaders is to arrange them in a sterile triangular sponge and insert them into an Endoring II (Jordco), an autoclavable device, which includes a millimetre ruler and optional gel-wells for medicaments and lubricants (see Figure 6-1). This arrangement facilitates ergonomic working conditions, with the instruments always close to the working field, and eliminates the need to reach for instrument on the bracket table and tray.

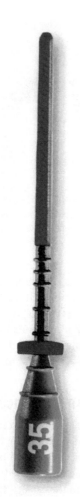

FIGURE 6-43 Thermafil obturator, a plastic carrier-based device coated with gutta-percha.

recently, systems made entirely from different densities of gutta-percha have been developed (e.g. GuttaCore, Dentsply; GuttaFusion, VDW), greatly simplifying the process of endodontic retreatment.[71]

DEVICES FOR MTA APPLICATION

Bioceramic cements, such as MTA, are now commonly used for sealing teeth with wide open apices, pulp capping and root perforation repairs.[72,73] These materials demand an array of instruments for their accurate application, including miniature gun systems, similar to amalgam carriers (e.g. MAP system, Produits Dentaires, Vevey, Switzerland; see Figure 10-36), and

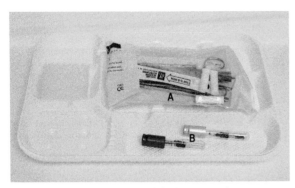

FIGURE 6-45 (A) Plastic tray containing instruments in a transparent autoclave bag; (B) files can be stored and sterilized in Pyrex glass test tubes.

STERILIZATION OF ENDODONTIC INSTRUMENTS

Infection control is the responsibility of the whole dental team. Universal precautions must be deployed at all times to prevent the risks of disease transmission within the dental surgery,[74] and all instruments coming into contact with patients must be cleaned and sterilized according to local best practice. In the United Kingdom, fears over the transmission of prion proteins associated with variant Creutzfeldt-Jakob Disease (vCJD)[75] have outlawed the reuse of endodontic files since 2007,[74,76] and all files must be disposed after a single use. Many endodontic instruments are now clearly marked for single use only, on the grounds of safety and fracture risk, in addition to issues of effective decontamination.[77]

Although there are financial implications, the single use of endodontic files is encouraged on the grounds of ensuring performance efficiency and reducing fracture risk. Many items such as files and paper points are routinely supplied by manufacturers, at no additional cost, in pre-sterilized blister packs for single use only.

Learning Outcomes

At the end of this chapter, the reader should be able to recognize and discuss a range of instruments and devices for:

- tooth isolation with a dental dam;
- safe access to the pulp space;
- retrieval of posts and other metallic obstructions from root canals;
- negotiation and shaping of root canals;
- irrigation and activation of irrigant solutions within root canals;
- filling root canals;
- sterilization and storage of endodontic instruments.

REFERENCES

1. Ahmed H, Cohen S, Lévy G, et al. Rubber dam application in endodontic practice: an update on critical educational and ethical dilemmas. Australian Dental Journal 2014;59: 457–63.
2. Chin SM, Ferguson JW, Bajurnows T. Latex allergy in dentistry. Review and report of case presenting as a serious reaction to latex dental dam. Australian Dental Journal 2004;49: 146–8.
3. Svec TA, Powers JM, Ladd GD. Hardness and stress corrosion of rubber dam clamps. Journal of Endodontics 1997;23: 397–8.
4. Bhuva B, Chong BS, Patel S. Rubber dam in clinical practice. ENDO (Lond, Engl) 2008;2:131–41.
5. Carr GB, Murgel CAF. The use of the operating microscope in endodontics. Dental Clinics of North America 2010;54: 191–214.
6. Smadi L, Khraisat A. Detection of a second mesiobuccal canal in the mesiobuccal roots of maxillary first molar teeth. Oral Surgery, Oral Medicine, Oral Pathology, Oral Radiology, and Endodontics 2007;103:77–81.
7. Gluskin AH, Ruddle CJ, Zinman EJ. Thermal injury through intraradicular heat transfer using ultrasonic devices: precautions and practical preventive strategies. Journal of the American Dental Association 2005;136:1286–93.
8. Wu M-K, van der Sluis LWM, Wesselink PR. The risk of furcal perforation in mandibular molars using Gates-Glidden drills with anticurvature pressure. Oral Surgery, Oral Medicine, Oral Pathology, Oral Radiology, and Endodontics 2005;99:378–82.
9. Stamos DE, Gutmann JL. Revisiting the post puller. Journal of Endodontics 1991;17:466–8.
10. Abbott PV. Incidence of root fractures and methods used for post removal. International Endodontic Journal 2002;35: 63–7.
11. Ruddle CJ. Nonsurgical retreatment. Journal Endodontics 2004;30:827–45.
12. Dickie J, McCrosson J. Post removal techniques. Part II. Dental Update 2014;41:76–84.
13. Anderson GC, Perdigão J, Hodges JS, et al. Efficiency and effectiveness of fiber post removal using 3 techniques. Quintessence International 2007;38:663–70.
14. Madarati AA, Hunter MJ, Dummer PM. Management of intracanal separated instruments. Journal of Endodontics 2013;39:569–81.
15. International Organization for Standardization (ISO). Dental root canal instruments – part 1: specification for files, reamers, barbed broaches, rasps, paste carriers, explorers and cotton broaches. ISO 3630–1: 1992. London: British Standards Institution; 1992.
16. Schäfer E. Root canal instruments for manual use: a review. Endodontics and Dental Traumatology 1997;13:51–64.

17. Young GR, Parashos P, Messer HH. The principles of techniques for cleaning root canals. Australian Dental Journal 2007;52(Suppl. 1):S52–63.

18. Schäfer E. Effects of four instrumentation techniques on curved canals: a comparison study. Journal of Endodontics 1996;22:685–9.

19. Allen MJ, Glickman GN, Griggs JA. Comparative analysis of endodontic pathfinders. Journal of Endodontics 2007;33: 723–6.

20. Pettiette MT, Metzger Z, Phillips C, et al. Endodontic complications of root canal therapy performed by dental students with stainless-steel K-files and nickel-titanium hand files. Journal of Endodontics 1999;25:230–4.

21. Tepel J, Schäfer E. Endodontic hand instruments: cutting efficiency, instrumentation of curved canals, bending and torsional properties. Endodontics and Dental Traumatology 1997;13:201–10.

22. Saunders EM. Hand instrumentation in root canal preparation. Endodontic Topics 2005;10:163–7.

23. Hülsmann M, Peters OA, Dummer PMH. Mechanical preparation of root canals: shaping goals, techniques and means. Endodontic Topics 2005;10:30–76.

24. Anderson ME, Price JW, Parashos P. Fracture resistance of electropolished rotary nickel titanium endodontic instruments. Journal of Endodontics 2007;33:1212–6.

25. Tripi TR, Bonaccorso A, Condorelli GG. Cyclic fatigue of different nickel-titanium endodontic rotary instruments. Oral Surgery, Oral Medicine, Oral Pathology, Oral Radiology, and Endodontics 2006;102:106–14.

26. Lee DH, Park B, Saxena A, et al. Enhanced surface hardness by boron implantation in Nitinol alloy. Journal of Endodontics 1996;22:543–6.

27. Rapisarda E, Bonaccorso A, Tripi TR, et al. The effect of surface treatments of nickel-titanium files on wear and cutting efficiency. Oral Surgery, Oral Medicine, Oral Pathology, Oral Radiology, and Endodontics 2000;89:363–8.

28. Schäfer E. Effect of physical vapor deposition on cutting efficiency of nickel-titanium files. Journal of Endodontics 2002;28:800–2.

29. Tripi TR, Bonaccorso A, Condorelli GG. Fabrication of hard coatings on NiTi instruments. Journal of Endodontics 2003;29:132–4.

30. Braga LC, Magalhães RR, Nakagawa RK, et al. Physical and mechanical properties of twisted or ground nickel-titanium instruments. International Endodontic Journal 2013;46:458–65.

31. Alapati SB, Brantley WA, Iijima M, et al. Metallurgical characterization of a new nickel-titanium wire for rotary endodontic instruments. Journal of Endodontics 2009;35:1589–93.

32. Otsuka K, Ren X. Physical metallurgy of Ti–Ni-based shape memory alloys. Progress in Materials Science 2005;50:511–678.

33. Haapasalo M, Shen Y. Evolution of nickel–titanium instruments: from past to future. Endodontic Topics 2013;29: 3–17.

34. Yared GM, Bou Dagher FE, Machtou P. Influence of rotational speed, torque and operator's proficiency on ProFile failures. International Endodontic Journal 2001;34:47–53.

35. Yared G, Eamli GA. Single file reciprocation: a literature review. ENDO (Lond, Engl) 2013;7:171–8.

36. Bartols A. Clinical experiences with Reciproc. ENDO (Lond, Engl) 2013;7:179–87.

37. Saber SEDM, Nagy MM, Schäfer E. Comparative evaluation of the shaping ability of WaveOne, Reciproc and OneShape single-file systems in severely curved root canals of extracted teeth. International Endodontic Journal 2015;48:109–14.

38. Rios Mde A, Villela AM, Cunha RS, et al. Efficacy of 2 reciprocating systems compared with a rotary retreatment system for gutta-percha removal. Journal of Endodontics 2014;40: 543–6.

39. Gergi R, Arbab-Chirani R, Osta N, et al. Micro-computed tomographic evaluation of canal transportation instrumented by different kinematics rotary nickel-titanium instruments. Journal of Endodontics 2014;40:1223–7.

40. Kazzi D, Horner K, Qualtrough AC, et al. A comparative study of three periapical radiographic techniques for endodontic working length estimation. International Endodontic Journal 2007;40:526–31.

41. Nekoofar MH, Ghandi MM, Hayes SJ, et al. The fundamental operating principles of electronic root canal length measurement devices. International Endodontic Journal 2006;39: 595–609.

42. Gordon MPJ, Chandler NP. Electronic apex locators. International Endodontic Journal 2004;37:425–37.

43. Altenburger MJ, Cenik Y, Schirrmeister JF, et al. Combination of apex locator and endodontic motor for continuous length control during root canal treatment. International Endodontic Journal 2009;42:368–74.

44. Peters OA, Schönenberger K, Laib A. Effects of four Ni-Ti preparation techniques on root canal geometry assessed by micro computed tomography. International Endodontic Journal 2001;34:221–30.

45. Haapasalo M, Qian W, Shen Y. Irrigation: beyond the smear layer. Endodontic Topics 2012;27:35–53.

46. Paqué F, Laib A, Gautschi H, et al. Hard-tissue debris accumulation analysis by high-resolution computed tomography scans. Journal of Endodontics 2009;35:1044–7.

47. Park E, Shen Y, Haapasalo M. Irrigation of the apical root canal. Endodontic Topics 2012;27:54–73.

48. Hülsmann M, Hahn W. Complications during root canal irrigation—literature review and case reports. International Endodontic Journal 2000;33:186–93.

49. Gulabivala K, Ng YL, Gilbertson M, et al. The fluid mechanics of root canal irrigation. Physiological Measurement 2010;31: R49–84.

50. van der Sluis LW, Versluis M, Wu MK, et al. Passive ultrasonic irrigation of the root canal: a review of the literature. International Endodontic Journal 2007;40:415–26.

51. Rödig T, Bozkurt M, Konietschke F, et al. Comparison of the Vibringe system with syringe and passive ultrasonic irrigation in removing debris from simulated root canal irregularities. Journal of Endodontics 2010;36:1410–3.

52. Rödig T, Döllmann S, Konietschke F, et al. Effectiveness of different irrigant agitation techniques on debris and smear layer removal in curved root canals: a scanning electron microscopy study. Journal of Endodontics 2010;36:1983–7.

53. Jiang LM, Lak B, Eijsvogels LM, et al. Comparison of the cleaning efficacy of different final irrigation techniques. Journal of Endodontics 2012;38:838–41.

54. Rödig T, Sedghi M, Konietschke F, et al. Efficacy of syringe irrigation, RinsEndo and passive ultrasonic irrigation in removing debris from irregularities in root canals with different apical sizes. International Endodontic Journal 2010;43: 581–9.

55. Susin L, Liu Y, Yoon JC, et al. Canal and isthmus debridement efficacies of two irrigant agitation techniques in a closed system. International Endodontic Journal 2010;43:1077–90.

56. Siqueira JF Jr, Rôças IN. Optimising single-visit disinfection with supplementary approaches: a quest for predictability. Australian Endodontic Journal 2011;37:92–8.

57. Peters CI, Koka RS, Highsmith S, et al. Calcium hydroxide dressings using different preparation and application modes: density and dissolution by simulated tissue pressure. International Endodontic Journal 2005;38:889–95.

58. Berry KA, Loushine RJ, Primack RD, et al. Nickel-titanium versus stainless-steel finger spreaders in curved canals. Journal of Endodontics 1998;24:752–4.

59. Schmidt KJ, Walker TL, Johnson JD, et al. Comparison of nickel-titanium and stainless-steel spreader penetration and accessory cone fit in curved canals. Journal of Endodontics 2000;26:42–4.

60. Briseno Marroquin B, Wolter D, Willershausen-Zönnchen B. Dimensional variability of nonstandardized greater taper finger spreaders with matching gutta-percha-points. International Endodontic Journal 2001;34:23–8.

61. Zmener O, Hilu R, Scavo R. Compatibility between standardized endodontic finger spreaders and accessory gutta-percha cones. Endodontics and Dental Traumatology 1996;12:237–9.

62. Bailey GC, Ng YL, Cunnington SA, et al. Root canal obturation by ultrasonic condensation of gutta-percha. Part II: an in vitro investigation of the quality of obturation. International Endodontic Journal 2004;37:694–8.

63. Lee FS, Van Cura JE, BeGole E. A comparison of root surface temperatures using different obturation heat sources. Journal of Endodontics 1998;24:617–20.

64. Ulusoy OI, Yilmazoğlu MZ, Görgül G. Effect of several thermoplastic canal filling techniques on surface temperature rise on roots with simulated internal resorption cavities: an infrared thermographic analysis. International Endodontic Journal 2015;48:171–6.

65. Yee FS, Marlin J, Krakow AA, et al. Three-dimensional obturation of the root canal using injection molded thermoplasticized dental gutta-percha. Journal of Endodontics 1977;3:168–74.

66. Cathro PR, Love RM. Comparison of MicroSeal and System B/Obtura II obturation techniques. International Endodontic Journal 2003;36:876–82.

67. Johnson WB. A new gutta-percha technique. Journal of Endodontics 1978;4:184–8.

68. Chu CH, Lo EC, Cheung GS. Outcome of root canal treatment using Thermafil and cold lateral condensation filling techniques. International Endodontic Journal 2005;38:179–85.

69. Hale R, Gatti R, Glickman GN, et al. Comparative analysis of carrier-based obturation and lateral compaction: a retrospective clinical outcomes study. International Journal of Dentistry 2012;2012:954675. doi: 10.1155/2012/954675.

70. Royzenblat A, Goodell GG. Comparison of removal times of Thermafil plastic obturators using ProFile rotary instruments at different rotational speeds in moderately curved canals. Journal of Endodontics 2007;33:256–8.

71. Beasley RT, Williamson AE, Justman BC, et al. Time required to remove guttacore, thermafil plus, and thermoplasticized gutta-percha from moderately curved root canals with protaper files. Journal of Endodontics 2013;39:125–8.

72. Bogen G, Kuttler S. Mineral trioxide aggregate obturation: a review and case series. Journal of Endodontics 2009;35:777–90.

73. Parirokh M, Torabinejad M. Mineral trioxide aggregate: a comprehensive literature review—Part III: Clinical applications, drawbacks, and mechanism of action. Journal of Endodontics 2010;36:400–13.

74. Department of Health (UK). Decontamination. Health Technical Memorandum 01-05: Decontamination in primary care dental practices, <https://www.gov.uk/government/uploads/system/uploads/attachment_data/file/170689/HTM_01-05_2013.pdf>; 2013.

75. Azarpazhooh A, Fillery ED. Prion disease: the implications for dentistry. Journal of Endodontics 2008;34:1158–66.

76. Cockcroft B. Advice for dentists on re-use of endodontic instruments and variant Creutzfeldt-Jakob Disease (vCJD). Letter from the Chief Dental Officer England, April 19, 2007. Department of Health, England; 2007.

77. Popovic J, Gasic J, Zivkovic S, et al. Evaluation of biological debris on endodontic instruments after cleaning and sterilization procedures. International Endodontic Journal 2010;43:336–41.

CHAPTER 7

Preparation of the Root Canal System

E. Schäfer

Chapter Contents

Summary

Root canal preparation allows for effective mechanical debridement and facilitates chemical disinfection of the root canal system. This chapter on the preparation of the root canal system will cover gaining access to the root canals, determining working length, root canal irrigation and preparation techniques, including hand and engine-driven instruments.

Introduction

The primary aim of root canal treatment, depending on pulpal status, is to maintain periradicular health by preventing infection of the root canal system or if already infected, to restore periradicular health by eliminating microorganisms and their byproducts from the root canal system.[1] This may involve the removal of necrotic pulp and tissue debris, removal of an inflamed pulp or in elective treatment, the removal of healthy pulp tissue.[2] Retreatment of failing cases is addressed in Chapter 14.

A greater awareness of the microbiota and pattern of colonization within the complexities of an infected root canal system and the development of newer techniques, instruments and materials have led to a biologically based rationale for root canal treatment:

- removal of all tissues, microorganisms, their byproducts and substrates from the root canal system;
- shaping of the root canal system to facilitate placement of irrigants, medicaments and a root canal filling;
- filling of the shaped canal system coupled with an adequate and timely coronal restoration.

The traditional 'endodontic triad' concept of cleaning, shaping and filling remains relevant as these three basic objectives must be achieved while ensuring

113

conservation of tooth structure and maintenance of canal shape.

Pretreatment Assessment

Before the initiation of the root canal treatment, clinical and radiographic examination may reveal relevant information, such as tooth angulation and rotation, in relation to the root canal system. The cemento-enamel junction provides an indication of the location level of the canal entrances, which is helpful when preparing the access cavity. Radiographs provide information about the presence of caries, the quality of the coronal restoration, the position and dimensions of the pulp chamber and the pulp horns, the existence of pulp stones or other intrapulpal calcifications and the number and the degree of curvatures of roots and canals; this topic is also covered in Chapter 3.

Preparation of the Tooth and Dental Dam

Before preparing the access cavity, caries and failing coronal restoration must be completely removed to prevent microbial microleakage, infected materials and restorative materials from being inadvertently introduced into the root canal system. Existing coronal restorations should only be retained if their marginal seal is considered satisfactory, free of caries and does not impede gaining access into the root canal system. If there is concern about restorability or that the quality of the marginal seal is satisfactory, the existing coronal restoration should be removed completely. Removal of existing restorations offers the advantages of confirmation that there is sufficient tooth substance remaining and allows for the detection of the presence of fracture lines or hairline cracks (Figure 7-1).

Unsupported cusps should be removed or protected by, for example, placing an orthodontic band around the tooth to prevent cusp fracture during and after root canal treatment. In some cases, after dismantling the coronal restoration, it may be necessary to place a provisional restoration to prevent microleakage, aid dental dam isolation and create a reservoir for the irrigant solution in the access cavity.

The maintenance of strict aseptic measures is a prerequisite for successful root canal treatment.

The tooth should be isolated from the oral environment to avoid ingress of saliva and entry of oral microorganisms into the root canal system; the easiest and most effective method is by use of a dental dam (see Chapter 6).[3] There is evidence that apart from protecting patients, the use of a dental dam leads to improvement in the outcome of root canal treatment.[4,5]

Access Cavity Preparation

The design of the access cavity is crucial to ensuring that the objectives of root canal treatment are met. A poorly designed access cavity may make it difficult to locate all the root canals, whereas unnecessary removal of tooth tissue results in a marked decrease in the fracture resistance of the tooth.[6] The design of the access cavity should reflect the anticipated position of the underlying root canal orifices (see Chapter 4). The relationship between the pulp chamber and external anatomical outline is assessed from preoperative radiographs. Careful alignment of the bur will reduce the possibility of causing a perforation, most commonly through the floor of the pulp chamber and into the furcation (Figure 7-2). In cases where the root canals may be difficult to locate, e.g. presence of pulp stones, or a small, or calcified, pulp chamber, it might be advisable to create an initial access cavity before dental dam application as it is easier to ensure proper bur alignment and prevent the removal of unnecessary amounts of sound dentine. However, this should not be an excuse not to use dental dam isolation, and all subsequent procedures must be carried out under dental dam isolation.

Since the pulp chamber is located in the centre of the tooth, an advisable approach is to start preparing the access cavity in the middle of the occlusal surface or in the direction of the most coronal pulp horn. After the initial vertical access into the pulp chamber, further horizontal preparation is required to completely remove the roof of the pulp chamber; a nonend cutting bur, such as the Endo-Z bur (Dentsply Maillefer, Ballaigues, Switzerland), may be used for this purpose to prevent damage to the pulp chamber floor (see also Chapters 4 and 6).

Preparation of the access cavity can be divided into three basic steps.[2,7]

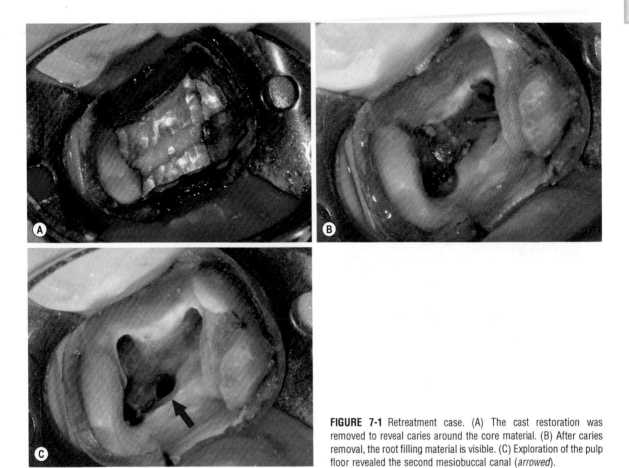

FIGURE 7-1 Retreatment case. (A) The cast restoration was removed to reveal caries around the core material. (B) After caries removal, the root filling material is visible. (C) Exploration of the pulp floor revealed the second mesiobuccal canal (*arrowed*).

1. Primary access cavity

The aim is to clean the whole pulp chamber, including the complete removal of hard tissues, such as pulp stones, that may impede straight-line access to the root canals (Figure 7-3). The colour of the dentine is an important and helpful feature; primary dentine of the pulp chamber walls is usually paler than the dentine of the chamber floor, whereas tertiary dentine is often yellowish or greyish in appearance. Differentiation of the various types of dentine is best achieved with the aid of good illumination and magnification (operating microscope or magnifying loupes) after carefully drying the access cavity (Figure 7-4). Fine ultrasonic tips, including diamond-coated varieties, allow careful and controlled removal of pulp calcifications and pulp chamber roof overhangs (Figure 7-5).

2. Secondary access cavity

After primary access cavity preparation, the pulp chamber should be soaked with sodium hypochlorite to dissolve tissues and disinfect the pulp chamber. The next step is to locate the root canal orifice/s. With the exception of single-rooted teeth, canal orifices are not located in the centre of the pulp chamber; rather, they are always positioned at the junction of the darker coloured horizontal floor of the pulp chamber and the lighter coloured vertical chamber walls. Identifying the floor-wall junction is important when searching for canal orifices. Dark developmental lines may be visible linking the canal orifices, which appear as a small area of opaque dentine against the chamber floor background. Useful methods to aid location of canal orifices include gentle exploration with a sharp probe

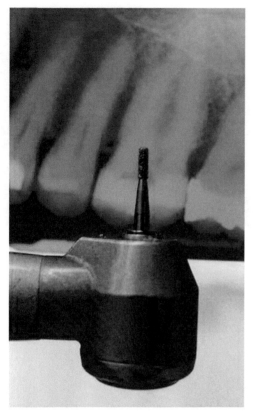

FIGURE 7-2 Alignment of the bur on the preoperative radiograph will help indicate the position and depth of the restoration and pulp chamber.

(Figure 7-6), staining with erythrosine, or methylene blue, dye and transilluminating the tooth.

3. Coronal canal enlargement and creation of straight-line access

Coronal flaring and the creation of straight-line access reduce the degree of canal curvature, allowing unimpeded passage of instruments in and out of the root canal. This reduces the restoring forces placed on the working instrument, minimizing the risk of canal straightening and instrument separation and the incidence of canal aberrations, such as zips, elbows and ledges during canal preparation.[8] In this step, the access cavity is refined and modified as necessary.

Working Length Determination

Regardless of treatment philosophy on the desired final endpoint of preparation, it is always necessary to ascertain the length of the root canal accurately to ensure adequate shaping, thorough disinfection and complete filling of the root canal system.[9] Evidence from two meta-analyses suggests that both underfilling and overfilling of the root canal is associated with a significant negative affect on prognosis.[10,11] Knowledge of the average length of teeth may be used to provide general guidance on working length. There are a number of widely accepted methods of working length determination.

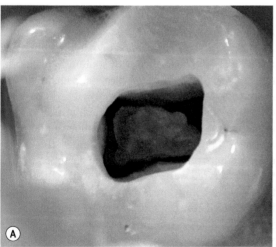
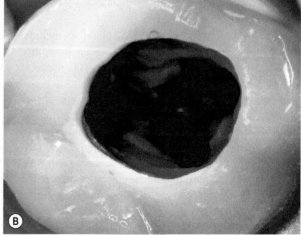

FIGURE 7-3 A pulp stone, adhering to the floor of the pulp chamber, impeding access to the root canal orifices (A). Straight-line access achieved following removal of the pulp stone (B).

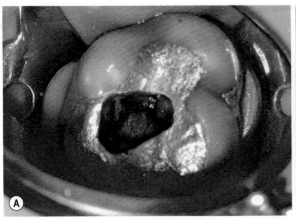
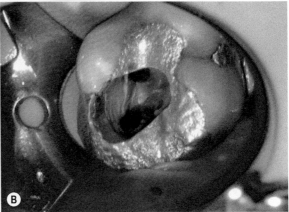

FIGURE 7-4 Inadequate access. (A) The pulp horns have been mistaken for the canal orifices and the roof of the pulp chamber is still *in situ;*. (B) Removal of the roof of the pulp chamber allows good visualization of the pulp floor.

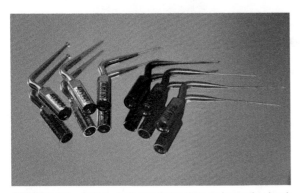

FIGURE 7-5 A selection of ultrasonic tips that can be used to break up calcific masses in the pulp space.

RADIOGRAPHIC METHOD

In this method, the working length is initially estimated by taking a measurement from an undistorted preoperative radiograph. A file, preferably ISO size 15 or larger so that it is easily discernible radiologically, is inserted into the canal to the estimated working length, and a radiograph is exposed. If the tip of the file is between 0 and 2 mm from the radiographic apex, it may be accepted as an accurate representation of tooth length. Depending on the desired final endpoint of preparation, the working length is adjusted accordingly. If adjustments of 2 mm or more are needed, the working length should be reconfirmed with an additional working length radiograph. The accuracy of the radiographic method in determining

the position of the apical constriction is reported to range from 30% to 82%.[12] Given that radiographic images are only two dimensional, the file may already be overextended beyond the apical foramen if its tip is located at the radiographic apex.[13] This method usually provides acceptable results; however, radiographs are frequently difficult to interpret, especially with posterior teeth. More important, the apical foramen may be at a distance from the radiographic apex further confusing interpretation. In such circumstances, additional methods of working length determination should be used.

ELECTRONIC APEX LOCATORS

Modern electronic apex locators measure the impedance of the root canal at different frequencies and are accurate to within 0.5 mm in >90% of cases.[14,15] Consequently, an apex locator can be more reliable than the radiographic method for determining working length.[16] The use of an apex locator allows for a reduction in the number of radiographs required during root canal treatment, avoiding unnecessary radiation. In a retrospective study, in which an apex locator was used solely to determine working length in infected teeth, a high success rate was achieved,[17] confirming their benefit. It is tempting to rely on just an electronic apex locator to determine working length; however, the radiographic method can provide further relevant information regarding root canal anatomy and help verify that the access to the root

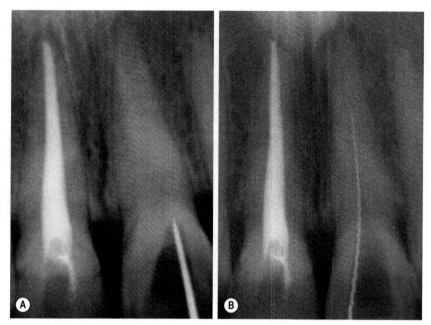

FIGURE 7-6 (A) In a tooth with an extensively calcified canal, a check radiograph with a probe in the base of the cavity will provide guidance for instrument progression. (B) A later radiograph confirms that the file is in the root canal.

canal system has been correctly prepared. Therefore, a combination of working length determination methods is advisable to improve the accuracy of canal length measurements.

PAPER POINT TECHNIQUE

The paper point technique[18,19] is based on the premise that when the contents of the root canal system are removed, the root canal should be dry, while the outside of the root canal system is hydrated from the periodontium or moist from granulation tissue, pus or blood. If a dry paper point is placed into a dried canal short of the apical foramen and withdrawn, it should remain dry. However, if a dry paper point is placed into a dried canal and inserted past the exit point of the canal, an apical section will be wet with fluid when it is withdrawn. The maximum depth a paper point can be inserted into the dried canal and still remain dry is considered to be the length of the root canal. Although it may be used to supplement, or reconfirm, canal length obtained by other methods, the paper point technique is inappropriate as a primary method for working length determination.

Root Canal Irrigation

In cases with radiographic and/or clinical signs of infection, the root canal system harbours microorganisms,[20] which are present in a planktonic form and as a biofilm adhering to the canal walls.[21] A primary aim of root canal treatment is to eliminate microorganisms in the root canal system.[22]

Mechanical instrumentation is able to significantly reduce the number of microorganisms in the root canal system, and there is no significant difference reported in the effectiveness between hand and rotary instrumentation.[23,24] However, current evidence suggests that predictable and complete elimination of microorganisms does not appear to be possible solely with hand, or even engine-driven, instruments.[25] Therefore, regardless of the instrumentation technique or system chosen, the use of irrigants is essential for thorough debridement of the root canal system. The aims of root canal irrigation are to[22,26]:

- reduce intraradicular microorganisms and neutralise endotoxins;
- dissolve vital or necrotic pulp tissue;

- lubricate the canal walls and instruments;
- facilitate removal of dentine particles and debris.

The main requirements of a root canal irrigant are:
- broad antimicrobial spectrum;
- nontoxic;
- tissue-dissolution capability;
- ability to penetrate into areas inaccessible to root canal instruments.

In addition, a root canal irrigant should have a low surface tension, is stable, inexpensive and easy to use. A plethora of irrigants have been used in root canal treatment over the years. The most widely used root canal irrigant is sodium hypochlorite (NaOCl), and current evidence strongly indicates that it is the irrigant of choice.[22] In concentrations of 1% to 5.25%, NaOCl dissolves vital and necrotic pulp tissue and organic components of both dentine and the smear layer.[27] The tissue-dissolving capability of NaOCl is superior to all other irrigants. Moreover, NaOCl is able to neutralize or inactivate lipopolysaccharides.[28] NaOCl displays a strong antimicrobial activity with comparatively short contact times and is more effective against the microbial biofilm compared with other irrigants.[29] The effectiveness of NaOCl has been shown to be dependent on the concentration and duration of exposure.

Care should be exercised at all times to prevent inadvertent and accidental extrusion of NaOCl into the periradicular tissues as this may result in tissue damage accompanied by varying degrees of pain, swelling and bruising. A detailed overview of complications during root canal irrigation with NaOCl has been published[30]; this topic is also discussed in Chapter 14.

Other root canal irrigants include chlorhexidine gluconate (CHX), which should be used in a concentration of 2%. CHX has a wide antimicrobial spectrum and is effective against gram-positive and gram-negative bacteria as well as yeasts[31]; it is less effective against gram-negative bacteria, which are predominantly found in primary endodontic infections.[32] Unlike NaOCl, CHX does not possess any tissue-dissolving ability and is unable to neutralize lipopolysaccharides. Another disadvantage of CHX is its antimicrobial activity that is strongly reduced by the presence of organic matters such as dentine, inflammatory exudates and serum albumin.[33] Therefore, CHX is inferior to NaOCl as a root canal irrigant.

Furthermore, mixing of NaOCl with CHX should be avoided as it will lead to the formation of a toxic, brownish precipitate of 4-chloraniline.[34]

Since both NaOCl and CHX are not able to remove the smear layer,[22] superficial layer consisting of dentine, pulp remnants and microorganisms that occlude the dentinal tubules, a chelating agent is required. Removal of the smear layer helps to open up dentinal tubules, eliminate embedded microorganisms and facilitate better penetration of the antimicrobial irrigant, to allow more extensive canal decontamination and improved canal cleanliness. Both ethylenediamine tetraacetic acid (EDTA) as a 17% solution (pH 7) and citric acid (10–20%) are able to remove the smear layer more effectively.[35] A suggested irrigation protocol is summarized in Figure 7-7. The issue of intracanal dressing is covered in Chapter 8.

Irrigation solutions are commonly delivered using specially designed endodontic needles and syringes. Flexible open-ended irrigation needles are recommended so that the needle can be bent according to the canal curvature. The needle is inserted into the canal to the level of the apical third. However, during the initial canal preparation, the needle may not reach this depth; therefore, it should be inserted to the binding point, pulled back out slightly so that it is loose in the canal and then the irrigant delivered gently and passively. As canal preparation proceeds, the needle will gradually reach deeper into the canal; at all times, the needle must not be jammed into the canal and the irrigant must not be delivered with unnecessary force. The smallest needle recommended for root canal irrigation is 30 gauge, with a diameter

Irrigation Protocol
- After access cavity preparation: flush the cavity and canal orifices with NaOCl; canals must always be kept wet with NaOCl during preparation
- Between instruments: NaOCl 2–5 mL/canal
- After shaping: NaOCl 5–10 mL/canal
- Removal of the smear layer: EDTA or citric acid 5 mL/canal
- NaOCl 2–5 mL/canal: optional activation (PUI)
- Optional: removal of NaOCl with NaCl or citric acid
- Optional: final irrigation with chlorhexidine 2–5 mL/canal

FIGURE 7-7 Suggested irrigation protocol. EDTA = ethylenediamine tetraacetic acid; PUI = passive ultrasonic activation.

of 0.3 mm, corresponding to ISO size 30. Thus, for effective irrigation, the apical preparation should be at least an ISO size 35 to 40, 0.02 taper or a size 25, 0.04 taper when using engine-driven instruments.[22]

Irrigants may also be delivered using ultrasonic devices; they have the added advantage of activating the irrigant to improve its action. Passive ultrasonic irrigation (PUI) after root canal preparation involves placing a small ultrasonically activated file into the root canal filled with NaOCl for three cycles of 20 seconds each to obtain the best possible results.[36] The action of PUI involves acoustic microstreaming and cavitation, resulting in improved removal of dentine debris, planktonic microorganisms and pulp tissue. As a result, the antimicrobial and tissue-dissolving efficiency of NaOCl is enhanced.

Root Canal Preparation

All root canal systems are curved in one or more planes, with the degree and extent of curvature varying from root to root. Irrespective of the instrumentation technique used, the apical part of the root canal system is usually the least well cleaned and prepared. The morphology of the apical root canal system is complex and highly variable.

Preparation of the root canal system requires considerable skill, particularly in cases with more severely curved canals or other complex anatomical features. Despite advances in instrument design, the experience and skills of the operator remains important. There is no replacement for practical instructions on root canal preparation in order to acquire the necessary skills and competency.

Currently, the available evidence is limited regarding the impact of maintenance of the original canal shape, during root canal preparation, on treatment outcome.[37] However, clinical studies indicated that better maintenance of the original canal shape resulted in increased success rates[38] and alterations of canal shape, such as ledging, were associated with reduced success rates.[39] It is therefore reasonable to select techniques and instruments that are best suited to maintaining the overall original canal curvature, even in severely curved root canals.

The major goals of mechanical root canal preparation are to[2]:

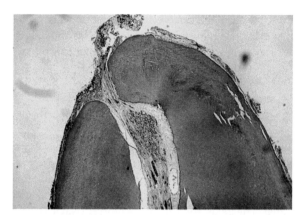

FIGURE 7-8 The anatomy of the apical constriction must be maintained during canal preparation.

- remove vital or necrotic tissue from the main root canal/s;
- create sufficient space for irrigation and medication;
- preserve integrity and location of the apical canal anatomy (Figure 7-8);
- avoid iatrogenic damage to the root canal system and structure;
- facilitate canal obturation;
- conserve sound root dentine to maintain function of the tooth.

In general and with minor differences, regardless of whether hand or engine-driven instruments are used, a 'coronal-to-apical' root canal preparation concept is commonly practised (Table 7-1).

HAND INSTRUMENTS

Hand instruments for preparing root canals are either manufactured from stainless steel, or nickel–titanium (NiTi), alloys; see Chapter 6. Stainless steel hand instruments are more rigid, have better cutting efficiency and wear resistance compared with their equivalent sized NiTi instruments, especially those in smaller sizes (ISO 06–15). Therefore, stainless steel hand instruments are best suited for creating a glide path as the low modulus of elasticity and greater flexibility of NiTi instruments mean that there is very limited tactile feedback when they are used inside a root canal. Tactile feedback is essential as it provides the operator with further relevant information regarding the degree of canal curvature, canal obstructions

TABLE 7-1 A Composite Protocol for Use with a 'Coronal-to-Apical' Root Canal Preparation Concept

Crown-down root canal preparation

① Access:
Create an unimpeded pathway to the pulp space and canal orifices using diamond or tungsten carbide fissures, or round burs; non-cutting tip bur and/or specialized ultrasonic tips.

② Coronal flaring:
Use Gates-Glidden burs or NiTi instruments designed to open the canal orifice and enlarge the coronal aspect of the root canal. Irrigate with sodium hypochlorite between each instrument change and throughout canal preparation.

③ Working length:
Establish working length using an apex locator and radiograph.

④ Glide path/pilot channel:
Use hand instruments and a filing or Balance-force action to create a pathway to working length.

⑤ Apical preparation and finishing:
Canal preparation continues with hand or engine-driven NiTi instruments in sequence, to working length, until the desired taper and apical size is achieved.

present, or whether the canal divides. Specially designed stainless steel files, such as C+ files (Dentsply Maillefer, Ballaigues, Switzerland) and C-Pilot files (VDW, Munich, Germany), are helpful for initial negotiation of sclerosed canals and/or severely curved root canals. These instruments have been heat tempered, have a modified tip geometry and exhibit greater buckling resistance compared with conventional stainless steel instruments. As a result, more pressure can be used to negotiate calcified canals with these instruments, and they provide excellent tactile feedback.[40,41]

Despite the many advantages of stainless steel instruments, a major disadvantage is that they are less flexible with increasing sizes. When a stainless steel instrument is used in a curved root canal, due to the restoring forces, it tends to straighten up, and this increases the likelihood of creating canal aberrations such as a zip or ledge. Regardless of the hand instrumentation technique used, the probability of canal straightening increases as the size of the stainless steel instrument or the degree of canal curvature increases.

Watch Winding, Circumferential Filing and Anticurvature Filing

Watch winding describes the manipulation of a hand file in a root canal in continuous clockwise and counterclockwise action, with slight apical pressure, to slowly advance the instrument apically. This technique, using a small size file, is usually performed in the initial negotiation of the root canal. Once the file has reached the desired length, circumferential filing, involving an in-out, push-pull filing action while simultaneously moving the file circumferentially around the canal walls, is used to instrument the root canal. Circumferential filing may be used to prepare straight or relatively straight canals. However, in a curved canal, circumferential filing will result in preferential removal of dentine from the inner curve of the root canal and the risk of a strip perforation. The mesial roots of mandibular molars and the mesiobuccal roots of maxillary molars are the teeth most at risk from this iatrogenic problem. Anticurvature filing[42] is a method for preparing a curved root canal in which more dentine is selectively removed from the outer, compared with the inner, curve of the root.

The Balanced Force Technique

The 'Balanced Force' technique was first described in 1985.[43] In the Balanced Force technique, flexible K files with noncutting tips are rotated a quarter-turn clockwise to engage dentine of the root canal wall. Apical pressure is applied, followed by a half turn of the file in the counterclockwise direction, which effectively 'cuts' the dentine that was engaged. The process can be repeated two or three times before removing the instrument to clean the flutes and irrigate the canal. Unlike many other techniques, files are not precurved when used in this manner. Compared with other hand instrumentation techniques, the Balanced Force concept was reported to allow preparation of curved canals with less canal straightening, associated with less apically extruded debris[44] and resulted in improved canal cleanliness.[45,46]

Patency Filing

During canal preparation, dentinal debris may build up, especially in the apical and curved parts of the canal. The resultant blockage impedes access of

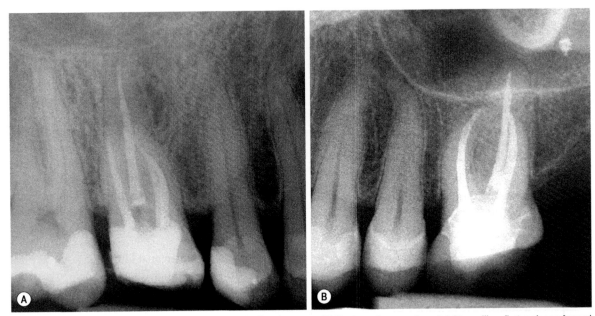

FIGURE 7-9 Root canal preparations using engine-driven NiTi instruments. (A) Root canal preparation of right maxillary first molar performed according to the Single-Length technique using a rotary NiTi system. (B) Root canal preparation of left maxillary first molar performed using a reciprocating Single-File system.

instruments and irrigants into the apical part of the canal; this may lead to difficulties in maintaining working length, canal transportation, ledge formation and potentially perforation. 'Apical patency' describes the concept of maintaining the apical constriction free of blockage. A patency file is defined as 'a small flexible K file which will passively move through the apical constricture without widening it'.[47] Therefore, patency filing involves the use of a patency file, usually set at 1 mm longer than the final working length to reduce the potential formation of a plug of infected dentinal debris in the apical 1 to 2 mm of the canal. Evidence to support this concept is equivocal.[48] Inoculating infected material beyond the apical constriction could result in postoperative discomfort or flare-ups. It is, however, important to make sure that the canal does not become blocked apically with infected debris during preparation; therefore, there is merit in recapitulating with a small instrument to keep the canal patent. Regular and copious irrigation will also help reduce apical packing of debris.

ENGINE-DRIVEN NICKEL–TITANIUM INSTRUMENTS

NiTi alloys exist in various crystallographic forms (austenite and martensite) and exhibit superelastic behaviour and shape memory. NiTi instruments are able to return to their original shape even after substantial deformation (up to 10%) once the load is removed, whereas with stainless steel instruments, deformation of just 1% results in permanent shape alteration. Since NiTi alloys are substantially more flexible than stainless steel alloys, this has made it possible to produce instruments with tapers greater than the standard ISO 0.02 (2% taper). NiTi engine-driven instruments are available in a range of tapers. Exploiting the properties of greater flexibility and superelastic behaviour, NiTi engine-driven instruments can more rapidly enlarge even severely curved canals, are able to maintain the original canal curvature far better than stainless steel instruments and can do it with fewer procedural errors (Figure 7-9).[2,8]

General rules when using engine-driven NiTi root canal instruments include the following:

- Instruments should be used with torque-controlled electric motors or handpieces to reduce the risk of instrument separation.
- A glide path should be created using either hand[41] or engine-driven (e.g. PathFile or Pro-Glider, Dentsply, Maillefer; ScoutRace, FKG, La

Chaux-de-Fonds, Switzerland; G-Files, Micro-Mega, Besançon, France) pathfinding-type instruments.[49,50]

- Most systems include orifice shapers/openers that are shorter, more tapered instruments designed for coronal flaring of the root canal before preparation of the rest of the canal.
- Instruments should never be forced apically, so excessive pressure on the instruments during preparation must be avoided.
- Instruments should be kept moving inside the canal.
- The predefined values of the motor with regard to torque and rotational speed should not be changed.
- Regular inspection should be carried out, when the instruments are withdrawn from the canal, to check for damages or signs of potential instrument separation.

Although modern engine-driven NiTi instruments are efficient and can improve the quality of canal preparation, they do not come into contact with all the canal walls; therefore, only relatively little dentine is removed, especially in the apical region.[51,52] Sufficient root canal irrigation is still essential for effective and thorough decontamination of the root canal system.

Advantages of NiTi instruments include:
- excellent shaping ability, even in severely curved root canals and complicated canal anatomies (e.g. S-shaped root canals, confluent canal systems; Figure 7-10);
- greater possible apical preparation sizes than with stainless steel hand instruments;
- ability to prepare more curved canals more evenly and to a greater taper;
- shorter preparation time, as fewer instruments are required;
- relatively shorter learning curve.

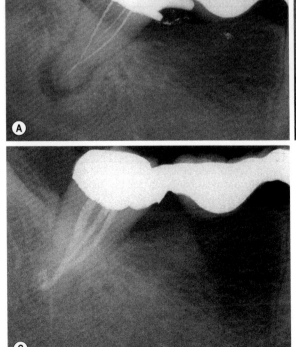
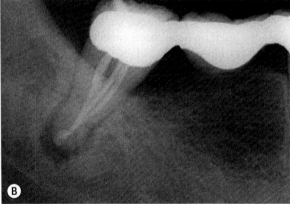

FIGURE 7-10 Confluent root canal system in a mandibular molar. (A) Working length radiograph showing apical confluence of all canals. (B) After root canal preparation using rotary NiTi instruments, the canals were obturated. (C) One-year follow-up radiograph indicating healing of the apical periodontitis.

Disadvantages include:

- potentially unpredictable instrument fracture;
- less tactile feedback during canal preparation;
- not suitable for helping bypass ledges as most NiTi instruments cannot be precurved;
- greater cost compared with stainless steel instruments.

Engine-driven NiTi instruments may be categorised into three main groups according to how they are used: Crown-Down approach, Single-Length technique and Single-File systems (Table 7-2).

CROWN-DOWN TECHNIQUE

In this technique the root canal is shaped in a coronal-to-apical direction. A predetermined sequence of instruments of different tapers (see Table 7-2) – usually from larger to smaller sizes – are required whereby each successively smaller instrument will be advanced slightly deeper into the root canal than the preceding instrument. The full working length is usually reached after usage of the third or fourth instrument of a particular sequence.

Advantages of the technique include:

- decreased frictional stress exerted on the instruments; taper lock less likely to occur;
- removal of infected coronal part, before entering the apical part, of the root canal;
- early coronal flaring, which significantly reduces alteration of the working length during canal preparation[53]; otherwise, as the canal is prepared, it is gradually straightened leading to alteration of the working length;
- improved access for irrigants into the apical part of the root canal, resulting in longer contact times between irrigation solutions and intracanal microorganisms;
- reduced risk of apical extrusion of debris into the periradicular tissue, as the working instrument is not tightly confined in the canal; however, this claim lacks good supporting evidence.

Disadvantages include:

- the need for comparatively more time and instruments, hence also cost, to fully shape a root canal;
- a longer learning curve, as with some systems, instrument sequences vary depending on the root canal anatomy, e.g. wide versus narrow and straight versus curved root canals.

TABLE 7-2 Different Concepts of Root Canal Preparation Using Engine-Driven Instruments with Representative Instrument System
Crown-Down Technique
ProFile (Dentsply Maillefer, Ballaigues, Switzerland)
ProTaper (Dentsply Maillefer, Ballaigues, Switzerland)
RaCe/BioRaCe (FKG, La-Chaux-de-Fonds, Switzerland)
FlexMaster (VDW, Munich, Germany)
HyFlex CM** (Coltène Whaledent, Altstätten, Switzerland)
Hero 642 (Micro-Méga, Besançon, France)
LightSpeed (LightSpeed Technology, San Antonio, TX, USA)
Single-Length Technique
Mtwo (VDW, Munich, Germany)
HyFlex EDM[†] (Coltène Whaledent, Altstätten, Switzerland)
ProTaper NEXT* (Dentsply Maillefer, Ballaigues, Switzerland)
ProTaper NEXT Gold[††] (Dentsply Maillefer, Ballaigues, Switzerland)
Single-File Systems
Rotary Motion
OneShape (Micro-Méga, Besançon, France)
F360/F6 SkyTaper (Brasseler Komet, Lemgo, Germany)
Reciprocating Motion
WaveOne* (Dentsply Maillefer, Ballaigues, Switzerland)
WaveOne Gold[††] (Dentsply Maillefer, Ballaigues, Switzerland)
Reciproc* (VDW, Munich, Germany)

*Made from M-wire NiTi; **made from CM-wire NiTi; [†]made by electrical discharge machining; [††]made from special heat-treated NiTi.

SINGLE-LENGTH TECHNIQUE

In this technique, following the coronal enlargement of the root canal uses orifice openers/shapers, or Gates-Glidden drills; all the instruments of a particular system (see Table 7-2) are used to the full working length. The sequence starts with the smallest size instrument and progressively larger sizes are all used to full working length. In this way, each instrument is creating a glide path for the next instrument.

Advantages of this technique include:

- easier to learn;
- fewer instruments required compared with the Crown-Down technique;
- easier and more rapid canal preparation compared with the Crown-Down technique.

Disadvantages include:

- the later introduction of irrigation solutions into the apical third of the canals compared with the Crown-Down technique;
- greater risk of infected coronal pulp tissue being transported into the apical part of the root canal.

SINGLE-FILE SYSTEMS

The currently available Single-File systems can be sub-divided into those used in full rotary motion, e.g. F360 (Brasseler, Lemgo, Germany) and OneShape (Micro-Méga, Besançon, France), and those used in reciprocating motion, e.g. Reciproc (VDW) and WaveOne (Dentsply Maillefer; see Table 7-2).

The Single-File systems F360 (Brasseler) and One-Shape (Micro-Mega) work in a clockwise, rotational motion. Unlike those in reciprocating motions, they do not require a specially programmed electronic motor. The currently available evidence suggests that their shaping ability in curved root canals is as good as that of the reciprocating Single-File systems and rotary Multiple-File NiTi systems.[54,55] In addition, there seems to be no increased risk of debris extrusion with rotary Single-File systems compared with rotary Multiple-File systems.[55]

The reciprocating motion of Single-File systems is usually in a counterclockwise (cutting) direction and then a clockwise (release) direction of movement of the instrument; the angle of the counterclockwise direction is greater than that of the reverse, clockwise, direction. The fact that the angle in the cutting direction is greater than that in the clockwise direction enables the instrument to continue to progress apically. These angles of movement are specific to the design of the particular instruments[56] and are programmed into an electronic motor, which is required.

The use of reciprocating Single-File systems Reciproc (VDW) and WaveOne (Dentsply Maillefer), both made from M-wire NiTi (see later), is associated with little to nearly no canal transportation even when shaping severely curved canals.[57–59] Evidence from all available studies indicates that these systems considerably reduce the working time for canal preparation compared with other engine-driven NiTi systems.[59] However, there are some controversies regarding the tendency of reciprocating instruments to cause dentinal defects, incomplete and complete cracks, and to extrude debris into the periradicular tissues.[59] Some studies have reported an increased risk of incomplete dentinal cracks in the apical part of the root canals and an increased tendency of apical debris extrusion with reciprocating instruments.[60,61] Others found either no difference in the incidence of cracks, or the amount of extruded debris between reciprocating and rotary NiTi instruments; yet others reported even better results for reciprocating instruments.[59]

Reciprocating instruments are able to cut dentine very effectively and to progress easily into narrow, or even sclerosed, root canals. However, to better control these instruments, to avoid instrument fractures and to reduce the stress generated, they should be used in a gentle up-and-down movement to maximum amplitude of 3 mm (Figure 7-11). One up-and-down movement is defined as one 'peck', and after three 'pecks' the instrument should be withdrawn and the canal copiously irrigated. The flutes of the instrument should

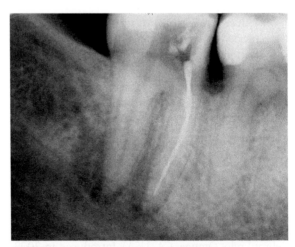

FIGURE 7-11 Fracture of a reciprocating NiTi file due to excessive force being applied and the failure to use the instrument in a gentle, up-and-down 'pecking' motion.

be cleaned and small hand instruments should be used to ensure that the canal is not blocked with debris or dentine chips.

Since the use of Single-File systems reduces canal preparation times by up to 60%,[58] there is a danger that less time is spent for irrigation and disinfection of the root canal system. To, at least, partially compensate for the reduced time and duration for the irrigant to work, a greater volume of the irrigant should be used, and additional activation of the irrigation solution is advisable. After completion of canal preparation, passive ultrasonic activation (PUI) of the irrigant, NaOCl is preferred, should be performed to improve chemical dissolution of residual debris and disinfection of the root canal system. With the use of Single-File systems, it is advisable to include further measures to improve canal cleanliness and disinfection.

In summary, advantages of the Single-File system include:

- considerably faster preparation; up to 60% reduction compared with the Single-Length technique;
- excellent shaping ability;
- reduced number of instruments;
- shorter learning curve.

Disadvantages include:

- inconclusive evidence regarding the increased risk of apical debris extrusion and creation of dentinal cracks associated with the use of reciprocating Single-File systems;
- reduced time for irrigation; special measures needed to improve canal cleanliness and disinfection, e.g. the use of passive ultrasonic activation (PUI) of the irrigant;
- reduced selection of available instrument sizes; as it is dependent on canal anatomy, further instruments might be required.

NEWER NICKEL–TITANIUM ALLOYS AND OTHER DEVELOPMENTS

To improve the properties of engine-driven NiTi root canal instruments, there have been several developments. Traditionally, NiTi instruments are manufactured by grinding wire blanks. The Twisted File (TF; SybronEndo, Orange, CA, USA), introduced in 2008, is manufactured by subjecting a NiTi blank in the austenitic phase to a thermal process to transform it into a different crystalline structure (R-phase), during which it is twisted and then converted back to the austenitic phase; this is claimed to enhance superelasticity and increased cyclic fatigue. More recently, the TF Adaptive system (SybronEndo) was released; used in combination with a dedicated motor (Elements Motor, SybronEndo) with 'Adaptive Motion Technology', the instrument is driven in rotary, or reciprocating, motion as it adjusts to intracanal torsional forces, depending on the amount of pressure applied.

Two special NiTi alloys have been introduced: M-wire and controlled memory (CM)-wire.[62] The M-wire alloy is a mixture of nearly equal amounts of two different NiTi phases, namely the R-phase and the austenite phase. Conventional NiTi alloy has an austenite structure[62–64] and its composition is about 55% nickel and 45% titanium in weight; whereas, M-wire consists of 55.8% nickel in weight with the addition of some iron. The alloy structure of M-wire is finer and more homogenous than that of austenite NiTi.[63] Instruments made from M-wire display a significantly increased fracture resistance and flexibility compared with austenite NiTi files. Representative instruments made from M-wire include ProTaper NEXT (Dentsply Maillefer), ProFile Vortex (Dentsply Tulsa, Tulsa, OK, USA), ProFile GT Series X (Dentsply Tulsa), Reciproc (VDW) and WaveOne (Dentsply Maillefer).

Another modification of NiTi, using a specific sequence of heat treatment, is the CM-wire. HyFlex CM (Coltène/Whaledent, Altstätten, Switzerland) instruments are made from CM-wire; this alloy is characterized by a lower percentage weight of nickel (52.1%) than conventional NiTi alloys.[64] These modifications result in increased flexibility and improved fatigue resistance. During root canal preparation, permanently deformed CM-wire instruments will regain their original shape when heated during sterilization at approximately 134°C.[65] Current evidence suggests that instruments made from these newer alloys, M-wire and CM-wire, maintain the original canal curvature well and caused almost no procedural errors even when preparing severely curved canals.[8]

Instead of grinding, the HyFlex EDM (Electrical Discharge Machining) instruments (Coltène/Whaledent) are manufactured using electro-erosion to improve surface hardness of the instruments; it is claimed that this results in increased cutting efficiency and reduced risk of instrument separation. Another innovation involves special heat treatment after grinding of the NiTi instruments; two representatives of NiTi instruments subjected to this heat treatment process are Pro-Taper NEXT Gold (Dentsply Maillefer) and WaveOne Gold (Dentsply Maillefer). It is claimed that this additional special heat treatment increases the flexibility and resistance to cyclic fatigue of the resultant NiTi instruments. However, independent scientific verifications of these claims are not yet available.

Learning Outcomes

After completion of this chapter, the reader should be able to describe and discuss the:
- steps to undertake to gain access to the root canal system;
- methods of determining working length;
- clinical relevance of root canal irrigation;
- advantages and disadvantages of root canal hand instruments;
- different concepts of engine-driven root canal preparation using NiTi instruments, including controversies associated with the use of Single-File systems, the benefits of newer NiTi alloys and other improvements.

REFERENCES

1. Ng YR, Mann V, Rahbaran S, et al. Outcome of primary root canal treatment: systematic review of the literature. International Endodontic Journal 2008;41:6–31.
2. Hülsmann M, Peters OA, Dummer P. Mechanical preparation of root canals: shaping goals, techniques and means. Endodontic Topics 2005;10:30–76.
3. Bhuva B, Chong BS, Patel S. Rubber dam in clinical practice. ENDO (Lond Engl) 2008;2:131–41.
4. Ahmad IA. Rubber dam usage for endodontic treatment: a review. International Endodontic Journal 2009;42:965–72.
5. Lin PY, Huang SH, Chang HJ, et al. The effect of rubber dam usage on the survival rate of teeth receiving initial root canal treatment: a nationwide population-based study. Journal of Endodontics 2014;40:1733–7.
6. Krishan R, Paqué F, Ossareh A, et al. Impacts of conservative endodontic cavity on root canal instrumentation efficacy and resistance to fracture assessed in incisors, premolars, and molars. Journal of Endodontics 2014;40:1160–6.
7. Bürklein S, Schäfer E. Minimally invasive endodontics. Quintessence International 2015;46:119–24.
8. Bürklein S, Schäfer E. Critical evaluation of root canal transportation by instrumentation. Endodontic Topics 2013;29:110–24.
9. Wu MK, Wesselink PR, Walton RE. Apical terminus location of root canal treatment procedures. Oral Surgery, Oral

Medicine, Oral Pathology, Oral Radiology and Endodontics 2000;89:99–103.
10. Kojima K, Inamoto I, Nagamatsu K, et al. Success rate of endodontic treatment of teeth with vital and nonvital pulps. A meta-analysis. Oral Surgery, Oral Medicine, Oral Pathology, Oral Radiology & Endodontics 2004;97:95–9.
11. Schaeffer MA, White RR, Walton RE. Determining the optimal obturation length: a meta-analysis of literature. Journal of Endodontics 2005;31:271–4.
12. Olson AK, Goerig AC, Cavataio RE, et al. The ability of the radiograph to determine the location of the apical foramen. International Endodontic Journal 1991;24:28–35.
13. ElAyouti A, Weiger R, Löst C. Frequency of overinstrumentation with an acceptable radiographic working length. Journal of Endodontics 2001;27:49–52.
14. Gordon MP, Chandler NP. Electronic apex locators. International Endodontic Journal 2004;37:425–37.
15. Martins JNR, Marques D, Mata A, et al. Clinical efficacy of electronic apex locators: systematic review. Journal of Endodontics 2014;40:759–77.
16. Cianconi L, Angotti V, Felici R, et al. Accuracy of three electronic apex locators compared with digital radiography: an ex vivo study. Journal of Endodontics 2010;36:2003–7.
17. Murakami M, Inoue S, Inoue N. Clinical evaluation of audiometric control root canal treatment: a retrospective study. Quintessence International 2002;33:465–74.
18. Rosenberg DB. The paper point technique. Part I. Dentistry Today 2003;22:80–6.
19. Rosenberg DB. The paper point technique. Part II. Dentistry Today 2003;22:627.
20. Trope M, Bergenholtz G. Microbiological basis for endodontic treatment: can a maximal outcome be achieved in one visit? Endodontic Topics 2002;1:40–53.
21. Siqueira JF. Endodontic infections: concepts, paradigms, and perspectives. Oral Surgery, Oral Medicine, Oral Pathology Oral Radiology & Endodontics 2002;94:281–93.
22. Zehnder M. Root canal irrigants. Journal of Endodontics 2006;32:389–98.
23. Siqueira JF Jr, Rocas IN, Santos SR, et al. Efficacy of instrumentation techniques and irrigation regiments in reducing the bacterial population within root canal. Journal of Endodontics 2002;28:181–4.
24. Chuste-Guillot MP, Badet C, Peli JF, et al. Effect of nickel-titanium rotary file techniques on infected root dentin reduction. Oral Surgery, Oral Medicine, Oral Pathology, Oral Radiology & Endodontics 2006;102:254–8.
25. Nair PW, Henry S, Cano V, et al. Microbial status of apical root canal system of human mandibular first molars with primary apical periodontitis after 'one-visit' endodontic treatment. Oral Surgery, Oral Medicine, Oral Pathology, Oral Radiology & Endodontics 2005;99:231–52.
26. Schäfer E. Irrigation of the root canal. ENDO (Lond Engl) 2007;1:11–27.
27. Naenni N, Thoma K, Zehnder M. Soft tissue dissolution capacity of currently used and potential endodontic irrigants. Journal of Endodontics 2004;30:785–7.
28. Silva IA, Leonardo MR, Assed S, et al. Histological study of the effect of some irrigating solutions on bacterial endotoxin in dogs. Brazilian Dental Journal 2004;15:109–14.
29. Clegg MS, Vertucci FJ, Walker C, et al. The effect of exposure to irrigant solutions on apical dentin biofilms in vitro. Journal of Endodontics 2006;32:434–7.

30. Hülsmann M, Hahn W. Complications during root canal irrigation – literature review and case reports. International Endodontic Journal 2000;33:186–93.

31. Haapasalo M, Endal U, Zandi H, et al. Eradication of endodontic infection by instrumentation and irrigation solutions. Endodontic Topics 2005;10:77–102.

32. Ringel AM, Patterson SS, Newton CW, et al. In vivo evaluation of chlorhexidine gluconate solution and sodium hypochlorite solution as root canal irrigants. Journal of Endodontics 1982;8:2004.

33. Portenier I, Haapasalo H, Rye A, et al. Inactivation of root canal medicaments by dentine, hydroxylapatite and bovine serum albumin. International Endodontic Journal 2001;34: 184–8.

34. Cintra LT, Watanabe S, Samuel RO, et al. The use of NaOCl in combination with CHX produces cytotoxic product. Clinical Oral Investigations 2014;18:935–40.

35. Zehnder M, Schmidlin P, Sener B, et al. Chelation in root canal therapy reconsidered. Journal of Endodontics 2005;31: 817–20.

36. van der Sluis L. Ultrasound in endodontics. ENDO (Lond Engl) 2007;1:29–36.

37. Schäfer E, Bürklein S. Impact of nickel-titanium instrumentation of the root canal on clinical outcomes: a focused review. Odontology/Journal of the Society of the Nippon Dental University 2012;100:130–6.

38. Pettiette MT, Delano O, Trope M. Evaluation of success rate of endodontic treatment performed by students with stainless-steel K-files and nickel-titanium hand files. Journal of Endodontics 2001;27:124–7.

39. Cheung GSP, Liu CSY. A retrospective study of endodontic treatment outcome between nickel-titanium rotary and stainless steel hand filing techniques. Journal of Endodontics 2009;35:938–43.

40. Allen MJ, Glickman GN, Griggs JA. Comparative analysis of endodontic pathfinders. Journal of Endodontics 2007;33: 723–6.

41. Lopes HP, Elias CN, Mangelli M, et al. Buckling resistance of pathfinding endodontic instruments. Journal of Endodontics 2012;38:402–4.

42. Abou-Rass M, Frank A, Glick D. The anticurvature filing method to prepare the curved root canal. Journal of the American Dental Association 1980;101:792–4.

43. Roane J, Sabala CL, Duncanson MG. The 'balanced force' concept for instrumentation of curved canals. Journal of Endodontics 1985;11:203–11.

44. Ferraz CC, Gomes NV, Gomes BP, et al. Apical extrusion of debris and irrigants using two hand and three engine-driven instrumentation techniques. International Endodontic Journal 2001;34:354–8.

45. Kyomen SM, Kaputo SM, White SN. Critical analysis of the balanced force technique in endodontics. Journal of Endodontics 1994;20:332–7.

46. Song YL, Bian Z, Fan B, et al. A comparison of instrument-centering ability within the root canal for three contemporary instrumentation techniques. International Endodontic Journal 2004;37:265–71.

47. Buchanan LS. Management of the curved root canal. Journal of the California Dental Association 1989;17:18–27.

48. Arias A, Azabal M, Hidalgo JJ, et al. Relationship between postendodontic pain, tooth diagnostic factors, and apical patency. Journal of Endodontics 2009;35:189–92.

49. D'Amario M, Baldi M, Petricca R, et al. Evaluation of a new nickel-titanium system to create the glide path in root canal preparation of curved canals. Journal of Endodontics 2013;39: 1581–4.

50. Elnaghy AM, Elsaka SE. Evaluation of the mechanical behaviour of PathFile and ProGlider pathfinding nickel-titanium rotary instruments. International Endodontic Journal 2015;48: 894–901.

51. Peters OA, Schonenberger K, Laib A. Effects of four Ni-Ti preparation techniques on root canal geometry assessed by micro computed tomography. International Endodontic Journal 2001;34:221–30.

52. Paqué F, Barbakow F, Peters OA. Root canal preparation with Endo-Eze AET: changes in root canal shape assessed by micro-computed tomography. International Endodontic Journal 2005;38:456–64.

53. Davis RD, Marshall JG, Baumgartner JC. Effect of early coronal flaring on working length change in curved canals using rotary nickel-titanium versus stainless steel instruments. Journal of Endodontics 2002;28:438–42.

54. Bürklein S, Benten S, Schäfer E. Quantitative evaluation of apically extruded debris with different single-file systems: Reciproc, F360 and OneShape versus Mtwo. International Endodontic Journal 2014;47:405–9.

55. Capar ID, Ertas H, Ok E, et al. Comparative study of different novel nickel-titanium rotary systems for root canal preparation in severely curved root canals. Journal of Endodontics 2014;40:852.

56. Fiedler A. Kinematics of 2 reciprocating endodontic motors: the difference between actual and set values. Journal of Endodontics 2014;40:990–4.

57. Paqué F, Zehnder M, De-Deus G. Microtomography-based comparison of reciprocating single-file F2 ProTaper technique versus rotary full sequence. Journal of Endodontics 2011;37: 1394–7.

58. Bürklein S, Hinschitza K, Dammaschke T, et al. Shaping ability and cleaning effectiveness of two single-file systems in severely curved root canals of extracted teeth: Reciproc and WaveOne versus Mtwo and ProTaper. International Endodontic Journal 2012;45:449–61.

59. Yared G, Ramli GA. Single file reciprocation: a literature review. ENDO (Lond Engl) 2013;7:171–8.

60. Bürklein S, Schäfer E. Apically extruded debris with reciprocating single-file and full-sequence rotary instrumentation systems. Journal of Endodontics 2012;38:850–2.

61. Bürklein S, Tsotsis P, Schäfer E. Incidence of dentinal defects after root canal preparation: reciprocating versus rotary instrumentation. Journal of Endodontics 2013;39:501–4.

62. Zhou H, Peng B, Zheng YF. An overview of the mechanical properties of nickel-titanium endodontic instruments. Endodontic Topics 2013;29:42–54.

63. Alapati SB, Brantley WA, Iijma M, et al. Metallurgical characterization of a new nickel-titanium wire for rotary endodontic instruments. Journal of Endodontics 2009;35:1589–93.

64. Gutmann JL, Gao Y. Alteration in the inherent metallic and surface properties of nickel-titanium root canal instruments to enhance performance, durability and safety: a focussed review. International Endodontic Journal 2012;45:113–28.

65. Bürklein S, Börjes L, Schäfer E. Comparison of preparation of curved root canals with Hyflex CM and Revo-S rotary nickel-titanium instruments. International Endodontic Journal 2014;47:470–6.

CHAPTER 8

Intracanal Medication

J. F. Siqueira Jr and I. N. Rôças

Chapter Contents

Summary

Endodontics may be considered to be concerned with the prevention or treatment of apical periodontitis, a disease with a microbial aetiology. The main phases of endodontic treatment, involving the elimination, or control, of infection are chemomechanical preparation and intracanal medication. The latter consists of applying a chemical agent into the root canal system to exert an intended pharmacological effect. Intracanal medication can be used for different purposes, but the most common indication is to enhance disinfection after chemomechanical procedures. Over the years, medicaments used for this purpose have changed from strong and toxic chemicals to more selective and effective agents, which are better tolerated by tissues. Calcium hydroxide is the most commonly recommended antimicrobial agent used for intracanal medication. However, this agent has some limitations and may be improved by the addition of another medicament, acting as a biologically active vehicle. Other substances such as chlorhexidine and antibiotics have also been used as intracanal medicaments.

Introduction

Endodontics is primarily involved with the prevention or treatment of apical periodontitis. Consequently, the favourable outcome of endodontic treatment can be defined by the absence of the signs and symptoms of apical periodontitis. Since bacterial infection of the root canal system is the primary cause of both primary and posttreatment apical periodontitis, the focus of endodontic treatment should be the prevention or eradication of infection (Figure 8-1).[1] Prevention is mainly related to asepsis and measures to ensure that pathogenic microorganisms are kept out of the operation field. When infection is present, its eradication or

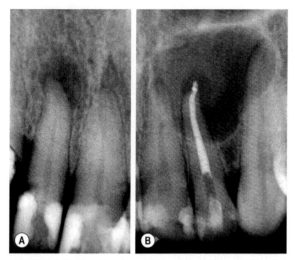

FIGURE 8-1 Teeth with primary (A) and posttreatment (B) apical periodontitis, which is primarily caused by intraradicular bacterial infection.

control depends on disinfection, which consists of eliminating pathogenic microorganisms, usually by chemical or physical means.

In everyday practice, clinicians basically manage two conditions requiring endodontic intervention: uninfected or infected root canal systems. The former condition is represented by teeth with vital pulps, which require root canal treatment electively or because of irreversible pulpitis. The latter condition is represented by teeth with necrotic pulps, with or without apical periodontitis, and previously root-treated teeth in need of retreatment because of post-treatment apical periodontitis.

Teeth with irreversible pulpitis are devoid of intra-radicular infection; if bacteria are present, they are generally located in the area of pulpal exposure or the coronal pulp. The radicular pulp may, or may not, be inflamed, but it is not infected.[2,3] It is generally accepted that teeth with vital pulps should be treated without delay, preferably in a single visit if feasible, to minimize the risk of microbial contamination of the root canal system.

Teeth with necrotic and infected pulps are a completely different issue. Intraradicular infection is the primary cause of both primary and posttreatment apical periodontitis.[4-7] Although asepsis remains important in these cases, effective elimination of

bacterial infection from the root canal system is paramount.[8,9]

The treatment outcome of infected teeth with apical periodontitis is between 10% and 25% lower than in teeth with no evidence of disease.[10-15] It should be emphasized that the treatment outcome of infected teeth, in the absence of detectable cultivable bacteria (negative culture) at the time of root filling, is very high and matches that of vital teeth.[16] Therefore, if a favourable treatment outcome with uninfected teeth is also to be achieved with infected teeth, the bacteriological conditions within the root canals should be rendered similar, which means maximal bacterial reduction must be attained before the root canal filling is placed.

The main steps of endodontic treatment involved with infection control are chemomechanical preparation and intracanal medication. Chemomechanical preparation plays an essential role in root canal disinfection since instruments and irrigants act primarily in the main canal, the largest area of the root canal system; consequently, this is where the highest bacteria density is harboured. Bacteria elimination from the root canal system is promoted by the mechanical action of instruments and the chemical antimicrobial action of irrigants. Although substantial amounts of bacteria are eliminated by chemomechanical preparation, studies have demonstrated detectable levels of bacteria still present in root canals after this phase, regardless of the type of irrigant used.[16-29] Since treatment outcome is improved if there is absence of detectable, cultivable bacteria at the time of root filling (Figure 8-2),[16,30-36] additional steps are considered necessary to enhance root canal disinfection. Several approaches have been proposed to optimize disinfection after the instrumentation and irrigation phase,[37] including single-visit strategies. However, intracanal medication is still required to obtain predictable, enhanced antimicrobial results. Therefore, the primary function of intracanal medication is to improve disinfection of the root canal system, acting on bacteria not eliminated by chemomechanical procedures. Moreover, there are some instances in which an intracanal medicament may be required for other reasons, including the induction of hard tissue formation, control of pain, persistent exudation or treat inflammatory root resorption.

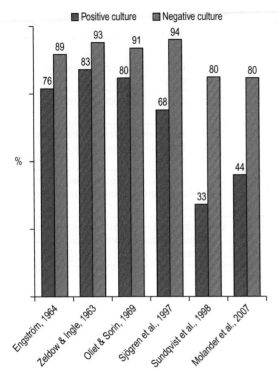

Positive culture ■ Negative culture

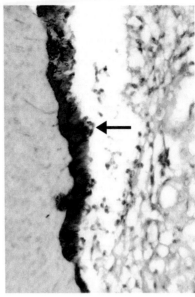

FIGURE 8-3 Bacterial biofilm (*arrowed*) adhering to the root canal wall.

FIGURE 8-2 Studies evaluating the endodontic treatment outcome of teeth showing a positive or negative culture of the canal at the time of root filling.

Microbiology of Endodontic Infections

APICAL PERIODONTITIS

Apical Periodontitis Is Caused by Bacterial Infection

Apical periodontitis is an inflammatory disease caused by bacterial infection of the root canal system.[4,5,7,38] Other microorganisms such as fungi, archaea and viruses have been found in association with apical periodontitis,[39–42] but bacteria are the main causative agents.[43] Apical periodontitis may be primary if the tooth had not been previously root treated or posttreatment if the tooth had been previously root treated.

Apical Periodontitis Is a Biofilm-Associated Disease

Bacteria in infected root canals associated with primary or posttreatment apical periodontitis exists mainly as a biofilm (Figure 8-3).[7] Biofilms are sessile, multicellular, microbial communities composed of microbial cells firmly attached to a hard or soft moist surface and enmeshed in a self-produced matrix of extracellular polymeric substances.[44,45] Occurrence of bacterial biofilms in infected root canals of teeth with apical periodontitis has been described by many studies.[6,46–48] However, their prevalence and their association with diverse presentations of apical periodontitis were demonstrated in a histobacteriological and histopathological study[7]; intraradicular biofilm arrangements were found in 80% of untreated canals and 74% of treated canals.

Biofilms were more frequently observed in the apical portion of canals of teeth with large lesions, especially those associated with a cyst. Extraradicular biofilms (see later) are very infrequent. Apical periodontitis seems to fulfill most of the established criteria used to determine whether a given infectious disease can be classified as being caused by biofilm communities.[7,49,50] Unfortunately, biofilm infections may be very difficult to eliminate.[51]

TYPES OF ENDODONTIC INFECTIONS

Endodontic infections are classified according to the anatomical location as intraradicular or extraradicular infection (Table 8-1). The former can be subdivided, according to the time bacteria gained entry into the

TABLE 8-1 **Types of Endodontic Infections**

Type	Definition	Effects
Intraradicular	Infection located within root canal system	Cause of primary and posttreatment apical periodontitis
Primary	Caused by microorganisms that invade and colonize necrotic pulp	Main cause of primary apical periodontitis
Persistent	Caused by microorganisms that are members of primary infection which persisted despite treatment	Main cause of posttreatment apical periodontitis as well as persistent exudation and symptoms
Secondary	Caused by microorganisms that gained entry into root canal system during or after treatment; usually a contamination problem	One of the causes of posttreatment apical periodontitis and persistent exudation and symptoms
Extraradicular	Infection initiated in root canal system but spreads to periradicular tissues; usually symptomatic	One of the causes of posttreatment apical periodontitis and persistent exudation and symptoms

root canal system, into three categories: primary, secondary or persistent infections.[52]

Primary Intraradicular Infections

Primary intraradicular infections are caused by bacteria that initially invade and colonize the necrotic pulp tissue (initial infection) and are the cause of primary apical periodontitis. Primary infections are characterized by a mixed consortium and composed of 10 to 30 bacterial species per canal[53]; however, recent studies using next generation DNA sequencing technologies have reported a greater number of bacterial species.[54,55] The bacterial load varies from 10^3 to 10^8 cells per infected canal.[56–58] There is a significant difference in the composition of bacterial communities associated with symptomatic and asymptomatic disease, with more species found in acute abscess cases.[54,59,60] Anaerobic species are the most prevalent and abundant bacteria encountered in primary infections; examples include black-pigmented gram-negative rods (*Prevotella* and *Porphyromonas* species), *Fusobacterium nucleatum, Treponema* species, *Dialister* species, *Pseudoramibacter alactolyticus, Propionibacterium* species, *Parvimonas micra, Tannerella forsythia, Filifactor alocis, Eubacterium* species and *Olsenella* species.[5,57,59,61–69] Some as-yet-uncultivated and uncharacterized bacterial species have also been detected in high prevalence.[63,66,70]

Persistent and Secondary Intraradicular Infections

Although the terms *persistent* and *secondary infections* have been used interchangeably, they are not synonymous. A persistent intraradicular infection is caused by bacteria associated with the primary infection, which had survived intracanal antimicrobial procedures. A secondary intraradicular infection is caused by microorganisms that were not present in the primary infection but were introduced in the root canal system at some stage after intervention, so called because it is secondary to intervention. A secondary infection is usually a contamination problem caused either by a breach in the aseptic chain, or by coronal leakage.

Persistent and secondary infections are, for the most part, clinically indistinguishable. Exceptions include infection-related complications, for example, acute exacerbations arising after the treatment of noninfected teeth and emergent posttreatment apical periodontitis lesions which were absent at the time of treatment but appeared on the follow-up radiograph. Both situations are typical examples of secondary infections.

Both persistent and secondary infections can be responsible for several clinical problems, including persistent exudation, persistent symptoms, interappointment flare-ups and treatment failure, characterized by posttreatment apical periodontitis.[16,34,35,55,71–74]

Studies evaluating the microbiota in root canal-treated teeth with posttreatment apical periodontitis revealed species that are associated with either a persistent, or a secondary, infection, which represent the possible cause of the disease. *Enterococcus faecalis* is a facultative bacteria most frequently detected in root canal-treated teeth.[73–78] Other species commonly found in association with posttreatment endodontic disease include *Streptococcus* species, *P. alactolyticus, Propionibacterium* species, *P. micra, F. alocis,* and *Dialister* species.[73,74,78] Yeasts, especially *Candida albicans,* can also be found more frequently in secondary infections than in primary infections.[34,79] Identification of nonoral species such as *Pseudomonas aeruginosa* and enteric rods in treated canals is strongly suggestive of a secondary infection. The number of microbial species present in adequately treated canals with posttreatment disease is lower than in inadequately treated or untreated canals.[34,59,62,72,73,80]

Extraradicular Infections

Extraradicular infections are characterized by bacterial invasion of the inflamed periradicular tissues and are a sequel to intraradicular infection. Extraradicular infections may be dependent on or independent of intraradicular infection; the existence of the latter condition remains to be proven. Except for acute and chronic apical abscesses, it is still controversial whether asymptomatic apical periodontitis lesions can harbour bacteria for very long, beyond the initial tissue invasion.

The Need to Enhance Disinfection

Culture-dependent or culture-independent (molecular) and histobacteriological studies have revealed that bacteria can persist in the root canal system after chemomechanical preparation in 40% to 60% of cases.[17,19,27,28,81–83] Bacteria surviving the effects of instruments and irrigants are usually located in areas that are difficult or impossible to reach during chemomechanical preparation.[6,82,84–86]

UNTOUCHED ROOT CANAL WALLS

Studies using microcomputed tomography and histobacteriological methods have shown that some areas of the main root canal system remain untouched by instruments (Figure 8-4).[82,87–90] This usually occurs

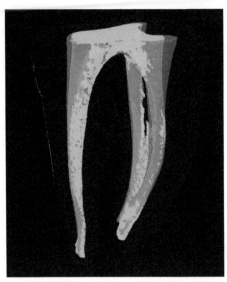

FIGURE 8-4 Microcomputed tomographic scan showing areas of the canal that remained untouched after chemomechanical preparation using rotary instruments (light green: preinstrumentation scan; dark green: postinstrumentation scan).

because the size of the apical preparation is smaller than the original canal diameter and/or the canal morphology is irregular, flattened, kidney-shaped, or oval in cross-section.[86,91] Different preparation techniques may leave at least 35% of the root canal surface area untouched[87]; this percentage may be worse in oval canals, where rotary instruments may only be in contact with 40% of the apical root canal walls.[91] If untouched canal walls are covered by a bacterial biofilm, there is a risk that bacteria will persist after chemomechanical preparation, especially if sodium hypochlorite irrigant did not manage to reach these areas or is not present in the canal for a sufficiently long duration to eliminate the biofilm.

ISTHMUSES, LATERAL CANALS AND APICAL RAMIFICATIONS

Bacterial infection in the canal may propagate in these very commonly occurring and anatomically varied areas.[3,85,92] Isthmuses have been observed at the apical 3 mm of 80% to 90% of molar roots.[93] Ramifications may be observed anywhere along the length of the root, but they occur more frequently in the apical portion and in posterior teeth.[94] In approximately 75% of teeth, ramifications are found in the apical third of the root.[3,95] Higher frequencies at 80% or more are observed for molars and maxillary premolars.[3]

DENTINAL TUBULES

Bacterial invasion of the dentinal tubules can occur in approximately 70% to 80% of canals in teeth with apical periodontitis (Figure 8-5).[96,97] Even though a shallow depth of penetration is more common *in vivo,* bacterial cells can still be observed penetrating approximately 300 µm in some teeth.[48] Bacterial cells penetrating deep into tubules are unlikely to be eliminated by chemomechanical preparation procedures.

Irrigant solutions, such as sodium hypochlorite and chlorhexidine, have pronounced antimicrobial activities and generally are effective against a large spectrum of microbial species found in infected root canals. However, the effectiveness is mostly observed when contact between irrigant and microbial cells are optimal. In clinical practice, the irrigant needs to diffuse to reach the aforementioned areas, but the short duration they remain in the canal during preparation procedures is a major limiting factor. Antimicrobial irrigating solutions usually remain in the root canal system for a shorter time period (10–30 minutes)

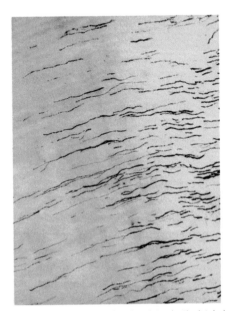

FIGURE 8-5 Dense bacterial infiltration into dentinal tubules in a tooth with apical periodontitis.

compared with an interappointment intracanal medicament (7 or more days). The substantial time difference can alter the effectiveness of bacterial elimination, especially if the antimicrobial agent is expected to reach areas distant from the main root canal by diffusion.

Antimicrobial Agents

HISTORY

The role of infection as the cause of apical periodontitis was first suggested in 1894 by the Willoughby Dayton Miller's classic study.[98] In the years that followed, the recognition of the microbial aetiology of endodontic problems resulted in the use of strong disinfecting agents during root canal treatment. Popular medications at that time included formaldehyde-containing substances[99] and phenolic[100] and iodoform-based pastes.[101] Later, antibiotic formulations were also recommended for intracanal medication.[102,103] In addition to infection control, medicaments were also used for pain control in endodontics; these include eugenol[104] and antiinflammatory drugs such as corticosteroids.[105,106] The cytotoxicity of most of these medicaments[107,108] led, over the years, to the search for substances with less adverse effects and the cessation of usage of many of these toxic compounds.

Of the substances currently recommended for intracanal medication, calcium hydroxide is most widely accepted and commonly used. Chlorhexidine and antibiotics have also been suggested for some situations (Table 8-2).

CALCIUM HYDROXIDE

Properties

Calcium hydroxide, a strong base (pH = 12.4), was introduced to dentistry in 1920 by Bernhard Hermann.[109] However, it was not until the 1980s that it became very popular given the excellent results reported from bacteriological studies.[17] Calcium hydroxide is an inorganic compound, and the most common presentation is in the form of an odourless white powder. In the presence of water, it dissociates into hydroxyl and calcium ions. Most of its biological effects are related to its alkaline pH and due to the hydroxyl ions.[110]

TABLE 8-2 Types of Intracanal Medicaments

Type	Examples	Usage and Indication
Aldehydes	Formocresol	Not recommended
	Tricresol formalin	Not recommended
	Glutaraldehyde	Not recommended
Phenols	Camphorated phenol	Not recommended
	Camphorated paramonochlor ophenol	Not recommended alone; biologically active vehicle for calcium hydroxide
	Eugenol	Pain control
Antibiotics	Penicillin	Not recommended
	Minocycline	Constituent of triple antibiotic paste
	Metronidazole	Constituent of triple antibiotic paste
	Ciprofloxacin	Constituent of triple antibiotic paste
	Clindamycin	Not recommended alone. Constituent of Odontopaste
	Doxycycline	Constituent of MTAD irrigant
	Demeclocycline	Constituent of Ledermix in association with a corticosteroid
Halogens	Sodium hypochlorite	Incompletely instrumented canals
	Iodine potassium iodide	Used by some; biologically active vehicle for calcium hydroxide
	Iodoform	Used by some
Others	Calcium hydroxide	Widely used
	Chlorhexidine	Used alone or as a biologically active vehicle for calcium hydroxide
Antiinflammatory drugs	Corticosteroids, nonsteroidal antiinflammatory drugs	Pain prevention and control

To exert its maximal effects, calcium hydroxide has to be placed into the entire length of the prepared canal. Although some clinicians have developed methods of placing calcium hydroxide powder into the canal, placement is easier, more reliable and the canal better filled when calcium hydroxide is mixed with a liquid, gel, creamy carrier or vehicle. Since the effects of calcium hydroxide are pH-dependent, the ideal vehicle should enable the ionic dissociation of calcium hydroxide, which will vary depending on the type of vehicle used. Calcium hydroxide vehicles have been classified, according to consistency and ability to permit its dissociation, into aqueous, viscous and oily vehicles (Table 8-3).[111] It is questionable if viscous or oily vehicles are of any value since they do not permit rapid dissociation and consequently, a high release of hydroxyl ions. As the effects of calcium hydroxide are dependent on the pH reached around where it has been placed, if the ionic release is slow, it may be unable to exert its intended effects.

Vehicles for calcium hydroxide may also be classified as being inert, or biologically active, from an antimicrobial standpoint (see Table 8-3).[1] Inert vehicles are, for the most part, biocompatible but do not significantly influence the antimicrobial properties of calcium hydroxide; these include distilled water, saline, anaesthetic solution, and glycerine. On the other hand, biologically active vehicles may provide additional effects to the calcium hydroxide, including improved or additive antimicrobial properties; these vehicles include camphorated paramonochlorophenol, chlorhexidine and iodine potassium iodide.

In laboratory studies, most endodontic bacteria are eliminated after a short period of exposure to calcium hydroxide, as a result of its high pH level.[17,112-114] When calcium hydroxide is in direct contact with the test bacteria in solution, the concentration of hydroxyl ions is very high and reaches levels incompatible with the survival of most bacterial species. The lethal effects of hydroxyl ions are caused by its action on bacterial lipids, proteins and DNA, leading to subsequent damage to the cellular apparatus and drastically altering cellular functions.[110] Calcium hydroxide can also inactivate some bacterial virulence factors, including

TABLE 8-3	Classification of Calcium Hydroxide Vehicles
Type	**Examples**
Classification Based on Consistency and Solubility	
Aqueous	Distilled water
	Saline
	Dental anaesthetic solution
	Anionic detergent solution
Viscous	Glycerine
	Polyethyleneglycol
	Propyleneglycol
Oily	Camphorated paramonochlorophenol
	Olive oil
	Silicone oil
Classification Based on Antimicrobial Effects	
Inert	Saline
	Distilled water
	Dental anaesthetic solution
	Glycerine
	Propyleneglycol
	Polyethyleneglycol
Biologically active	Camphorated paramonochlorophenol
	Chlorhexidine
	Iodine potassium iodide
	Ledermix
	Odontopaste

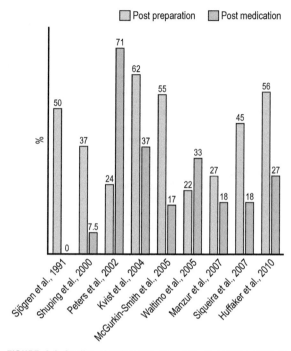

FIGURE 8-6 Studies showing the incidence of positive cultures after chemomechanical preparation and intracanal medication with calcium hydroxide paste in inert vehicles.

lipopolysaccharides (endotoxins) and the lipoteichoic acid.[115–118]

Antimicrobial Effectiveness in Endodontic Therapy

The maximal effects of calcium hydroxide on bacteria are observed when the concentration of hydroxyl ions is sufficiently high and reaches lethal levels. In clinical practice, such conditions are not easy to achieve because direct contact between calcium hydroxide and bacteria is not always possible.

Clinical studies revealed that the effectiveness of calcium hydroxide in significantly improving disinfection after chemomechanical preparation is somewhat inconsistent (Figure 8-6).[18,21,25,35,81,119,120] This indicates that calcium hydroxide has limitations when it comes to intracanal disinfection. In addition to the difficulties of achieving optimal contact between medicament and bacteria colonizing the intricacies of the

root canal system, the medicament has to diffuse to areas distant from the main root canal; these may help explain the limitations of calcium hydroxide in predictably disinfecting the root canal system.

Calcium hydroxide owes its biocompatibility to its low water solubility and diffusibility[8]; hence, its cytotoxic effect is limited to the tissue area in which it is in direct contact. On the other hand, the same low solubility and diffusibility make it difficult for calcium hydroxide to promote a rapid and significant increase in pH to eliminate bacteria present in dentinal tubules, tissue remnants, ramifications and isthmuses.

The killing of bacteria by calcium hydroxide depends on the availability of hydroxyl ions in solution, which is much higher in the main root canal, where it is placed. As calcium hydroxide diffuses to other areas in the root canal system, the concentration of hydroxyl ions decreases as a result of the action of tissue buffering systems (bicarbonate and phosphate), acids, proteins and carbon dioxide.[110] Furthermore, its antimicrobial effects are significantly reduced in the presence of serum and dentine.[121–123] Consequently, calcium hydroxide is a slow-working antimicrobial agent and requires prolonged exposure to allow for saturation of the buffering ability of dentine and tissue remnants. Long-term use, preferably with changes of the calcium hydroxide, is necessary to maximize disinfection of the root canal system. Another option is to combine calcium hydroxide with biologically active vehicles.

Another factor that may interfere with calcium hydroxide antimicrobial effectiveness is the presence of resistant species in the root canal system. Resistance to calcium hydroxide has been reported for some microbial species, such as *E. faecalis* and *Candida*,[17,112,124–126] which are commonly found in root-treated teeth with posttreatment disease.[34,72–75,78]

Combination with Biologically Active Vehicles

As a result of the limitations discussed earlier, calcium hydroxide is not expected to promote complete disinfection in all cases.[110] In an attempt to overcome the limitations of calcium hydroxide in inert vehicles, studies have investigated combining calcium hydroxide with a biologically active vehicle, or another antibacterial agent, such as camphorated paramonochlorophenol or chlorhexidine (Figure 8-7).[114,125,127,128]

In vitro studies have reported that calcium hydroxide combined with camphorated paramonochlorophenol as a biologically active vehicle has a broader antimicrobial spectrum and eliminates resistant microorganisms. It has a larger radius of antimicrobial action,

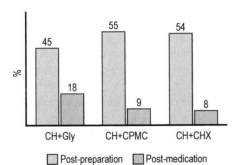

FIGURE 8-7 Studies showing the incidence of positive cultures after chemomechanical preparation and intracanal medication with calcium hydroxide (CH) in an inert, glycerine (Gly) or biologically active, camphorated paramonochlorophenol (CPMC) or chlorhexidine (CHX) vehicles.

eliminates microorganisms located in regions more distant from the locality where it was placed, kills microorganisms faster and is less affected by serum and necrotic tissue than mixtures of calcium hydroxide in inert vehicles.[110,114,123,125,129–131] Glycerine is added to the calcium hydroxide paste to dilute the camphorated paramonochlorophenol and to facilitate both handling and removal of the mixture from the canal. Although camphorated paramonochlorophenol exhibits high toxicity when used alone, satisfactory biocompatibility results have been observed in animal studies with this combination.[132,133] Clinical studies evaluating the incidence of postoperative pain,[134] bacterial reduction[22,28] and long-term treatment outcomes[135] have reported optimal results when using an antibacterial protocol that includes a 7-day interappointment medication with a combination of calcium hydroxide, camphorated paramonochlorophenol and glycerine.

Chlorhexidine has also been proposed as a biologically active vehicle in combination with calcium hydroxide. *In vitro* studies have shown conflicting results for this combination, with some reporting that the antimicrobial effects were higher than calcium hydroxide alone,[136] whereas others found no significant difference.[128,130,137–139] The antibacterial efficacy of chlorhexidine may be significantly reduced after it is mixed with calcium hydroxide.[130,136,139] Clinical data have also been inconsistent; some studies have found no significant difference between calcium hydroxide alone, or mixed with chlorhexidine, in terms of bacterial reduction[120,140]; whereas other studies have reported satisfactory results for this mixture not only in terms of bacterial elimination[23,58,141,142] but also in lipopolysaccharide inactivation.[142]

Calcium hydroxide combined with chlorhexidine has a high pH, similar to calcium hydroxide in water.[128,141] The antimicrobial activity of chlorhexidine is influenced by pH; the optimum is pH 5.5 to 7.0. At a higher pH, it precipitates and may not be available to act as an antimicrobial agent.[141] Despite the expected greater loss of chlorhexidine when mixed with calcium hydroxide, the combined antimicrobial effects may still be of significance, as revealed by clinical studies.[23,141,58,142] The antibacterial effects of this combination may be related to small residues of active chlorhexidine still present in the mixture and/or due to the high pH of the mixture itself.

A combination of calcium hydroxide with Ledermix (Haupt Pharma GmbH, Wolfratshausen, Germany), a steroid (triamcinolone)/antibiotic (demeclocycline) compound, has been recommended to take advantage of the action of the individual ingredients.[143] Odontopaste (Australian Dental Manufacturing, Kenmore Hills, Brisbane, Queensland, Australia), another steroid (triamcinolone)/antibiotic (clindamycin) preparation, has also been combined with calcium hydroxide as an intracanal medication. However, studies have demonstrated that when Ledermix or Odontopaste is mixed with calcium hydroxide, it resulted in a significant loss of antibiotic activity[144] and rapid destruction of the steroid component.[145]

OTHER INTRACANAL MEDICAMENTS

In the past, several toxic substances, including aldehydes (formocresol, tricresol formalin, glutaraldehyde) and phenols (camphorated phenol or paramonochlorophenol, cresatin, eugenol), have been used as intracanal medicaments. Most are toxic to host tissues, some are allergenic and may even be carcinogenic; some are ineffective in clinical practice. Consequently, the use of most of these substances has been discontinued, and they are no longer recommended. Apart from calcium hydroxide, other medicaments in use include chlorhexidine and antibiotics.

Chlorhexidine

Chlorhexidine is a cationic bis-biguanide, insoluble in water, and is formulated with either gluconic or acetic acid to form water-soluble digluconate, or diacetate, salts. It has been widely used as a topical antiseptic solution, and effective concentrations range from 0.12% to 2%. Chlorhexidine is highly effective against several gram-positive and gram-negative oral bacterial species as well as yeasts.[146–149] Chlorhexidine's properties include substantivity,[150,151] which is the ability to be adsorbed into the tissues and be released slowly over an extended period, remaining active even after its removal; it also exhibits low irritancy to living tissues.[152,153] However, chlorhexidine is not a tissue solvent and cases of hypersensitivity have been reported.[154]

Depending on the concentration, chlorhexidine may be bacteriostatic or bactericidal. At lower concentrations, chlorhexidine penetrates and disrupts the bacterial cytoplasmic membrane resulting in leakage of cytoplasmic components, a bacteriostatic effect. At higher bactericidal concentrations, chlorhexidine enters the bacterial cytoplasm via the damaged membranes and interacts with phosphated entities to form irreversible precipitates,[147,155] killing the cell.

As an intracanal medicament, chlorhexidine has been shown *in vitro* to be more effective than calcium hydroxide in disinfecting dentinal tubules.[130,139,156–158] However, clinical studies found no difference in the incidence of postoperative pain in treatment, or retreatment, cases after intracanal medication with either chlorhexidine or calcium hydroxide.[159] Likewise, no significant differences were observed for the antimicrobial effects of 7-day intracanal medication with calcium hydroxide, 2% chlorhexidine, or a combination of both.[120,160] However, a study[161] reported that a 14-day dressing with calcium hydroxide produced significantly better antimicrobial results than with 2% chlorhexidine gel. No significant improvement in disinfection after chemomechanical preparation was observed after a final rinse with a commercially available mixture of a tetracycline isomer, an acid and a detergent (BioPure MTAD, Dentsply Tulsa Dental, Tulsa, OK, USA) followed by intracanal medication with 2% chlorhexidine gel.[162] Treatment protocols using either 2% chlorhexidine liquid, or calcium hydroxide, as interappointment dressings resulted in similar long-term outcomes.[163]

Antibiotics

Antibiotics are naturally occurring substances of microbial origin, or synthetic, or semisynthetic, substances that exhibit antimicrobial activity in low concentrations by killing, or inhibiting the growth of, selective microorganisms. Antibiotics exert their actions on specific groups of microorganisms, and its range of effectiveness is termed its *spectrum*. The spectrum is broad when the antibiotic is effective against a wide variety of gram-positive and gram-negative bacteria; the spectrum is small when it acts against a reduced number of susceptible species. Since antibiotics used systemically, or topically, are usually successful in treating infections in the body, their use as topical antimicrobial agents in root canal treatment was suggested.

The main concerns about using antibiotics as intracanal medicaments include the possibility of:

- Sensitization. The patient is sensitized to that drug and becomes predisposed to further allergic reactions when in contact with the same drug for another purpose. This is more critical with penicillins, cephalosporins and sulphonamide, for which severe and common allergic reactions have been reported.
- Development of resistant strains. The inappropriate use of antibiotics is to be discouraged and avoided because of the risks of developing resistant bacterial strains that may cause diseases that are difficult or even impossible to treat.[164] The kinetics of antibiotics applied topically in the root canal is not known; whether it can reach and affect the resident host microbiota is unclear. Bacterial strains carrying antibiotic resistance genes in endodontic infections have been detected.[165–167] If the same antibiotic is used topically in the canal, these resistant strains may selectively survive and cause persistent infections; this is especially true for penicillins, tetracyclines, and macrolides. From a therapeutic standpoint, if a persistent infection caused by antibiotic resistant strains becomes acute, it may render ineffective, when required the use of systemic antibiotics.
- Limited spectrum. No antibiotic is effective against all endodontic pathogens. Endodontic infections are characterized by multispecies communities with a large interindividual variability in the bacterial species composition.[168] Compared with the disinfectants discussed in this chapter, antibiotics have a more restricted spectrum of activity and hence may be ineffective against all pathogens involved.

Penicillin was proposed as an intracanal medication more than half a century ago as part of Grossman's polyantibiotic paste.[102] However, the risks of sensitization and the presence of beta-lactamase producing bacterial strains in the root canal resulted in a lack of justification for its continued use as an interappointment dressing.

Tetracycline is widely used in periodontics and has been included in some formulations for endodontic use. For instance, Ledermix contains a tetracycline derivative (demeclocycline) and a corticosteroid (triamcinolone).[106] Biopure MTAD (Dentsply, Tulsa

Dental) is an irrigating solution containing a mixture of tetracycline derivative (doxycycline), an acid (citric acid) and a detergent (Tween 80) and has been recommended for canal disinfection and smear layer removal.[169,170] In a clinical study, no significant improvement in disinfection was observed when MTAD was used as a final rinse.[162] Furthermore, the detection of tetracycline-resistant genes in endodontic bacteria means its use and effectiveness is questionable.[165–167]

Minocycline, also a tetracycline derivative, along with metronidazole and ciprofloxacin, are constituents of triple antibiotic paste,[171,172] recommended as intracanal medication in regenerative endodontic procedures for immature teeth with necrotic pulps and apical periodontitis.[173,174] Although good results have been reported for the use of triple antibiotic paste in such cases, for safety and effectiveness, there is still a need to establish and to control the concentrations of the antibiotics, to ensure that it is adequate.[175]

Clindamycin has a good spectrum of activity against endodontic pathogens. It has been tested as an interappointment dressing,[176] but its effects were limited and not better than calcium hydroxide. Odontopaste is a zinc oxide–based preparation containing a corticosteroid (triamcinolone) and an antibiotic (clindamycin); it has been marketed as an alternative to Ledermix.

Endodontic Treatment in Single or Multiple Visits

Single-visit treatment implies performing chemomechanical procedures and placing a permanent root canal filling at the very same appointment. The decision as to whether the root canal treatment can be completed in one, or more, visits depends primarily on the condition of the pulp and the periradicular tissues. Other factors such as the clinician's experience and skills, technical difficulties and patient compliance may also influence this decision.

Whenever possible, noninfected vital teeth should be treated in a single visit. Infected teeth, especially if apical periodontitis is present, should be approached differently. As discussed earlier, it is questionable whether chemomechanical procedures alone will predictably achieve adequate disinfection in all cases; especially, if infection is present in anatomic areas inaccessible to instruments and irrigants.

A debatable issue in clinical endodontic practice is whether a medicament that remains in the root canal between appointments will significantly improve disinfection and enhance periradicular tissue healing. Chemomechanical procedures are highly effective, and therefore, of crucial importance in the control of root canal infection.[17,24,27,177,178] However, residual bacteria have been detected in 40% to 60% of the canals even after chemomechanical preparation when sodium hypochlorite, or chlorhexidine, was used as an irrigant.[17,19,20,22,23,26,27,56,81,179,180]

There is a paucity of well-controlled clinical studies comparing the outcome of the endodontic treatment of teeth with apical periodontitis performed in one, or more, visits. Some studies have reported that two, or more, visits, with calcium hydroxide as the intracanal medication, resulted in an outcome 10% to 20% higher than with one-visit treatment (Figure 8-8).[10,16,181–184]

Nonetheless, other studies showed virtually no difference,[185] or an approximate 10% more favourable outcome, with single-visit treatment (see Figure 8-8).[186–188] Systematic reviews on single- versus multiple-visit treatments[189–191] showed no significant differences in treatment outcome but data available have been, so far, insufficient for definitive conclusions. A study[192] using a large sample size composed of teeth treated by only one operator indicated that treatment performed in two, or more, visits using calcium hydroxide for intracanal medication resulted in a significantly higher favourable outcome rate compared with cases treated in a single visit; this is consistent with studies showing that the best protocol for infection control involves the use of an intracanal medication in a two-visit treatment approach.[18,19,25,81,82] Numerous histological studies in animals have also reported a significantly better outcome for treatments performed in two visits rather than one visit.[133,193–196] However, treatment in more than two visits should be avoided whenever possible as it predisposes to the development of secondary infections[197] and reduced survival of the treated teeth.[198]

Other Indications for Intracanal Medication

Apart from enhancing disinfection in routine cases of primary or posttreatment apical periodontitis, intracanal medication has also been recommended for other situations.

PREVENT ROOT CANAL CONTAMINATION

In vital teeth, in cases where treatment could not be completed in a single visit, an intracanal medicament is placed to act as a physico-chemical barrier to protect against, or at least delay, microbial contamination of the canal between appointments. Contamination might occur as a result of microleakage or breakage of the temporary restoration.

PAIN CONTROL

Pain of endodontic origin is associated with inflammation and is usually caused by infection. Therefore, pain control using intracanal medicaments is related to infection control. The use of antiinflammatory drugs,

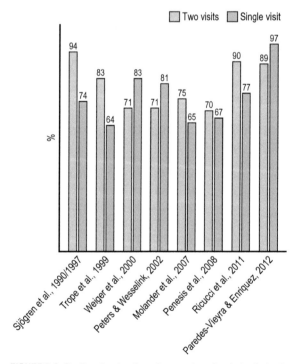

FIGURE 8-8 Studies showing the outcome rates of endodontic treatment performed in one or two/multiple visits.

such as corticosteroids[199] or nonsteroidal drugs,[200] has been recommended in some cases, but it is advisable to limit their use only for infection-free, vital cases. Antiinflammatory drugs can also be used for the prevention of pain in cases where it is most anticipated. Examples included a vital tooth that had not been completely instrumented, or had been overinstrumented. Teeth with persistent symptoms after chemomechanical procedures are usually associated with persistent infection and should be managed similar to cases with persistent exudation.

CONTROL PERSISTENT EXUDATION

The presence of a persistent exudate in the canal after chemomechancial preparation is highly suggestive of recalcitrant infection, especially if the exudate is purulent. However, occurrence of a serous exudate, a condition clinically referred to as a 'weeping' canal, may be caused by infection, but it can also be associated with a relatively large, opened apical foramen, natural or overinstrumented, in communication with a pocket cyst.

Intracanal medication is used in these cases to act indirectly on the inflammatory process by helping to eliminate its primary cause, i.e., residual microorganisms in the apical part of the canal. Topical intracanal use of antiinflammatory drugs, such as corticosteroids, which act directly on inflammation, are not generally recommended in these cases because their action is on the effect rather than the cause, usually microorganisms involved in persistent, or secondary, infections.

IMPROVE ROOT CANAL CLEANLINESS

In teeth with aberrant internal anatomy, due to internal resorption or developmental anomalies, calcium hydroxide can be used to help clean areas untouched by instruments because it can dissolve organic matter[201,202]; soft tissue pretreated with calcium hydroxide is more rapidly dissolved by sodium hypochlorite.[201] It is recommended that calcium hydroxide be packed into the root canal irregularities, and at the subsequent visit, it is removed using files in conjunction with copious sodium hypochlorite irrigation. Ultrasonic activation of the sodium hypochlorite irrigant can also improve cleaning of these less easily accessible areas.

CONTROL INFLAMMATORY ROOT RESORPTION

In teeth with external inflammatory root resorption, calcium hydroxide has been used to resolve the resorptive process. External inflammatory root resorption is due to intraradicular infection and can be associated with chronic apical periodontitis, or following traumatic injury to the tooth (Figure 8-9). Inflammatory resorption of the root surface may progress rapidly and lead to significant tooth tissue loss in a matter of months if left untreated.[203] In such cases, root canal treatment, including calcium hydroxide intracanal medication, is usually effective.[182,204,205]

On the other hand, external noninflammatory root resorption, or replacement resorption, observed after replantation of avulsed teeth, may proceed irrespective of treatment or medicament used.[206] In such cases, calcium hydroxide is apparently ineffective[207,208]; long-term use of calcium hydroxide may even contribute to increasing the likelihood of replacement resorption.[209,210] Since the cells involved and the biochemical mechanisms of root resorption are basically the same, the difference in outcome when using calcium hydroxide is suggestive that it does not act directly on the resorptive process itself, i.e., by neutralizing osteoclast acids, creating unfavourable conditions for osteoclast

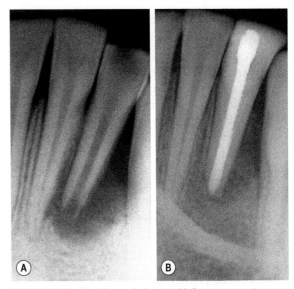

FIGURE 8-9 Tooth with an apical external inflammatory root resorption associated with apical periodontitis. Before (A) and after (B) treatment with long-term calcium hydroxide medication. (Reproduced courtesy of RGD Carvalho.)

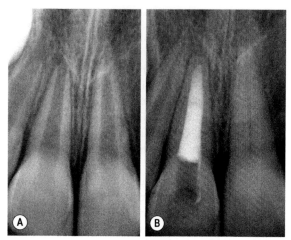

FIGURE 8-10 Immature tooth with pulp necrosis and apical periodontitis. Before (A) and after (B) apexification procedure using calcium hydroxide. (Reproduced courtesy of RGD Carvalho.)

enzymes, or killing osteoclasts itself. Instead, the good results with calcium hydroxide medication, in cases of external inflammatory root resorption, are related to its antimicrobial effects on bacteria located within dentinal tubules and other anatomical irregularities, which induce and maintain inflammation and the resorptive process.[205]

INDUCTION OF HARD TISSUE FORMATION

In immature teeth with necrotic pulps and open apices, calcium hydroxide may again be used, after chemomechanical preparation, to help eliminate infection (Figure 8-10). It also serves as a long-term dressing to maintain the environment free of microorganisms until repair of the periradicular tissues ensues and an apical barrier is achieved by the formation of a cementum-like hard tissue. Alternative treatment modalities for immature teeth with necrotic pulps and apical periodontitis include the use of bioceramic materials, such as the mineral trioxide aggregate (MTA), or regenerative endodontic procedures.

Suggested Clinical Procedures

NONINFECTED (VITAL) CASES

After access cavity preparation under dental dam isolation, pulp extirpation, copious sodium hypochlorite irrigation and chemomechanical preparation are carried out; if time and clinical conditions permit, the root canal should be obturated during the same visit. If this is not possible, calcium hydroxide paste in an inert vehicle should be placed and root canal filling scheduled for the next visit. With these cases, efforts should always be made to complete chemomechanical cleaning and shaping early, preferably at the first visit. Where it was not possible to complete instrumentation, in selected cases, a corticosteroid medicament may be placed to prevent postoperative pain.

INFECTED (NECROTIC OR RETREATMENT) CASES

Ideally, teeth with infected root canals and apical periodontitis should be treated in two visits. At the first appointment, the root canals should be completely cleaned and shaped in the presence of copious and frequent irrigation of 0.5% to 5% sodium hypochlorite solution. Then, the smear layer is removed by flushing the canal with an aqueous solution of ethylenediaminetetraacetic acid (EDTA). Passive ultrasonic activation of the sodium hypochlorite irrigant (Chapter 7) or a final rinse with chlorhexidine may be carried out to improve canal disinfection.[58,211,212] Next, calcium hydroxide paste, in a biologically active vehicle if desired, is placed into the entire length of the prepared root canal. The use of an additive medicament with calcium hydroxide is especially relevant in retreatment cases, because of the increased risk of the presence of microbial species, such as *E. faecalis*[112] and *C. albicans*,[126] which are resistant to calcium hydroxide. At the second appointment, the calcium hydroxide dressing is removed and the root canal filled.

If canal preparation cannot be completed at the first visit, there may be no room for placement of calcium hydroxide; tissue remnants can significantly dampen its effects anyway. With these cases, following final irrigation with sodium hypochlorite, excess solution is removed by aspiration and the root canal is then coronally sealed. Root canal preparation will have to be completed at the second appointment, followed by placement of calcium hydroxide intracanal medication.

APPLICATION OF CALCIUM HYDROXIDE MEDICAMENT

There are many commercially available calcium hydroxide products and some are packaged in a syringe to facilitate placement. However, a Lentulo spiral filler is an efficient instrument for the placement of calcium hydroxide paste.[213,214] The largest Lentulo spiral filler that reaches to within 2 to 3 mm short of the working length without binding to the canal walls is selected. Operated in a low-speed handpiece, two or three applications of calcium hydroxide paste are placed into the canal.

Learning Outcomes

After reading this chapter, the reader should be able to explain and discuss the:
- indications for using intracanal medication in endodontic treatment;
- properties and modes of action of different intracanal medicaments;
- different types of endodontic infections and cite the most important associated microbial species;
- way bacteria colonize the root canal system;
- different clinical conditions based on presence or absence of infection and how to manage them properly;
- clinical antimicrobial effectiveness during the different phases of endodontic treatment and the need for enhanced canal disinfection to achieve a favourable treatment outcome.

REFERENCES

1. Siqueira JF Jr. Treatment of endodontic infections. London: Quintessence Publishing; 2011.
2. Langeland K. Tissue response to dental caries. Endodontics and Dental Traumatology 1987;3:149–71.
3. Ricucci D, Siqueira JF Jr. Fate of the tissue in lateral canals and apical ramifications in response to pathologic conditions and treatment procedures. Journal of Endodontics 2010; 36:1–15.
4. Kakehashi S, Stanley HR, Fitzgerald RJ. The effects of surgical exposures of dental pulps in germ-free and conventional laboratory rats. Oral Surgery, Oral Medicine, and Oral Pathology 1965;20:340–9.
5. Sundqvist G. Bacteriological studies of necrotic dental pulps [Odontological Dissertation no.7]. Umea, Sweden: University of Umea; 1976.
6. Ricucci D, Siqueira JF Jr, Bate AL, et al. Histologic investigation of root canal-treated teeth with apical periodontitis: a retrospective study from twenty-four patients. Journal of Endodontics 2009;35:493–502.
7. Ricucci D, Siqueira JF Jr. Biofilms and apical periodontitis: study of prevalence and association with clinical and histopathologic findings. Journal of Endodontics 2010;36:1277–88.
8. Siqueira JF Jr. Strategies to treat infected root canals. Journal of the California Dental Association 2001;29:825–37.
9. Orstavik D. Root canal disinfection: a review of concepts and recent developments. Australian Endodontic Journal 2003;29:70–4.
10. Sjögren U, Hagglund B, Sundqvist G, et al. Factors affecting the long-term results of endodontic treatment. Journal of Endodontics 1990;16:498–504.
11. Hoskinson SE, Ng YL, Hoskinson AE, et al. A retrospective comparison of outcome of root canal treatment using two different protocols. Oral Surgery, Oral Medicine, Oral Pathology, Oral Radiology, and Endodontics 2002;93:705–15.
12. Chugal NM, Clive JM, Spångberg LS. Endodontic infection: some biologic and treatment factors associated with outcome. Oral Surgery, Oral Medicine, Oral Pathology, Oral Radiology, and Endodontics 2003;96:81–90.
13. Orstavik D, Qvist V, Stoltze K. A multivariate analysis of the outcome of endodontic treatment. European Journal of Oral Sciences 2004;112:224–30.
14. de Chevigny C, Dao TT, Basrani BR, et al. Treatment outcome in endodontics: the Toronto study – phase 4: initial treatment. Journal of Endodontics 2008;34:258–63.
15. Cheung GS, Liu CS. A retrospective study of endodontic treatment outcome between nickel-titanium rotary and stainless steel hand filing techniques. Journal of Endodontics 2009; 35:938–43.
16. Sjögren U, Figdor D, Persson S, et al. Influence of infection at the time of root filling on the outcome of endodontic treatment of teeth with apical periodontitis. International Endodontic Journal 1997;30:297–306.
17. Byström A, Sundqvist G. The antibacterial action of sodium hypochlorite and EDTA in 60 cases of endodontic therapy. International Endodontic Journal 1985;18:35–40.
18. Shuping GB, Ørstavik D, Sigurdsson A, et al. Reduction of intracanal bacteria using nickel-titanium rotary instrumentation and various medications. Journal of Endodontics 2000; 26:751–5.
19. McGurkin-Smith R, Trope M, Caplan D, et al. Reduction of intracanal bacteria using GT rotary instrumentation, 5.25% NaOCl, EDTA, and Ca(OH)$_2$. Journal of Endodontics 2005;31:359–63.
20. Paquette L, Legner M, Fillery ED, et al. Antibacterial efficacy of chlorhexidine gluconate intracanal medication *in vivo*. Journal of Endodontics 2007;33:788–95.
21. Siqueira JF Jr, Guimarães-Pinto T, Rôças IN. Effects of chemomechanical preparation with 2.5% sodium hypochlorite and intracanal medication with calcium hydroxide on cultivable bacteria in infected root canals. Journal of Endodontics 2007;33:800–5.
22. Siqueira JF Jr, Magalhães KM, Rôças IN. Bacterial reduction in infected root canals treated with 2.5% NaOCl as an irrigant and calcium hydroxide/camphorated paramonochlorophenol paste as an intracanal dressing. Journal of Endodontics 2007;33:667–72.
23. Siqueira JF Jr, Paiva SS, Rôças IN. Reduction in the cultivable bacterial populations in infected root canals by a chlorhexidine-based antimicrobial protocol. Journal of Endodontics 2007;33:541–7.
24. Siqueira JF Jr, Rôças IN, Paiva SS, et al. Bacteriologic investigation of the effects of sodium hypochlorite and chlorhexidine

during the endodontic treatment of teeth with apical periodontitis. Oral Surgery, Oral Medicine, Oral Pathology, Oral Radiology, and Endodontics 2007;104:122–30.

25. Huffaker SK, Safavi K, Spångberg LS, et al. Influence of a passive sonic irrigation system on the elimination of bacteria from root canal systems: a clinical study. Journal of Endodontics 2010;36:1315–8.

26. Rôças IN, Siqueira JF Jr. Identification of bacteria enduring endodontic treatment procedures by a combined reverse transcriptase-polymerase chain reaction and reverse-capture checkerboard approach. Journal of Endodontics 2010;36: 45–52.

27. Rôças IN, Siqueira JF Jr. Comparison of the *in vivo* antimicrobial effectiveness of sodium hypochlorite and chlorhexidine used as root canal irrigants: a molecular microbiology study. Journal of Endodontics 2011;37:143–50.

28. Rôças IN, Siqueira JF Jr. *In vivo* antimicrobial effects of endodontic treatment procedures as assessed by molecular microbiologic techniques. Journal of Endodontics 2011;37: 304–10.

29. Paiva SS, Siqueira JF Jr, Rôças IN, et al. Supplementing the antimicrobial effects of chemomechanical debridement with either passive ultrasonic irrigation or a final rinse with chlorhexidine: a clinical study. Journal of Endodontics 2012;38: 1202–6.

30. Zeldow BI, Ingle JI. Correlation of the positive culture to the prognosis of endodontically treated teeth: a clinical study. Journal of the American Dental Association 1963;66: 9–13.

31. Engström B, Hard AF, Segerstad L, et al. Correlation of positive cultures with the prognosis for root canal treatment. Odontologisk Revy 1964;15:257–70.

32. Oliet S, Sorin SM. Evaluation of clinical results based upon culturing root canals. Journal of the British Endodontic Society 1969;3:3–6.

33. Heling B, Shapira J. Roentgenologic and clinical evaluation of endodontically treated teeth with or without negative culture. Quintessence International 1978;11:79–84.

34. Sundqvist G, Figdor D, Persson S, et al. Microbiologic analysis of teeth with failed endodontic treatment and the outcome of conservative re-treatment. Oral Surgery, Oral Medicine, Oral Pathology, Oral Radiology, and Endodontics 1998;85:86–93.

35. Waltimo T, Trope M, Haapasalo M, et al. Clinical efficacy of treatment procedures in endodontic infection control and one year follow-up of periapical healing. Journal of Endodontics 2005;31:863–6.

36. Fabricius L, Dahlén G, Sundqvist G, et al. Influence of residual bacteria on periapical tissue healing after chemomechanical treatment and root filling of experimentally infected monkey teeth. European Journal of Oral Sciences 2006;114: 278–85.

37. Siqueira JF Jr, Rôças IN. Optimising single-visit disinfection with supplementary approaches: a quest for predictability. Australian Endodontic Journal 2011;37:92–8.

38. Möller AJR, Fabricius L, Dahlén G, et al. Influence on periapical tissues of indigenous oral bacteria and necrotic pulp tissue in monkeys. Scandinavian Journal of Dental Research 1981; 89:475–84.

39. Slots J, Sabeti M, Simon JH. Herpesviruses in periapical pathosis: an etiopathogenic relationship? Oral Surgery, Oral Medicine, Oral Pathology, Oral Radiology, and Endodontics 2003; 96:327–31.

40. Siqueira JF Jr, Sen BH. Fungi in endodontic infections. Oral Surgery, Oral Medicine, Oral Pathology, Oral Radiology, and Endodontics 2004;97:632–41.

41. Vianna ME, Conrads G, Gomes BPFA, et al. Identification and quantification of archaea involved in primary endodontic infections. Journal of Clinical Microbiology 2006;44:1274–82.

42. Ferreira DC, Paiva SS, Carmo FL, et al. Identification of herpesviruses types 1 to 8 and human papillomavirus in acute apical abscesses. Journal of Endodontics 2011;37:10–6.

43. Siqueira JF Jr, Rôças IN. Diversity of endodontic microbiota revisited. Journal of Dental Research 2009;88:969–81.

44. Donlan RM, Costerton JW. Biofilms: survival mechanisms of clinically relevant microorganisms. Clinical Microbiology Reviews 2002;15:167–93.

45. Costerton JW. The biofilm primer. Berlin, Heidelberg: Springer-Verlag; 2007.

46. Nair PNR. Light and electron microscopic studies of root canal flora and periapical lesions. Journal of Endodontics 1987;13: 29–39.

47. Molven O, Olsen I, Kerekes K. Scanning electron microscopy of bacteria in the apical part of root canals in permanent teeth with periapical lesions. Endodontics and Dental Traumatology 1991;7:226–9.

48. Siqueira JF Jr, Rôças IN, Lopes HP. Patterns of microbial colonization in primary root canal infections. Oral Surgery, Oral Medicine, Oral Pathology, Oral Radiology, and Endodontics 2002;93:174–8.

49. Parsek MR, Singh PK. Bacterial biofilms: an emerging link to disease pathogenesis. Annual Review of Microbiology 2003; 57:677–701.

50. Hall-Stoodley L, Stoodley P. Evolving concepts in biofilm infections. Cellular Microbiology 2009;11:1034–43.

51. Costerton JW, Stewart PS, Greenberg EP. Bacterial biofilms: a common cause of persistent infections. Science 1999;284: 1318–22.

52. Siqueira JF Jr. Endodontic infections: concepts, paradigms, and perspectives. Oral Surgery, Oral Medicine, Oral Pathology, Oral Radiology, and Endodontics 2002;94:281–93.

53. Siqueira JF Jr, Rôças IN. Exploiting molecular methods to explore endodontic infections, Part II. Redefining the endodontic microbiota. Journal of Endodontics 2005;31:488–98.

54. Santos AL, Siqueira JF Jr, Rôças IN, et al. Comparing the bacterial diversity of acute and chronic dental root canal infections. PLoS ONE 2011;6:e28088.

55. Hong BY, Lee TK, Lim SM, et al. Microbial analysis in primary and persistent endodontic infections by using pyrosequencing. Journal of Endodontics 2013;39:1136–40.

56. Vianna ME, Horz HP, Gomes BP, et al. *In vivo* evaluation of microbial reduction after chemo-mechanical preparation of human root canals containing necrotic pulp tissue. International Endodontic Journal 2006;39:484–92.

57. Sakamoto M, Siqueira JF Jr, Rôças IN, et al. Bacterial reduction and persistence after endodontic treatment procedures. Oral Microbiology and Immunology 2007;22:19–23.

58. Paiva SS, Siqueira JF Jr, Rôças IN, et al. Clinical antimicrobial efficacy of NiTi rotary instrumentation with NaOCl irrigation, final rinse with chlorhexidine and interappointment medication: a molecular study. International Endodontic Journal 2013;46:225–33.

59. Sakamoto M, Rôças IN, Siqueira JF Jr, et al. Molecular analysis of bacteria in asymptomatic and symptomatic endodontic

infections. Oral Microbiology and Immunology 2006;21: 112–22.

60. Siqueira JF Jr, Rôças IN, Rosado AS. Investigation of bacterial communities associated with asymptomatic and symptomatic endodontic infections by denaturing gradient gel electrophoresis fingerprinting approach. Oral Microbiology and Immunology 2004;19:363–70.

61. Baumgartner JC, Falkler WA Jr. Bacteria in the apical 5 mm of infected root canals. Journal of Endodontics 1991;17: 380–3.

62. Sundqvist G. Associations between microbial species in dental root canal infections. Oral Microbiology and Immunology 1992;7:257–62.

63. Munson MA, Pitt Ford T, Chong B, et al. Molecular and cultural analysis of the microflora associated with endodontic infections. Journal of Dental Research 2002;81: 761–6.

64. Gomes BP, Pinheiro ET, Gade-Neto CR, et al. Microbiological examination of infected dental root canals. Oral Microbiology and Immunology 2004;19:71–6.

65. Siqueira JF Jr, Rôças IN. Uncultivated phylotypes and newly named species associated with primary and persistent endodontic infections. Journal of Clinical Microbiology 2005;43: 3314–19.

66. Rôças IN, Siqueira JF Jr. Root canal microbiota of teeth with chronic apical periodontitis. Journal of Clinical Microbiology 2008;46:3599–606.

67. Sakamoto M, Siqueira JF Jr, Rôças IN, et al. Diversity of spirochetes in endodontic infections. Journal of Clinical Microbiology 2009;47:1352–7.

68. Siqueira JF Jr, Rôças IN. Distinctive features of the microbiota associated with different forms of apical periodontitis. Journal of Clinical Microbiology 2009;doi:10.3402/jom. v3401i3400.2009.

69. Ribeiro AC, Matarazzo F, Faveri M, et al. Exploring bacterial diversity of endodontic microbiota by cloning and sequencing 16S rRNA. Journal of Endodontics 2011;37:922–6.

70. Rôças IN, Neves MA, Provenzano JC, et al. Susceptibility of as-yet-uncultivated and difficult-to-culture bacteria to chemomechanical procedures. Journal of Endodontics 2014;40: 33–7.

71. Lin LM, Pascon EA, Skribner J, et al. Clinical, radiographic, and histologic study of endodontic treatment failures. Oral Surgery, Oral Medicine, and Oral Pathology 1991;71: 603–11.

72. Pinheiro ET, Gomes BP, Ferraz CC, et al. Microorganisms from canals of root-filled teeth with periapical lesions. International Endodontic Journal 2003;36:1–11.

73. Siqueira JF Jr, Rôças IN. Polymerase chain reaction-based analysis of microorganisms associated with failed endodontic treatment. Oral Surgery, Oral Medicine, Oral Pathology, Oral Radiology, and Endodontics 2004;97:85–94.

74. Rôças IN, Siqueira JF Jr. Characterization of microbiota of root canal-treated teeth with posttreatment disease. Journal of Clinical Microbiology 2012;50:1721–4.

75. Rôças IN, Siqueira JF Jr, Santos KR. Association of *Enterococcus faecalis* with different forms of periradicular diseases. Journal of Endodontics 2004;30:315–20.

76. Fouad AF, Zerella J, Barry J, et al. Molecular detection of *Enterococcus* species in root canals of therapy-resistant endodontic infections. Oral Surgery, Oral Medicine, Oral Pathology, Oral Radiology, and Endodontics 2005;99: 112–8.

77. Sedgley C, Nagel A, Dahlen G, et al. Real-time quantitative polymerase chain reaction and culture analyses of *Enterococcus faecalis* in root canals. Journal of Endodontics 2006;32: 173–7.

78. Gomes BP, Pinheiro ET, Jacinto RC, et al. Microbial analysis of canals of root-filled teeth with periapical lesions using polymerase chain reaction. Journal of Endodontics 2008; 34:537–40.

79. Peciuliene V, Reynaud AH, Balciuniene I, et al. Isolation of yeasts and enteric bacteria in root-filled teeth with chronic apical periodontitis. International Endodontic Journal 2001;34:429–34.

80. Sakamoto M, Siqueira JF Jr, Rôças IN, et al. Molecular analysis of the root canal microbiota associated with endodontic treatment failures. Oral Microbiology and Immunology 2008;23: 275–81.

81. Sjögren U, Figdor D, Spångberg L, et al. The antimicrobial effect of calcium hydroxide as a short-term intracanal dressing. International Endodontic Journal 1991;24:119–25.

82. Vera J, Siqueira JF Jr, Ricucci D, et al. One- versus two-visit endodontic treatment of teeth with apical periodontitis: a histobacteriologic study. Journal of Endodontics 2012;38: 1040–52.

83. Rôças IN, Lima KC, Siqueira JF Jr. Reduction in bacterial counts in infected root canals after rotary or hand nickel-titanium instrumentation – a clinical study. International Endodontic Journal 2013;46:681–7.

84. Walton RE. Histologic evaluation of different methods of enlarging the pulp canal space. Journal of Endodontics 1976;2:304–11.

85. Nair PN, Henry S, Cano V, et al. Microbial status of apical root canal system of human mandibular first molars with primary apical periodontitis after 'one-visit' endodontic treatment. Oral Surgery, Oral Medicine, Oral Pathology, Oral Radiology, and Endodontics 2005;99:231–52.

86. Siqueira JF Jr, Araujo MC, Garcia PF, et al. Histological evaluation of the effectiveness of five instrumentation techniques for cleaning the apical third of root canals. Journal of Endodontics 1997;23:499–502.

87. Peters OA, Schönenberger K, Laib A. Effects of four Ni-Ti preparation techniques on root canal geometry assessed by micro-computed tomography. International Endodontic Journal 2001;34:221–30.

88. Paque F, Ganahl D, Peters OA. Effects of root canal preparation on apical geometry assessed by micro-computed tomography. Journal of Endodontics 2009;35:1056–9.

89. Siqueira JF Jr, Alves FR, Versiani MA, et al. Correlative bacteriologic and micro-computed tomographic analysis of mandibular molar mesial canals prepared by self-adjusting file, Reciproc, and Twisted File systems. Journal of Endodontics 2013;39:1044–50.

90. Versiani MA, Leoni GB, Steier L, et al. Micro-computed tomography study of oval-shaped canals prepared with the self-adjusting file, Reciproc, WaveOne, and ProTaper universal systems. Journal of Endodontics 2013;39:1060–6.

91. Wu M-K, van der Sluis LWM, Wesselink PR. The capability of two hand instrumentation techniques to remove the inner layer of dentine in oval canals. International Endodontic Journal 2003;36:218–24.

92. Ricucci D, Siqueira JF Jr. Apical actinomycosis as a continuum of intraradicular and extraradicular infection: case report and critical review on its involvement with treatment failure. Journal of Endodontics 2008;34:1124–9.

93. Kim S, Kratchman S. Modern endodontic surgery concepts and practice: a review. Journal of Endodontics 2006;32: 601–23.
94. De Deus QD. Frequency, location, and direction of the lateral, secondary, and accessory canals. Journal of Endodontics 1975;1:361–6.
95. Vertucci FJ. Root canal anatomy of the human permanent teeth. Oral Surgery, Oral Medicine, and Oral Pathology 1984; 58:589–99.
96. Peters LB, Wesselink PR, Buijs JF, et al. Viable bacteria in root dentinal tubules of teeth with apical periodontitis. Journal of Endodontics 2001;27:76–81.
97. Matsuo T, Shirakami T, Ozaki K, et al. An immunohistological study of the localization of bacteria invading root pulpal walls of teeth with periapical lesions. Journal of Endodontics 2003;29:194–200.
98. Miller WD. An introduction to the study of the bacterio-pathology of the dental pulp. Dental Cosmos 1894;36:505–28.
99. Buckley JP. The rational treatment of putrescent pulps and their sequelae. Dental Cosmos 1906;48:537–44.
100. Walkhoff O. Ein beitrag der pharmakologic der chlorophenol-Kanpfer-preparate. Zhnrztl Rdsch 1929;965.
101. Walkhoff O. Mein System der Medikamentösen Behandlung Schwerer Erkrankungen der Zahnpulpa und des Periodontiums. Berlin, Germany: Hermann Meusser; 1928.
102. Grossman LI. Polyantibiotic treatment of pulpless teeth. Journal of the American Dental Association 1951;43: 265–8.
103. Nygaard-Östby B. Introduction to endodontics. Oslo, Norway: Universitetsforlaget Oslo; 1971.
104. Markowitz K, Moynihan M, Liu M, et al. Biologic properties of eugenol and zinc oxide-eugenol. A clinically oriented review. Oral Surgery, Oral Medicine, and Oral Pathology 1992;73:729–37.
105. Schroeder A. Cortisone in dental surgery. International Dental Journal 1962;12:356–73.
106. Ehrmann EH. The effect of triamcinolone with tetracycline on the dental pulp and apical periodontium. Journal of Prosthetic Dentistry 1965;15:144–52.
107. Spångberg L, Engstrom B, Langeland K. Biologic effects of dental materials. III. Toxicity and antimicrobial effect of endodontic antiseptics in vitro. Oral Surgery, Oral Medicine, and Oral Pathology 1973;36:856–71.
108. Spångberg L, Rutberg M, Rydinge E. Biologic effects of endodontic antimicrobial agents. Journal of Endodontics 1979;5: 166–75.
109. Hermann BW. Calciumhydroxyd als mittel zum behandeln und füllen von zahnwurzelkanälen. Würzburg: Med. Diss; 1920. 48p.
110. Siqueira JF Jr, Lopes HP. Mechanisms of antimicrobial activity of calcium hydroxide: a critical review. International Endodontic Journal 1999;32:361–9.
111. Fava LR, Saunders WP. Calcium hydroxide pastes: classification and clinical indications. International Endodontic Journal 1999;32:257–82.
112. Byström A, Claesson R, Sundqvist G. The antibacterial effect of camphorated paramonochlorophenol, camphorated phenol and calcium hydroxide in the treatment of infected root canals. Endodontics and Dental Traumatology 1985;1: 170–5.
113. Georgopoulou M, Kontakiotis E, Nakou M. In vitro evaluation of the effectiveness of calcium hydroxide and paramonochlo-rophenol on anaerobic bacteria from the root canal. Endodontics and Dental Traumatology 1993;9:249–53.
114. Siqueira JF Jr, de Uzeda M. Influence of different vehicles on the antibacterial effects of calcium hydroxide. Journal of Endodontics 1998;24:663–5.
115. Safavi KE, Nichols FC. Effect of calcium hydroxide on bacterial lipopolysaccharide. Journal of Endodontics 1993;19: 76–8.
116. Jiang J, Zuo J, Chen SH, et al. Calcium hydroxide reduces lipopolysaccharide-stimulated osteoclast formation. Oral Surgery, Oral Medicine, Oral Pathology, Oral Radiology, and Endodontics 2003;95:348–54.
117. Tanomaru JM, Leonardo MR, Tanomaru Filho M, et al. Effect of different irrigation solutions and calcium hydroxide on bacterial LPS. International Endodontic Journal 2003;36: 733–9.
118. Baik JE, Kum KY, Yun CH, et al. Calcium hydroxide inactivates lipoteichoic acid from Enterococcus faecalis. Journal of Endodontics 2008;34:1355–9.
119. Peters LB, van Winkelhoff AJ, Buijs JF, et al. Effects of instrumentation, irrigation and dressing with calcium hydroxide on infection in pulpless teeth with periapical bone lesions. International Endodontic Journal 2002;35:13–21.
120. Manzur A, Gonzalez AM, Pozos A, et al. Bacterial quantification in teeth with apical periodontitis related to instrumentation and different intracanal medications: a randomized clinical trial. Journal of Endodontics 2007;33:114–8.
121. Portenier I, Haapasalo H, Rye A, et al. Inactivation of root canal medicaments by dentine, hydroxylapatite and bovine serum albumin. International Endodontic Journal 2001;34: 184–8.
122. Haapasalo M, Qian W, Portenier I, et al. Effects of dentin on the antimicrobial properties of endodontic medicaments. Journal of Endodontics 2007;33:917–25.
123. Oliveira JC, Alves FR, Uzeda M, et al. Influence of serum and necrotic soft tissue on the antimicrobial effects of intracanal medicaments. Brazilian Dental Journal 2010;21:295–300.
124. Haapasalo M, Ørstavik D. In vitro infection and disinfection of dentinal tubules. Journal of Dental Research 1987;66: 1375–9.
125. Siqueira JF Jr, de Uzeda M. Disinfection by calcium hydroxide pastes of dentinal tubules infected with two obligate and one facultative anaerobic bacteria. Journal of Endodontics 1996;22:674–6.
126. Waltimo TM, Siren EK, Ørstavik D, et al. Susceptibility of oral Candida species to calcium hydroxide in vitro. International Endodontic Journal 1999;32:94–8.
127. Waltimo TM, Ørstavik D, Siren EK, et al. In vitro susceptibility of Candida albicans to four disinfectants and their combinations. International Endodontic Journal 1999;32:421–9.
128. Siren EK, Haapasalo MP, Waltimo TM, et al. In vitro antibacterial effect of calcium hydroxide combined with chlorhexidine or iodine potassium iodide on Enterococcus faecalis. European Journal of Oral Sciences 2004;112:326–31.
129. Gomes BP, Ferraz CC, Garrido FD, et al. Microbial susceptibility to calcium hydroxide pastes and their vehicles. Journal of Endodontics 2002;28:758–61.
130. Siqueira JF Jr, Rôças IN, Lopes HP, et al. Elimination of Candida albicans infection of the radicular dentin by intracanal medications. Journal of Endodontics 2003;29:501–4.
131. Menezes MM, Valera MC, Jorge AO, et al. In vitro evaluation of the effectiveness of irrigants and intracanal medicaments on

microorganisms within root canals. International Endodontic Journal 2004;37:311–9.

132. Grecca FS, Leonardo MR, da Silva LA, et al. Radiographic evaluation of periradicular repair after endodontic treatment of dog's teeth with induced periradicular periodontitis. Journal of Endodontics 2001;27:610–2.

133. Silveira AM, Lopes HP, Siqueira JF Jr, et al. Periradicular repair after two-visit endodontic treatment using two different intracanal medications compared to single-visit endodontic treatment. Brazilian Dental Journal 2007;18:299–304.

134. Siqueira JF Jr, Rôças IN, Favieri A, et al. Incidence of postoperative pain after intracanal procedures based on an antimicrobial strategy. Journal of Endodontics 2002;28:457–60.

135. Siqueira JF Jr, Rôças IN, Riche FN, et al. Clinical outcome of the endodontic treatment of teeth with apical periodontitis using an antimicrobial protocol. Oral Surgery, Oral Medicine, Oral Pathology, Oral Radiology, and Endodontics 2008;106: 757–62.

136. Gomes BP, Vianna ME, Sena NT, et al. *In vitro* evaluation of the antimicrobial activity of calcium hydroxide combined with chlorhexidine gel used as intracanal medicament. Oral Surgery, Oral Medicine, Oral Pathology, Oral Radiology, and Endodontics 2006;102:544–50.

137. Evans MD, Baumgartner JC, Khemaleelakul SU, et al. Efficacy of calcium hydroxide: chlorhexidine paste as an intracanal medication in bovine dentin. Journal of Endodontics 2003;29: 338–9.

138. Podbielski A, Spahr A, Haller B. Additive antimicrobial activity of calcium hydroxide and chlorhexidine on common endodontic bacterial pathogens. Journal of Endodontics 2003;29: 340–5.

139. Schafer E, Bossmann K. Antimicrobial efficacy of chlorhexidine and two calcium hydroxide formulations against *Enterococcus faecalis*. Journal of Endodontics 2005;31:53–6.

140. Vianna ME, Horz HP, Conrads G, et al. Effect of root canal procedures on endotoxins and endodontic pathogens. Oral Microbiology and Immunology 2007;22:411–8.

141. Zerella JA, Fouad AF, Spångberg LS. Effectiveness of a calcium hydroxide and chlorhexidine digluconate mixture as disinfectant during retreatment of failed endodontic cases. Oral Surgery, Oral Medicine, Oral Pathology, Oral Radiology, and Endodontics 2005;100:756–61.

142. de Oliveira LD, Carvalho CA, Carvalho AS, et al. Efficacy of endodontic treatment for endotoxin reduction in primarily infected root canals and evaluation of cytotoxic effects. Journal of Endodontics 2012;38:105–7.

143. Abbott PV, Hume WR, Heithersay GS. Effects of combining Ledermix and calcium hydroxide pastes on the diffusion of corticosteroid and tetracycline through human tooth roots *in vitro*. Endodontics and Dental Traumatology 1989;5:188–92.

144. Athanassiadis M, Jacobsen N, Nassery K, et al. The effect of calcium hydroxide on the antibiotic component of Odontopaste and Ledermix paste. International Endodontic Journal 2013;46:530–7.

145. Athanassiadis M, Jacobsen N, Parashos P. The effect of calcium hydroxide on the steroid component of Ledermix and Odontopaste. International Endodontic Journal 2011;44:1162–9.

146. Stanley A, Wilson M, Newman HN. The *in vitro* effects of chlorhexidine on subgingival plaque bacteria. Journal of Clinical Periodontology 1989;16:259–64.

147. Denton GW. Chlorhexidine. In: Block SS, editor. Disinfection, sterilization, and preservation. Philadelphia: Lea & Febiger; 1991. p. 276–7.

148. Ohara P, Torabinejad M, Kettering JD. Antibacterial effects of various endodontic irrigants on selected anaerobic bacteria. Endodontics and Dental Traumatology 1993;9:95–100.

149. Vianna ME, Gomes BP, Berber VB, et al. *In vitro* evaluation of the antimicrobial activity of chlorhexidine and sodium hypochlorite. Oral Surgery, Oral Medicine, Oral Pathology, Oral Radiology, and Endodontics 2004;97:79–84.

150. Basrani B, Santos JM, Tjaderhane L, et al. Substantive antimicrobial activity in chlorhexidine-treated human root dentin. Oral Surgery, Oral Medicine, Oral Pathology, Oral Radiology, and Endodontics 2002;94:240–5.

151. Rosenthal S, Spångberg L, Safavi K. Chlorhexidine substantivity in root canal dentin. Oral Surgery, Oral Medicine, Oral Pathology, Oral Radiology, and Endodontics 2004;98:488–92.

152. Yesilsoy C, Whitaker E, Cleveland D, et al. Antimicrobial and toxic effects of established and potential root canal irrigants. Journal of Endodontics 1995;21:513–5.

153. Tanomaru Filho M, Leonardo MR, Silva LAB, et al. Inflammatory response to different endodontic irrigating solutions. International Endodontic Journal 2002;35:735–9.

154. Beaudouin E, Kanny G, Morisset M, et al. Immediate hypersensitivity to chlorhexidine: literature review. European Annals of Allergy and Clinical Immunology 2004;36: 123–6.

155. McDonnel G, Russell AD. Antiseptics and disinfectants: activity, action, and resistance. Clinical Microbiology Reviews 1999;12:147–79.

156. Krithikadatta J, Indira R, Dorothykalyani AL. Disinfection of dentinal tubules with 2% chlorhexidine, 2% metronidazole, bioactive glass when compared with calcium hydroxide as intracanal medicaments. Journal of Endodontics 2007;33: 1473–6.

157. Delgado RJ, Gasparoto TH, Sipert CR, et al. Antimicrobial effects of calcium hydroxide and chlorhexidine on Enterococcus faecalis. Journal of Endodontics 2010;36:1389–93.

158. Delgado RJ, Gasparoto TH, Sipert CR, et al. Antimicrobial activity of calcium hydroxide and chlorhexidine on intratubular *Candida albicans*. International Journal of Oral Science 2013;5:32–6.

159. Gama TG, de Oliveira JC, Abad EC, et al. Postoperative pain following the use of two different intracanal medications. Clinical Oral Investigations 2008;12:325–30.

160. Vianna ME, Horz HP, Conrads G, et al. Comparative analysis of endodontic pathogens using checkerboard hybridization in relation to culture. Oral Microbiology and Immunology 2008;23:282–90.

161. Teles AM, Manso MC, Loureiro S, et al. Effectiveness of two intracanal dressings in adult Portuguese patients: a qPCR and anaerobic culture assessment. International Endodontic Journal 2014;47:32–40.

162. Malkhassian G, Manzur AJ, Legner M, et al. Antibacterial efficacy of MTAD final rinse and two percent chlorhexidine gel medication in teeth with apical periodontitis: a randomized double-blinded clinical trial. Journal of Endodontics 2009;35: 1483–90.

163. Tervit C, Paquette L, Torneck CD, et al. Proportion of healed teeth with apical periodontitis medicated with two percent chlorhexidine gluconate liquid: a case-series study. Journal of Endodontics 2009;35:1182–5.

164. Pallasch TJ. Global antibiotic resistance and its impact on the dental community. Journal of the California Dental Association 2000;28:215–33.

165. Jungermann GB, Burns K, Nandakumar R, et al. Antibiotic resistance in primary and persistent endodontic infections. Journal of Endodontics 2011;37:1337–44.

166. Rôças IN, Siqueira JF Jr. Antibiotic resistance genes in anaerobic bacteria isolated from primary dental root canal infections. Anaerobe 2012;18:576–80.

167. Rôças IN, Siqueira JF Jr. Detection of antibiotic resistance genes in samples from acute and chronic endodontic infections and after treatment. Archives of Oral Biology 2013;58:1123–8.

168. Siqueira JF Jr, Rôças IN. Community as the unit of pathogenicity: an emerging concept as to the microbial pathogenesis of apical periodontitis. Oral Surgery, Oral Medicine, Oral Pathology, Oral Radiology, and Endodontics 2009;107:870–8.

169. Torabinejad M, Khademi AA, Babagoli J, et al. A new solution for the removal of the smear layer. Journal of Endodontics 2003;29:170–5.

170. Torabinejad M, Shabahang S, Aprecio RM, et al. The antimicrobial effect of MTAD: an *in vitro* investigation. Journal of Endodontics 2003;29:400–3.

171. Hoshino E, Kurihara-Ando N, Sato I, et al. *In-vitro* antibacterial susceptibility of bacteria taken from infected root dentine to a mixture of ciprofloxacin, metronidazole and minocycline. International Endodontic Journal 1996;29:125–30.

172. Sato I, Ando-Kurihara N, Kota K, et al. Sterilization of infected root-canal dentine by topical application of a mixture of ciprofloxacin, metronidazole and minocycline in situ. International Endodontic Journal 1996;29:118–24.

173. Banchs F, Trope M. Revascularization of immature permanent teeth with apical periodontitis: new treatment protocol? Journal of Endodontics 2004;30:196–200.

174. Windley IIIW, Teixeira F, Levin L, et al. Disinfection of immature teeth with a triple antibiotic paste. Journal of Endodontics 2005;31:439–43.

175. Diogenes AR, Ruparel NB, Teixeira FB, et al. Translational science in disinfection for regenerative endodontics. Journal of Endodontics 2014;40:S52–7.

176. Molander A, Reit C, Dahlen G. Microbiological evaluation of clindamycin as a root canal dressing in teeth with apical periodontitis. International Endodontic Journal 1990;23:113–8.

177. Byström A, Sundqvist G. Bacteriologic evaluation of the efficacy of mechanical root canal instrumentation in endodontic therapy. Scandinavian Journal of Dental Research 1981;89:321–8.

178. Card SJ, Sigurdsson A, Ørstavik D, et al. The effectiveness of increased apical enlargement in reducing intracanal bacteria. Journal of Endodontics 2002;28:779–83.

179. Leonardo MR, Tanomaru Filho M, Silva LA, et al. In vivo antimicrobial activity of 2% chlorhexidine used as a root canal irrigating solution. Journal of Endodontics 1999;25:167–71.

180. Kvist T, Molander A, Dahlen G, et al. Microbiological evaluation of one- and two-visit endodontic treatment of teeth with apical periodontitis: a randomized, clinical trial. Journal of Endodontics 2004;30:572–6.

181. Friedman S, Lost C, Zarrabian M, et al. Evaluation of success and failure after endodontic therapy using a glass ionomer cement sealer. Journal of Endodontics 1995;21:384–90.

182. Trope M, Moshonov J, Nissan R, et al. Short vs. long-term calcium hydroxide treatment of established inflammatory root resorption in replanted dog teeth. Endodontics and Dental Traumatology 1995;11:124–8.

183. Molander A, Warfvinge J, Reit C, et al. Clinical and radiographic evaluation of one- and two-visit endodontic treatment of asymptomatic necrotic teeth with apical periodontitis: a randomized clinical trial. Journal of Endodontics 2007;33:1145–8.

184. Trope M, Delano EO, Ørstavik D. Endodontic treatment of teeth with apical periodontitis: single vs. multivisit treatment. Journal of Endodontics 1999;25:345–50.

185. Penesis VA, Fitzgerald PI, Fayad MI, et al. Outcome of one-visit and two-visit endodontic treatment of necrotic teeth with apical periodontitis: a randomized controlled trial with one-year evaluation. Journal of Endodontics 2008;34:251–7.

186. Weiger R, Rosendahl R, Lost C. Influence of calcium hydroxide intracanal dressings on the prognosis of teeth with endodontically induced periapical lesions. International Endodontic Journal 2000;33:219–26.

187. Peters LB, Wesselink PR. Periapical healing of endodontically treated teeth in one and two visits obturated in the presence or absence of detectable microorganisms. International Endodontic Journal 2002;35:660–7.

188. Paredes-Vieyra J, Enriquez FJ. Success rate of single- versus two-visit root canal treatment of teeth with apical periodontitis: a randomized controlled trial. Journal of Endodontics 2012;38:1164–9.

189. Sathorn C, Parashos P, Messer HH. Effectiveness of single-versus multiple-visit endodontic treatment of teeth with apical periodontitis: a systematic review and meta-analysis. International Endodontic Journal 2005;38:347–55.

190. Figini L, Lodi G, Gorni F, et al. Single versus multiple visits for endodontic treatment of permanent teeth: a cochrane systematic review. Journal of Endodontics 2008;34:1041–7.

191. Su Y, Wang C, Ye L. Healing rate and post-obturation pain of single- versus multiple-visit endodontic treatment for infected root canals: a systematic review. Journal of Endodontics 2011;37:125–32.

192. Ricucci D, Russo J, Rutberg M, et al. A prospective cohort study of endodontic treatments of 1,369 root canals: results after 5 years. Oral Surgery, Oral Medicine, Oral Pathology, Oral Radiology, and Endodontics 2011;112:825–42.

193. Katebzadeh N, Hupp J, Trope M. Histological periapical repair after obturation of infected root canals in dogs. Journal of Endodontics 1999;25:364–8.

194. Tanomaru Filho M, Leonardo MR, da Silva LA. Effect of irrigating solution and calcium hydroxide root canal dressing on the repair of apical and periapical tissues of teeth with periapical lesion. Journal of Endodontics 2002;28:295–9.

195. Holland R, Otoboni Filho JA, de Souza V, et al. A comparison of one versus two appointment endodontic therapy in dogs' teeth with apical periodontitis. Journal of Endodontics 2003;29:121–4.

196. De Rossi A, Silva LA, Leonardo MR, et al. Effect of rotary or manual instrumentation, with or without a calcium hydroxide/1% chlorhexidine intracanal dressing, on the healing of experimentally induced chronic periapical lesions. Oral Surgery, Oral Medicine, Oral Pathology, Oral Radiology, and Endodontics 2005;99:628–36.

197. Siren EK, Haapasalo MP, Ranta K, et al. Microbiological findings and clinical treatment procedures in endodontic cases selected for microbiological investigation. International Endodontic Journal 1997;30:91–5.

198. Cheung GS. Survival of first-time nonsurgical root canal treatment performed in a dental teaching hospital. Oral Surgery,

Oral Medicine, Oral Pathology, Oral Radiology, and Endodontics 2002;93:596–604.

199. Moskow Aea. Intracanal use of a corticosteroid solution as an endodontic anodyne. Oral Surgery, Oral Medicine, and Oral Pathology 1984;58:600.

200. Negm MM. Management of endodontic pain with nonsteroidal anti-inflammatory agents: a double-blind, placebo-controlled study. Oral Surgery, Oral Medicine, and Oral Pathology 1989;67:88–95.

201. Hasselgren G, Olsson B, Cvek M. Effects of calcium hydroxide and sodium hypochlorite on the dissolution of necrotic porcine muscle tissue. Journal of Endodontics 1988;14:125–7.

202. Andersen M, Lund A, Andreasen JO, et al. *In vitro* solubility of human pulp tissue in calcium hydroxide and sodium hypochlorite. Endodontics and Dental Traumatology 1992;8:104–8.

203. Donaldson M, Kinirons MJ. Factors affecting the time of onset of resorption in avulsed and replanted incisor teeth in children. Dental Traumatology 2001;17:205–9.

204. Trope M. Root resorption due to dental trauma. Endodontic Topics 2002;1:79–100.

205. Barnett F. The role of endodontics in the treatment of luxated permanent teeth. Dental Traumatology 2002;18:47–56.

206. Ørstavik D. Intracanal medication. In: Pitt Ford TR, editor. Harty's endodontics in clinical practice. Oxford, UK: Wright; 1997. p. 106–22.

207. Dumsha T, Hovland EJ. Evaluation of long-term calcium hydroxide treatment in avulsed teeth – an *in vivo* study. International Endodontic Journal 1995;28:7–11.

208. Thong YL, Messer HH, Siar CH, et al. Periodontal response to two intracanal medicaments in replanted monkey incisors. Dental Traumatology 2001;17:254–9.

209. Lengheden A, Blomlof L, Lindskog S. Effect of immediate calcium hydroxide treatment and permanent root-filling on periodontal healing in contaminated replanted teeth. Scandinavian Journal of Dental Research 1991;99:139–46.

210. Lengheden A, Blomlof L, Lindskog S. Effect of delayed calcium hydroxide treatment on periodontal healing in contaminated replanted teeth. Scandinavian Journal of Dental Research 1991;99:147–53.

211. Carver K, Nusstein J, Reader A, et al. *In vivo* antibacterial efficacy of ultrasound after hand and rotary instrumentation in human mandibular molars. Journal of Endodontics 2007;33:1038–43.

212. Alves FR, Almeida BM, Neves MA, et al. Disinfecting oval-shaped root canals: effectiveness of different supplementary approaches. Journal of Endodontics 2011;37:496–501.

213. Sigurdsson A, Stancill R, Madison S. Intracanal placement of Ca(OH)2: a comparison of techniques. Journal of Endodontics 1992;18:367–70.

214. Torres CP, Apicella MJ, Yancich PP, et al. Intracanal placement of calcium hydroxide: a comparison of techniques, revisited. Journal of Endodontics 2004;30:225–7.

CHAPTER 9

Root Canal Filling

N. P. Chandler

Chapter Contents

Summary

In recent years, several newer root canal filling materials have been introduced, the focus being to improve on the perceived deficiencies of currently available materials and obturation techniques, while achieving savings in both time and cost. Most developments aim to replace gutta-percha with a variety of other materials as the core filling material. Newer root canal sealers have also been introduced to complement these systems. All core materials are available in sizes corresponding to the taper of modern root canal preparation, including engine-driven instruments, as part of matched systems. Single-cone root fillings may now provide an acceptable result in selected cases. After its successful application in immature teeth and apical surgery, Mineral trioxide aggregate (MTA) has an increasing role as a root canal filling material, either in sealers or on its own. The ideal root canal filling material is yet to be developed, and some root canal shapes remain a challenge to fill. The aims of this chapter are to describe the fundamental principles of canal filling using gutta-percha and to provide an overview of relevant alternative methods.

Introduction

The entire root canal system should be filled following cleaning and shaping. The objectives of root canal filling are to:

- prevent any microorganisms, which remain in the root canal system from proliferating and passing into the periapical tissues via the apical foramen and other pathways;
- seal the pulp chamber and root canal system from coronal microleakage to prevent microorganisms and/or toxins entering the canal system;

- prevent percolation of periapical exudate and possibly microorganisms into the pulp space via the apical foramen and other pathways;
- prevent percolation of gingival exudate and microorganisms into the pulp space via lateral/furcation canals opening into the gingival sulcus or through exposed, patent dentinal tubules around the cervical neck of the tooth.

The quality of the root canal filling depends on the complexity of the root canal system, the efficacy of canal preparation, the materials and techniques used and the skill and experience of the operator. Filling root canals does not represent the end of root canal treatment, as restoration of the clinical crown to prevent leakage into the pulp space, the next step, is critical to long-term success.[1] There is evidence that the quality of the coronal seal affects the prognosis of root canal treatment.[2]

Many materials and techniques have been used to fill root canals. The most popular material is gutta-percha combined with a sealer because it is versatile and can be used in a variety of techniques.

Canal Anatomy

Pulp anatomy is complex with many root canals having apical deltas, lateral canals and other aberrations; accessory canals, fins and anastomoses are not uncommon, especially in posterior teeth. These, together with the consequences of physiological and pathological dentine deposition and procedural problems during canal preparation, present challenges. The original anatomy of the root canal system often has a major influence on the techniques used to fill canals and on the quality of the final result.

Access and Canal Preparation

The aims of preparation are to clean and shape the root canal system. Access and preparation have been discussed in Chapters 4 and 7, respectively. Regardless of the root filling method, greater emphasis must be made on the process of cleaning and shaping the root canal. Time and care spent during preparation will facilitate root canal filling. The quality of canal preparation with modern instruments is related to the quality of adaption of the root filling when studied in three dimensions using contemporary tomography techniques.[3] As well as removing microorganisms and debris from the root canal system, preparation produces the desired canal shape to receive the root filling. Cleaning of the canal may be achieved with irrigants and removal of dentine from the canal walls. Creation of an inappropriate canal shape will make it difficult to introduce root filling materials along the length of the canal, resulting in a poorly condensed filling with voids. Thus, the ability to fill canals predictably is significantly dependent on the adequacy of access and the quality of the root canal preparation.

The method of root canal filling will be dictated by the preparation technique and shaping objectives. Some operators prefer to create an apical stop at the dentine-cementum junction, where a natural apical constriction is believed to exist; hence instrumentation does not extend beyond the apical foramen.[4] With this canal shape, the filling technique of choice is cold lateral condensation of gutta-percha. Other operators create a continuously tapering canal shape where the smallest diameter is at the foramen.[5] With this shape, a variety of warm gutta-percha techniques are more appropriate; otherwise, the lack of an apical stop will predispose the master gutta-percha cone, used in lateral condensation, to being distorted and pushed beyond the foramen when a spreader is introduced.

Criteria for Filling

Root canal filling is often delayed for one or more visits after preparation to allow interappointment medicaments placed in the canal to act on the microbiota and for clinical signs and symptoms to resolve.[6] Unfortunately, delaying root canal filling may lead to loss of, or microleakage through, the provisional restoration. Also, all medicaments have limited antimicrobial activity and duration of effectiveness. Under the right circumstances, modern root canal preparation techniques are effective in eliminating microorganisms, so in selected cases, root canal preparation and filling may be completed in one visit.

The decision as to when to fill root canals is controversial and debatable. Advocates for immediate filling of canals after preparation believe that their regimen for eliminating microorganisms by preparing a continuously tapering canal shape[5] and the extensive use of sodium hypochlorite and ethylenediamine-tetraacetic acid (EDTA), or alternative irrigation, is effective. It has been argued that the root canal system is likely to be sufficiently cleared of microorganisms and substrate to allow immediate filling.[7] Meanwhile, there is strong evidence that delaying root canal filling and use an intracanal medicament will reduce the microbial population and endotoxins present.[8,9] It will encourage more rapid resolution of apical periodontitis and provide an improved prognosis.[10–12] To further confuse the issue, there has been research reporting no difference between the healing rate of one-visit, or two-visit, root canal treatment incorporating calcium hydroxide medication.[13]

Logically, teeth with noninfected pulps and no sign of apical periodontitis can be prepared and filled in one visit, whereas infected cases with apical periodontitis should be treated cautiously, with additional appointments to allow an intracanal medicament to further reduce the microbial population (see Chapter 8). Interestingly, although patients might prefer treatment in a single visit, they may well opt for further treatment visits if a higher success rate can be offered.[14] Irrespective of the number of treatment visits, it is essential that the root canal can be properly dried before filling; otherwise, it is likely to influence the effectiveness of the seal.[15]

Materials Used to Fill Root Canals

Many materials have been used to fill root canals. Historically, these ranged from feathers and wood sticks, precious metals to amalgam and dental cements. The requirements for a root canal filling material have been specified for many years. Many materials have proved to be inadequate, impractical or biologically unacceptable.

A radiographically dense appearance with an absence of voids is desirable at the end of treatment, but no materials or techniques are entirely predictable for filling and sealing canals. Some voids are likely in all root fillings.[16]

Sealers

A root canal sealer is used in combination with the core root canal filling material, e.g. gutta-percha. The primary role of the sealer is to obliterate the irregularities between the root canal wall and the core material. Almost all of today's root canal filling techniques use a sealer to enhance the seal of the root canal filling.[17]

Root canal sealers are used for the following purposes:
- cementing (luting) the core material to the canal;
- filling the discrepancies between the root canal walls and core material;
- acting as a lubricant;
- acting as an antimicrobial agent;
- acting as a marker for accessory canals, resorptive defects, root fractures and other spaces into which the main core material may not penetrate.

The requirements and characteristics of an ideal sealer are[18]:
- nonirritating to periapical tissues;
- insoluble in tissue fluids;
- dimensionally stable;
- providing a hermetic seal;
- radiopaque;
- bacteriostatic;
- sticky with good adhesion to the canal wall once set;
- good penetration into dentinal tubules;
- easily mixed;
- nonstaining to dentine;
- good working time;
- easily removable if necessary.

No current material satisfies all these requirements, but many work well in clinical practice. Along with providing a satisfactory seal, it must be well tolerated by the periapical tissues and be relatively easy to handle. Some sealers are toxic when freshly prepared[19]; however, their toxicity is reduced substantially after setting.[20] Thus, although sealers produce varying degrees of periapical inflammation, it is normally only temporary and depending on composition, it does not appear to prevent tissue healing.

Most sealers are absorbed to some extent when exposed to tissue fluid,[21] so the volume of sealer must be kept to a minimum with the core material forming the bulk of the root filling. The core material should force the sealer into inaccessible areas and into irregularities along the root canal walls. Excess sealer should ideally flow back into the access cavity, but some gutta-percha techniques tend to force sealer apically and

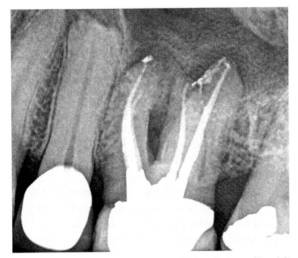

FIGURE 9-1 Sealer extrusion from the palatal root of a maxillary left first molar. The canals, including the second mesiobuccal, are filled with condensed gutta-percha. (Reproduced courtesy of R. Roy.)

laterally via the foramen and accessory canals.[22] (Figure 9-1) The passage of sealer into the periapical tissues is not encouraged, but there is equivocal evidence that it will reduce the success rate of treatment provided that canal preparation and filling have been performed with care. Clinical experience suggests that most excess sealer in the periapical region is absorbed with time but large volumes of extruded sealer must be avoided.

The depth of penetration of sealers into dentinal tubules is variable.[23,24] Techniques such as employing ultrasound can promote dentinal tubule penetration.[25] Although all sealers have their advantages and disadvantages, there has been only limited research to suggest that selection might influence treatment outcome.[12] Future improvements in sealers might involve a search for materials with better dentinal tubule penetration, slight expansion, resistance to degradation and an enhanced ability to adhere to dentine, whatever its condition.

Sealers in use today can be divided into six groups based on their constituents:

- zinc oxide–eugenol sealers;
- calcium hydroxide sealers;
- resin sealers;
- glass ionomer sealers;
- silicone-based sealers;
- calcium silicate/MTA-based sealers.

ZINC OXIDE–EUGENOL SEALERS

Most zinc oxide–eugenol sealers are based on Grossman's formula.[26] Commercial products include Tubli-Seal (SybronEndo, Orange, CA, USA), Pulp Canal Sealer (SybronEndo) and Roth Sealer (Roth International Ltd, Chicago, IL, USA). Modified formulations with extended working times are available.

Once set, zinc oxide–eugenol sealers are relatively weak and porous and are susceptible to decomposition in tissue fluids, particularly when extruded into the periapical tissues. All zinc oxide–eugenol cements are cytotoxic and the cellular response may last longer than those produced by other materials.[20] However, these problems are not usually apparent clinically, and zinc oxide–eugenol materials are probably the most commonly used sealers. The various zinc oxide–eugenol sealers have a range of setting times and flow characteristics, so the choice of formulation is dependent on the case. Difficult canals that need some time to fill require a sealer with an extended working time. If heat is applied during root canal filling, its influence on the setting time of sealers should also be taken into account.

CALCIUM HYDROXIDE SEALERS

Calcium hydroxide sealers have been developed on the assumption that they preserve the vitality of the pulp stump and stimulate healing and hard tissue formation at the apical wound.[27] Laboratory research has demonstrated their sealing ability to be similar to zinc oxide–eugenol sealers[28]; however, it remains to be seen whether they maintain their integrity during long-term exposure to tissue fluids since calcium hydroxide is soluble and may leach out and weaken the remaining cement.

Commercial products include Sealapex (SybronEndo), a calcium hydroxide-containing polymeric resin, Apexit Plus (Ivoclar Vivadent, Schaan, Liechtenstein) and epoxy-based Acroseal (Septodont, Saint-Maur-des-fossés Cedex, France).

RESIN-BASED SEALERS

Resin-based materials have been available for many years. The first resin sealer, AH 26 (Dentsply DeTrey, Konstanz, Germany), a powder and liquid, consisted of an epoxy resin base which set slowly when mixed with an activator. It has good sealing and adhesive properties and antibacterial activity. However, it initially produces a severe inflammatory reaction,[20] which subsides after some weeks; the material is then well tolerated by the periapical tissues. The resin has strong allergenic and mutagenic potential, and cases of contact allergy and paraesthesia[29] have been reported. The material releases formaldehyde,[30] which explains its strong antibacterial effect.[31] AH 26 has largely been superseded by AH Plus (Dentsply DeTrey), a two-paste system formulated to polymerize with minimal formaldehyde release. AH Plus is also less cytotoxic, with a thinner film thickness and lower solubility. The use of AH Plus in warm gutta-percha techniques results in chemical changes which adversely affect its physical properties[32,33] with its setting time reduced and its film thickness increased.[34]

EndoREZ (Ultradent, South Jordan, UT, USA) is a urethane dimethacrylate (UDMA)-based resin sealer. It is recommended for use with EndoREZ points (Ultradent) and methacrylate resin-coated gutta-percha points so that there is bonding between the root filling, sealer and root canal dentine. A 10-year study of this sealer used with lateral condensation of gutta-percha cones suggests the material may be recommended as an alternative to other sealers.[35] With this sealer, the susceptibility to interfacial biofilm proliferation depends on the etching system used.[36] The application of a separate adhesive layer may improve the bond strength of UDMA sealers to dentine.[37] Other resin sealers include Hybrid Root SEAL (Sun Medical Co. Ltd., Moriyama City, Shiga, Japan) or MetaSEAL (Parkell, Edgewood, NY, USA), both of the same chemical formulation and are based on 4-methacryloethyl trimellitate anhydride (4-META).

The choice of canal irrigants and irrigation protocols should be considered when resin-based sealers are selected as the final rinse can have a positive influence on adhesion to dentine.[38,39]

GLASS IONOMER SEALERS

The ability of glass ionomers to adhere to dentine would appear to provide many advantages if used as a sealer. Its endodontic potential was recognized soon after its introduction as a restorative material,[40] but it was many years before a sealer was formulated and now it is no longer easily available.

Activ GP glass ionomer sealer (Brasseler, Savannah, GA, USA) is used with Activ GP points (Brasseler). These gutta-percha points are impregnated and coated with the glass ionomer. The sealer is meant to adhere chemically and micromechanically to the points and also bond to dentine (a form of monoblock, see later).

SILICONE-BASED SEALERS

RoekoSeal (Coltène/Whaledent, Alstätten, Switzerland) is a polydimethylsiloxane-based sealer said to expand slightly on setting (0.2%) and is highly radiopaque; the claimed advantages include good sealing ability[41] and excellent biocompatibility.[42]

GuttaFlow (Coltène/Whaledent) is a modification of RoekoSeal. GuttaFlow contains particles of gutta-percha less than 30 µm in size and and also expands slightly (0.2%) on curing, according to the manufacturer. The material is considered to be almost insoluble. It is used with a single master gutta-percha cone, without mechanical compaction, although lateral or vertical condensation techniques are acceptable. Its flow is significantly better into lateral grooves and depressions in the apical regions of root canals than lateral condensation or warm compaction with AH 26 sealer.[43] It is effective in filling oval-shaped canals.[44] Its sealing qualities are similar to lateral compaction, or the System B technique with AH 26.[45] All traces of irrigants must be thoroughly rinsed from the canal with water, or isopropyl alcohol, before introducing the material. GuttaFlow has a working time of 15 minutes and a setting time of about 30 minutes; GuttaFlow FAST has a 5-minute working time and a 10-minute set. A potential concern is extrusion of material beyond the apex,[43] although its cytotoxicity is lower than some other sealers.

CALCIUM SILICATE/MINERAL TRIOXIDE AGGREGATE-BASED SEALERS

The most recent innovations in sealers are the calcium silicate/MTA-based materials. These materials are considered to be biocompatible and promote the deposition of hydroxyapatite crystalline deposits from amorphous calcium-phosphate precursors along the surface of the root canal.[46–49] These new 'bioceramic' sealers include ProRoot Endo sealer (Dentsply Maillefer, Ballaigues, Switzerland), MTA Fillapex (Angelus, Londrina, Brazil) and MTA Obtura (Angelus),

Endo-CPM-Sealer (EGEO S.R.L., Buenos Aires, Argentina), EndoSequence BC sealer (Brasseler USA, Savannah, GA, USA), TotalFill BC sealer (FKG, La-Chaux-de-Fonds, Switzerland) and iRoot SP sealer (Innovative Bioceramix Inc, Vancouver, BC, Canada).

ProRoot Endo sealer (Dentsply Maillefer) is a calcium silicate-based endodontic sealer designed to be used in conjunction with a root filling material in either the cold lateral, warm vertical, or carrier-based, filling techniques. The major components of the powder are tricalcium silicate and dicalcium silicate, with the inclusion of calcium sulphate as the setting retardant, bismuth oxide as a radiopacifier and a small amount of tricalcium aluminate. The liquid is an aqueous polyvinyl-pyrrolidone homopolymer.[46] After storage in a simulated body fluid, the sealer demonstrated the formation of spherical amorphous calcium-like phases and apatite-like phases. An experimental MTA sealer with a water-soluble polymer revealed the release of calcium ions in solution that encouraged the deposition of calcium phosphate crystals when in contact with water, or a physiological solution.[47,50,51]

iRoot SP sealer is another newer calcium silicate-based sealer. The mineralization phenomenon also occurs with EndoSequence BC Sealer,[52] Endo-CPM-Sealer[53] and MTA Fillapex.[48] Calcium silicate-based sealers are characterized by a high viscosity and small particle size. These allow excellent adaptation to dentine and they have shown superior bond strengths at the middle and apical third of extracted teeth.[54–56] Endosequence BC sealer has been shown to increase the force to fracture of root-filled premolar teeth.[57]

Entombment of any remaining bacteria is a key objective of all root filling material; a recent study[58] reported entombment by MTA. This seems to be a feature unique to the material, with amorphous structures and intratubular crystal growth contributing to the effect. The favourable properties of calcium silicate/MTA-based sealers may provide improved results in conventional canal obturation, whereas the entombment effect could have a major positive influence on the outcome of retreatment cases. A disadvantage of MTA-based sealers is their slow set, but this may be overcome with developments in setting accelerators.

Smear Layer

The smear layer, comprising both organic and inorganic components, is found on the root canal walls after canal instrumentation.[59] It is composed largely of particulate dentine debris created by endodontic instruments during root canal preparation; it also contains pulpal remnants and microorganisms. With further instrumentation, the material is forced against the canal walls, forming a friable and loosely adherent layer. The smear layer is typically 1 to 2 µm thick, although it can also be found within the dentinal tubules for up to 40 µm.

The smear layer has received much attention, not only because it may harbour microorganisms already in the canal but also because it may create an avenue for the leakage of microorganisms and act as a substrate for microbial proliferation. It may be broken down by bacterial action to provide a pathway for leakage. In addition, the smear layer has the potential to influence the adaptation of sealer against the root canal walls and its tubular penetration, thereby increasing the likelihood of leakage.[24,60] Indeed, it has been shown that most leakage occurs between the sealer and the wall of the root canal.[61]

Smear layer removal before filling would appear to be desirable as it would eliminate microorganisms and allow for better adaptation of sealer. However, this procedure has been questioned since opening the tubules might increase the diffusion of potentially irritant root filling materials through the tubules to the root surface,[62] allow microorganisms trapped in the tubules to escape,[63] or to proliferate within the tubules and potentially increase leakage. Sealers vary in their tubule penetration,[23,24] and while penetration is considered an advantage, there seems to be a lack of correlation between penetration and seal in nonbonded root fillings.[64] The key method of smear layer removal involves 17% EDTA as a chelating agent together with sodium hypochlorite to dissolve the organic component.[59]

Gutta-Percha

Gutta-percha has been used inside root canals for about 140 years and is the most widely used root filling material. Gutta-percha is a form of rubber obtained from tropical trees of the *Sapotaceae* family. Endodontic gutta-percha is a *trans-* isomer of polyisoprene, which exists in two crystalline forms, the α- and β-phases. The α-phase occurs naturally and the β-phase arises during refining; the two are interchangeable depending on temperature. Use of the α-phase has increased with the popularity of thermoplastic techniques. Gutta-percha is mixed with other materials to produce a blend that can be used effectively within the root canal. Commercial gutta-percha cones contain gutta-percha (19–22%), zinc oxide (59–75%), various waxes, colouring agents, antioxidants and metal salts to provide radiopacity. There is considerable variation in the physical properties of commercially available cones and obturating products.[65]

Gutta-percha cones are:
- inert;
- dimensionally stable;
- nonallergenic to almost all individuals;
- antibacterial;
- nonstaining to dentine;
- radiopaque;
- compactable;
- softened by heat;
- softened by organic solvents;
- removable from the root canal when necessary.

However, the disadvantages are:
- lack of rigidity;
- lack of adhesion to dentine.

Gutta-percha points may be sterilized in sodium hypochlorite solution.[66]

CANAL FILLING WITH GUTTA-PERCHA

The objective of root canal filling is to completely fill the root canal system in an attempt to seal the canal from leakage apically and coronally. Gutta-percha is versatile and can be used in a variety of techniques, but a sealer is always necessary to cement the material to the canal wall and to fill minor irregularities.

Over the years, many newer filling techniques have been described, accompanied by claims of greater efficacy, reduced leakage, or time and money saving. Unfortunately, newer does not necessarily mean better, and sadly, there is still only little evidence from clinical trials to suggest that there are significant differences between root canal filling techniques and treatment outcome. It is prudent to wait for the published results

of laboratory and clinical studies before investing and learning a newer, untested technique.

Methods for filling canals using gutta-percha can, broadly, be divided into three main groups:
- cold gutta-percha;
- heat-softened gutta-percha;
- solvent-softened gutta-percha.

COLD GUTTA-PERCHA TECHNIQUES

Cold gutta-percha techniques are simple to master as they are not complicated by the need to soften the material with heat or solvents; hence, they do not require expensive devices or equipment. However, cold gutta-percha cannot be effectively compacted into all the irregularities in a root canal system, so this is the role of the sealer. Lateral condensation is the most popular method of root filling with cold gutta-percha.

Lateral Condensation

With the advent of the standardized preparation technique,[67] the method of filling root canals with a single, full-length gutta-percha cone and sealer became popular. The concept was simple and attractive; the root canal was prepared to a round cross-sectional shape of a standard size with reamers and filled with a gutta-percha cone of the same diameter. Unfortunately, a round canal shape was rarely achieved, especially in curved roots, and the single cone required large amounts of sealer to fill the intervening gaps resulting in increased leakage.[68] It was also clear that discrepancies in size and taper between gutta-percha cones and equivalent numbered instruments were prevalent. While many clinicians appreciated these problems and adopted other filling techniques, others continued to fill canals using this method (Figure 9-2).

Current canal preparation techniques produce a flared canal with a flowing conical shape and cannot be filled adequately with a single 0.02 taper gutta-percha cone. Gutta-percha cones with ISO standardized tip sizes but with varying tapers, e.g. 0.04 or 0.06 tapers, are available (Figure 9-3). These cones with increased taper can fill funnel-shaped canals more effectively because they are more likely to correspond to the canal shape created by instruments with similar taper. In a laboratory study on curved canals, a single tapered cone technique has been found to be

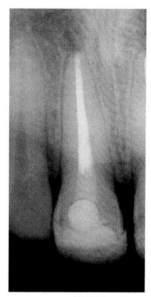

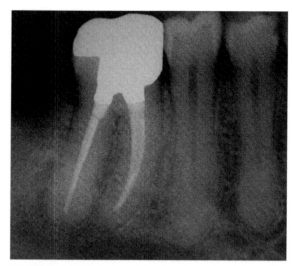

FIGURE 9-4 Mandibular right first molar. The mesial canals are filled with 0.04 taper, size 40 gutta-percha cones and the distal canal with a 0.06 taper, size 40 cone. Canal entrances are covered with IRM (Dentsply) and an amalgam intradicular core for the coronal restoration. (Reproduced courtesy of D. Violich.)

FIGURE 9-2 Maxillary central incisor filled with laterally condensed gutta-percha.

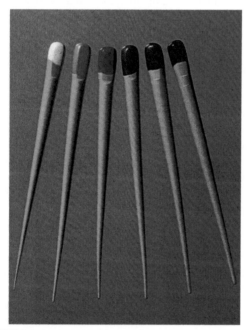

FIGURE 9-3 Gutta-percha cones, 0.06 taper with standardized 15 to 40 tip sizes (left to right).

comparable with lateral condensation in terms of the amount of gutta-percha occupying the root canal space; the technique is also faster than lateral condensation.[69] A clinical example shows radiographically acceptable results (Figure 9-4).

Lateral condensation of cold gutta-percha is taught and practised throughout the world and is the technique of choice for many clinicians. It is simple and rapid to carry out. It can be used in virtually all cases where canal preparation results in an apical stop and is the standard against which most newer techniques are compared. It allows excellent length control and can be used with a wide choice of sealers. Lateral condensation involves the placement of a master (primary) gutta-percha cone to the terminus of the preparation followed by placing additional (accessory) gutta-percha cones alongside (Figure 9-5). The use of a standardized master cone provides the possibility of a predictable fit at the apex, while the accessory cones fill the intervening space, produced as a result of the flared canal shape. The root filling, therefore, consists of numerous cones cemented together and to the canal wall by sealer; there is no merging of the cones into a homogeneous mass of gutta-percha (Figure 9-6). The technique is not recommended when the canal has no

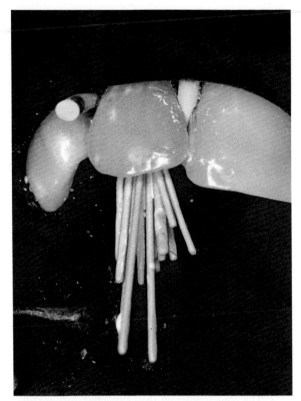

FIGURE 9-5 Maxillary left canine with multiple gutta-percha cones in place during lateral condensation.

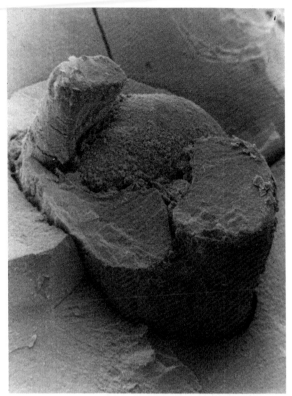

FIGURE 9-6 Scanning electron micrograph of a section of a root with laterally condensed gutta-percha *in situ*. Close adaptation of the cones to the wall of the canal and the limited space occupied by sealer or voids is evident. The circular cross-section of the cones have been modified by spreader insertion. (Reproduced courtesy of B. Tidmarsh.)

apical stop, and files can easily pass through the foramen (when the canal has a continuous taper with the foramen being the narrowest).

A spreader is inserted alongside the master cone to improve its adaptation at the terminus of the preparation and to create the space for the accessory gutta-percha cones. When inserted to within 1 mm of the terminus to condense the master cone apically and laterally, the result will be considerably less leakage than if the spreader had only entered part of the way into the canal.[70] The need to advance the spreader well into the root canal is one of the main reasons for flaring canals. A narrow, parallel shape will not allow the spreader to influence the adaptation of the apical region of the master gutta-percha cone. Narrow canal preparations also risk removing the master gutta-percha cone when withdrawing the spreader as it might pierce the cone instead of condensing the material.

The requirements for successful lateral condensation are:

- a flared canal preparation with an apical stop;
- a well-fitting master gutta-percha cone;
- spreader/s of the appropriate size and taper;
- accessory cones, which match the dimensions of the spreader/s;
- an appropriate sealer.

The master gutta-percha cone must fit the full length of the preparation, be tight at the end-point of the canal preparation (ideally present some resistance to withdrawal or 'tug-back'), and not be able to pass through the foramen.

The size of the master gutta-percha cone should correspond to the master apical file used to prepare the apical stop. The selected cone is held with tweezers

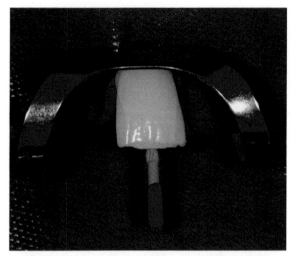

FIGURE 9-7 Master gutta-percha cone notched at the working length corresponding to the chosen incisal edge reference point.

at the correct working length and then inserted into the canal. Ideally, the cone should:

- pass down to the full working length;
- be impossible to push beyond this depth;
- fit tightly, giving some resistance to withdrawal (tug-back).

The tweezers are squeezed slightly to mark the cone (Figure 9-7). A 'cone-fit' radiograph may be taken to confirm the correct depth in relation to the terminus of the preparation and the radiographic apex. If the canal length is correctly estimated, the cone should be at the right depth and position, and the canal filling procedure can proceed. However, a number of problems can occur either as a result of technical difficulties during canal preparation or because of size discrepancies in the gutta-percha cones and/or instruments. Most of these problems can be easily addressed, but they require some thought to ensure that the problem is identified.

Gutta-Percha Cone Reaches the Working Length but Is Loose

This may occur for a number of reasons.

- The gutta-percha cone was smaller than expected. During manufacture, a tolerance of ±0.05 mm is allowed at d_1, so that it is possible for a gutta-percha cone with the correct size to be smaller than the master apical file size and prepared

canal. The solution may be to remove 1 mm increments from the tip of the cone with a scalpel to increase the tip diameter or to select a larger gutta-percha cone.
- The end-point of preparation was wider than expected. File sizes may vary; the tolerance can be ±0.02 mm at d_1, so the canal can be wider than anticipated. The solution is the same as that described above.

Gutta-Percha Cone Passes Beyond Working Length or Through Foramen

This can occur when the apical stop is inadequate or when the cone selected is too small. If the stop is not sufficiently definite, then the cone will pass more deeply and through the foramen. The solution is either to remove 1 mm increments from the gutta-percha cone until it binds in the canal at the working length, or to consider further canal preparation.

Gutta-Percha Cone Does Not Reach the Working Length

This is the most common problem, for a number of reasons:

- The cone was larger than expected. Just as cones can be smaller than the nominal size and appear loose, they can also be larger. If a cone is a short distance (<2 mm) away from the endpoint of the preparation, it may be possible to try a selection of cones of the same size and find one that fits.
- The canal was not widened sufficiently at the endpoint or the canal taper was too narrow. The solution is to revisit the canal preparation; increasing the taper along the length of the canal may also be necessary.
- Dentine debris is blocking the apical region of the canal, usually as a result of insufficient irrigation. Passive ultrasonic irrigation may be helpful to remove a blockage.[71]

Selection of Spreaders and Accessory Gutta-Percha Cones

Once the master gutta-percha cone has been chosen, it is important to select and try-in the spreader to ensure that it can pass to within 1 mm of the termination of the preparation. There is a correlation between spreader penetration and the quality of seal. Spreaders should be precurved for curved canals and a silicone stop used to mark their depth of insertion. Nickel–titanium spreaders, which are more flexible, are also available. To reduce the risk of root fracture due to excessive condensation pressures, finger rather than hand-held spreaders may be used.[72,73]

Spreaders come in standardized 0.02 tapers, the same as for most hand files. Nonstandardized spreaders have relatively small diameters at the tip but a range of tapers ranging from extrafine through fine, medium to large; some manufacturers use letters rather than words to denote the degree of taper, e.g. A, B, C or D. Spreaders with a standardized taper are manufactured in a range of ISO diameters.

When nonstandardized spreaders are used, the cones should also be nonstandardized. However, standardized spreaders require standardized accessory gutta-percha cones. In this way, the cone will fill the space created by the corresponding spreader. It is also beneficial to use instruments and materials from the same manufacturer to ensure more accurate sizing.

The size of the spreader, and thus, cones are determined by the size of the canal. Large canals with a substantial taper are more efficiently filled with larger taper cones, whereas smaller canals with narrower tapers should be filled with finer cones. On most occasions, an extrafine, or fine, spreader is required along with matching accessory gutta-percha cones.

Completion of Lateral Condensation

1. The master gutta-percha cone, spreader, accessory cones and sealer should be organized to ensure they can be handled efficiently.
2. The canal should be dried with paper points.
3. The sealer should be mixed and smeared onto the canal wall using either a hand file rotated counterclockwise, by coating a paper point and inserting it into the canal and/or by coating the master cone itself. Large volumes of sealer introduced with engine-driven devices may be hazardous.
4. The master cone should be 'buttered' lightly with sealer and then inserted immediately to the full working length.
5. The spreader is then placed alongside the master cone and pushed apically with controlled force until it reaches the appropriate depth,

1 mm from the endpoint of preparation. These forces can be considerable,[72,73] and the direction of force should be apical with no lateral action, which risks root fracture. Apical pressure is applied in a constant manner for 10 to 20 seconds to compact the gutta-percha in an apical and lateral direction. In curved canals, the spreader may be precurved and applied either lateral to or on the outer aspect of the master cone or a nickel–titanium spreader may be used.

6. The first accessory gutta-percha cone is inserted into the space created by the spreader.
7. The spreader is then reinserted without delay. It should not go down to the full working length.
8. A second accessory gutta-percha cone is inserted into the space created.
9. This sequence of spreader use and cone insertion continues until the canal is full, with the number of accessory cones required varying from canal to canal (Figure 9-8). If a postretained restoration is planned, lateral condensation can cease when the apical 5 to 6 mm have been filled.

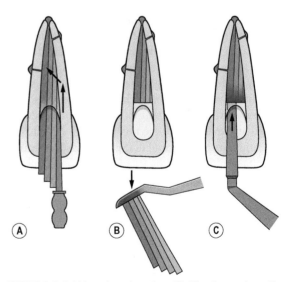

FIGURE 9-8 Cold lateral condensation. (A) After the master gutta-percha cone is fitted, accessory cones are added and condensed until there is no longer space for the spreader. (B) A heated instrument is used to sever the gutta-percha cones and (C) vertically condensed. (Based on an original drawing by M. Monteith.)

10. If the final coronal restoration is not postretained, the excess gutta-percha emerging from the canal entrance should be removed with a hot instrument and condensed vertically with a plugger to promote a satisfactory seal. The gutta-percha should be reduced to below the gingival level, particularly in anterior teeth, in order to maintain the translucency of the crown and to prevent the possibility of sealer staining the dentine. In all cases, having the root filling confined to well within the root and protected by an orifice barrier material and suitable restoration will reduce the risk of microleakage.

When a postretained restoration is planned, gutta-percha can be removed immediately leaving 4 to 5 mm of apical root filling undisturbed.[74] Post space preparation at this stage is advantageous as the operator is aware of the anatomy and canal length. A dental dam is already in place, and the required length of post is easily determined.

Lateral condensation is simple to carry out, rapid and has been used for many years with considerable success, even in quite demanding cases. However, since it is impossible for cold gutta-percha to flow into all the irregularities in the root canal system, parts of the canal must either remain unfilled,[75] or be filled only with sealer. The importance of cleaning anatomical irregularities in oval canals must be emphasized. Otherwise, they remain packed with debris and reduce the quality of the root filling; canals which are this shape present a challenge for most obturation methods.[76]

Innovative means of obturation using gutta-percha, aimed at reducing the time involved with lateral condensation, include SimpliFill (SybronEndo). A section of gutta-percha or Resilon (see later section on monoblocks) is held at the end of the SimpliFill disposable delivery device, which is inserted into the canal to the desired depth. An apical plug of root filling is left inside the canal by twisting to free the delivery device, which is then withdrawn; the remainder of the canal is then back filled if required.

The perceived deficiencies of lateral condensation have resulted in the development of techniques in which gutta-percha is softened by heat or solvents so that the core material can be condensed into anatomic irregularities. Some of these techniques are 'hybrids'

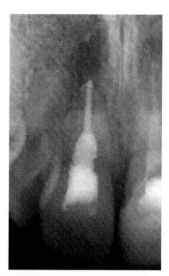

FIGURE 9-9 Hybrid technique used to root fill a maxillary right central incisor. Apical part filled using laterally condensed gutta-percha, and coronal part back filled with warm gutta-percha. (Reproduced courtesy of A. Soma.)

with the benefits of length control of lateral condensation and heat, softening used to rapidly fill the remainder of the canal (Figure 9-9). Other techniques involve heat to soften the whole length of gutta-percha in the root canal.

HEAT-SOFTENED GUTTA-PERCHA TECHNIQUES

For decades, the only technique that used heat-softened gutta-percha was warm vertical condensation,[77] but innovative methods for warming and condensing gutta-percha are now available. In some, cold gutta-percha is placed in the canal and warmed *in situ*; these can be referred to as intracanal heating techniques. Others rely on warming the gutta-percha outside and then delivering it into the canal; thus, they are called extracanal heating techniques.

For canals prepared with an apical stop, lateral condensation of gutta-percha is an excellent and popular method of filling and the one best suited for most operators. The heat-softened techniques are technically more demanding for inexperienced and nonspecialist operators, and caution is required. Practising on simulated canals in plastic models and on extracted teeth is very valuable and will aid familiarity.

Intracanal Heating Techniques

In these techniques, cold gutta-percha is placed in the canal and then heated to become soft and condensable. All of these techniques involve the use of a sealer. The popularity of these methods was limited until Schilder[77] described his method for filling canals using warm vertical condensation.

Warm Vertical Condensation. The aim of the Schilder technique[77] is to fill the canal with heat-softened gutta-percha packed with sufficient vertical pressure to force it to flow into the entire root canal system, including the accessory and lateral canals. The traditional technique requires a flared canal preparation with a definite apical stop. The flared canal accommodates the pluggers used to condense the gutta-percha and facilitates the flow of the material apically. Excessive widening of the canal at the apical stop is counterproductive and actually results in more apical leakage and an increased incidence of overextensions.[78]

The traditional technique uses spreaders heated with an open flame, but electrically heated devices (e.g. Touch 'n Heat, SybronEndo) are relatively inexpensive and convenient. The method produces homogeneous compact fillings with gutta-percha flowing into irregularities, apical deltas and lateral canals;[79] signs of sealer and gutta-percha extrusion into the apical and lateral periodontal ligaments are not infrequent.[80] However, no substantial improvement in the apical or coronal seal[81] has been demonstrated compared with cold lateral condensation. A review suggests that postoperative pain, filling quality and long-term outcomes are similar.[80] Despite the use of very hot instruments, the actual increase in temperature within the mass of gutta-percha is minimal, with no long-term adverse periodontal effects reported.[82] Intracanal heating of gutta-percha with ultrasonic devices has also been described[83] and is reported to save time.

Continuous Wave of Condensation Technique. In recent years, the traditional warm vertical condensation technique has been simplified with the use of electrically heated spreaders and pluggers (Touch 'n Heat, System B Heat Source, Elements 3 Unit, SybronEndo; BeeFill Pack, VDW, Munich, Germany); cordless versions are also available (System B Endodontic Cordless Pack, elementsfree cordless, SybronEndo; B&L SuperEndo Alpha II, B & L Biotech, Fairfax, VA, USA). These resulted in a revival of interest in warm condensation techniques.

The continuous wave of condensation technique[84] uses the System B type heat sources. There are two stages, down-packing and back-packing. In down-packing, heat is carried along the length of the master gutta-percha cone starting coronally and ending in apical 'corkage'. The apical and lateral movement of thermosoftened gutta-percha is referred to as a 'wave of condensation'. The temperature set at the tip of the plugger is controlled and maintained. Thus, the technique is simpler and more rapid than other techniques because down-packing is completed in a single, continuous vertical movement. Back-packing involves filling the middle and coronal portions of the canal and can be accomplished using thermoplasticized gutta-percha devices, e.g. injection systems, (see later) that can deposit increments of warm gutta-percha.

The continuous wave technique requires a smooth tapering canal shape with the smallest diameter at the foramen. A nonstandardized gutta-percha cone of similar taper is then selected and tried to ensure it achieves the correct length and fits snugly, with tug-back. This is essential to provide resistance during condensation and prevent extrusion of the gutta-percha cone. A radiograph should be taken to confirm the fit. Alternatively, a tapered gutta-percha point matching the instrument system, which prepared the canal may be used; this simplifies selection.

A plugger that matches the canal taper is chosen, attached to the heating device and then tried in the canal so that it stops 4 to 5 mm from the termination of the preparation, a position termed the *binding point*; this is marked with a silicone stop. It is important that the taper of the plugger matches the taper produced after canal preparation and that it does not contact the canal walls at this point. The pluggers can be pre-curved if required.

After the sealer application, the selected cone is positioned in the canal and the excess protruding out of the canal entrance removed with the heated plugger. The plugger is then placed on the point, activated (maximum power, 200°C) and driven down (down-packed) through the gutta-percha to the level

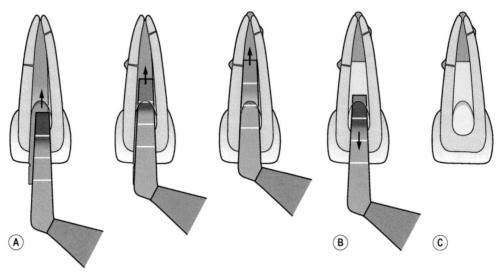

FIGURE 9-10 Continuous wave condensation. (A) Down-pack. (B) Separation and withdrawal. (C) Apical 4 to 5 mm 'corked' with gutta-percha. (Based on an original drawing by M. Monteith.)

of the binding point as indicated by the silicone stop (Figure 9-10). After 1 second, the activating button is released and further vertical pressure applied on the cooling plugger for another 10 seconds to counteract shrinkage. Finally, the heat source is activated for a further second, while apical pressure is maintained before the plugger is withdrawn. Most of the gutta-percha in the middle and coronal but not the apical portions is removed when the plugger is withdrawn; the apex is now 'corked'. The rest of the canal can be back filled using the same heating device, gutta-percha plugs with pluggers or more effectively with an injection device.

The continuous wave technique seems simple but the skills required take considerable time to master, particularly in teeth with confluent canal systems, so practise on extracted teeth is essential. Radiographs often show material forced into irregularities and lateral canals implying more complete filling with material, most likely sealer, extruded beyond the foramen (Figure 9-11). As achieving apical patency is an essential step when preparing canals with a continuous taper and due to the high hydraulic pressure involved with this technique, extrusion of root filling material is not uncommon. The passage of sealer into the periapical region is a concern as,

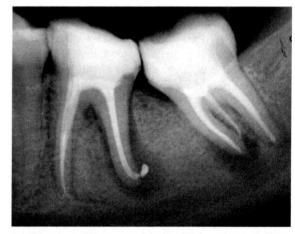

FIGURE 9-11 Sealer extrusion from the distal root of a mandibular left first molar. The second molar is an example of radix entomolaris. (Reproduced courtesy of M. Alghamdi.)

although it is likely to be absorbed, it may cause inflammation.

Vibration and Heat. A combination of heat and vibration may be used to condense gutta-percha using the RootBuddy (Nikinc Dental, Eindhoven, The Netherlands). This cordless instrument provides low frequency (100 Hz) pulses and heats to 350°C. It can be used for lateral and warm vertical condensation techniques with any core material. A master cone is heated in vibration mode and accessory cones then placed. Heated plugger tips, available in nickel–titanium or soft stainless steel, allow great flexibility in curved canals. This may provide improved condensation and homogeneity in tortuous canal systems, which would otherwise need canal enlargement for conventional warm obturation techniques.[85]

Rotating Condenser. The use of an engine-driven rotating compactor to soften and condense gutta-percha vertically and laterally was described by McSpadden.[86] A rotating stainless steel instrument was used to generate frictional heat within the canal to plasticize a cold cone and drive the thermomechanically plasticized material apically. The original instruments have been discontinued, but the Gutta-Condensor (Dentsply Maillefer), which operates at 8000 rpm in a high-torque handpiece, and Thermal Lateral Condensor (Brasseler) are available.

The original technique involved the condenser being activated in the canal, alongside the master gutta-percha cone, at approximately 12 000 rpm without apical pressure. The gutta-percha softens very rapidly and is driven apically by advancing the condenser to about 2 mm from the termination of the preparation. As the apical region filled, the condenser backs out of the canal and is slowly withdrawn while still rotating at the optimum speed. In large canals the procedure is repeated with additional gutta-percha cones to fill coronal deficiencies.

Following concerns about the unpredictable nature of the technique, particulary apical extrusion of root-filling material and instrument fracture, the method was modified.[87] A hybrid technique combined the predictability of lateral condensation near the apex with the speed and efficacy of the condenser in the remainder of the canal. A master cone is cemented, and lateral condensation of accessory points is carried out in the apical 3 to 4 mm before using the compactor in the rest of the canal.

Modern rotating condensers are manufactured from nickel–titanium, not just stainless steel, and used with gutta-percha that has been presoftened outside the mouth; these techniques are described later in this chapter.

Extracanal Heating Techniques

These rely on gutta-percha being warmed and softened out of the mouth before its insertion into the root canal.

Precoated Carriers. An approach to filling canals using a carrier to introduce thermally softened gutta-percha into the canal was described almost four decades ago.[88] The efficacy of this technique was based on the flow characteristics of a special α-phase gutta-percha and the ability of the carrier to transport and condense it.

The technique was commercially modified in 1989 and, initially, featured metal carriers, but plastics are now used (e.g. Thermafil Endodontic Obturators, Dentsply Tulsa Dental). The carrier is precoated with gutta-percha (obturator) and when warmed in a controlled manner in a dedicated oven, the material is sticky and adhesive with good flow characteristics. A series of instruments, plastic verifiers, are provided to check the diameter of the termination of the preparation and to simplify the selection of the correct size of obturator. Obturators are now made to match the conicity of the instrument system used to prepare the canal.

The technique for using precoated carriers is simple.[89] After preparation and drying, an uncoated carrier, or a verifier, of the estimated size is inserted to the full working length in the canal; a radiograph can confirm the position. The size of obturator is selected and the working length marked with a silicone stop (Figure 9-12). The canal is then coated with a small amount of sealer. The obturator is placed in the conditioning oven for the appropriate time, removed and immediately seated into the canal. It should not be inserted so that the tip of the carrier reaches the apical extent of preparation; the aim is to ensure the tip of the carrier is 0.5 mm from this point leaving the apical region filled only with gutta-percha and sealer. The canal length must be measured accurately, and the silicone stop on the obturator carefully positioned.

After the gutta-percha has cooled, the obturator is severed at the canal entrance and the handle discarded. Any excess gutta-percha in the chamber is removed and the remainder condensed vertically to

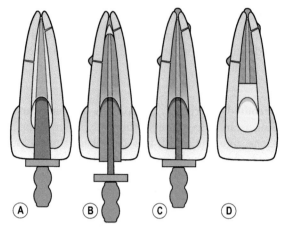

FIGURE 9-12 Precoated carrier obturation. (A) Verification of size with a blank carrier. (B) Selected carrier conditioned in oven, placed into canal and (C) inserted to length. (D) Excess removed. (Based on an original drawing by M. Monteith.)

enhance the coronal seal; additional gutta-percha can be introduced if the canal morphology dictates. A disadvantage of some of these devices, particularly when a postretained restoration is planned, is the fact that the shaft of the carrier remains in the root canal. Another disadvantage is that the heat-softened gutta-percha may be stripped from the carrier, and the apical portion of the canal is then occupied by the carrier instead of gutta-percha.

Most laboratory studies on precoated carriers suggest the technique is significantly faster than lateral condensation and produces fillings of similar radiographic appearance and an equivalent or better apical seal with both the original metal and plastic carriers. A minority of studies have reported that lateral condensation produced a better apical seal.[90–93] In laboratory studies, the use of precoated carriers has been associated with an increased incidence of sealer and gutta-percha extrusion, but this may be reduced by modern variable taper preparations.[94] A small scale study suggested that Thermafil (Dentsply Tulsa Dental) might be superior to lateral condensation when used by novice undergraduates.[95]

Voids have been found in all root fillings done with Thermafil and System B,[16] whereas a study found that Thermafil, System B and single-point cold gutta-percha fillings featured similar percentages of filling and void distribution.[96]

Concerns have been expressed about the problems of removing carriers should retreatment be necessary.[97,98] Newer Thermafil obturators (Dentsply Tulsa Dental) feature a v-shaped groove in the shaft of the carrier which is aimed at facilitating removal, and research shows they may be removed from moderately curved canals using rotary nickel–titanium files.[99]

There are also similar carrier-based systems on the market. GuttaFusion (VDW) is a system consisting of an outer coating of flowable gutta-percha on a carrier made entirely of cross-linked gutta-percha. The flowable coating maintains the characteristics of gutta-percha, and is claimed to avoid the stripping of material from the carrier. There is easy separation of the handle by bending it at the canal entrance, and the system facilitates removal of material to prepare a post space. The size of obturator is selected with the help of a verifier and obturators corresponding to engine-driven preparation files (Reciproc, VDW). A time-saving is reported compared with lateral condensation of gutta-percha.

GuttaCore (Dentsply Tulsa Dental) is another obturator system which uses a cross-linked gutta-percha core. The core is adequately strong, resists melting and is coated with conventional gutta-percha. The device aims to provide the same quality of obturation as Thermafil, but its removal with files is easier and faster if retreatment, or post space preparation, is necessary.[100] The canals to receive it should be prepared to the minimum size recommended. A thin layer of sealer is also recommended, placed in the coronal half of the canal, and of a type which is not too thick. A newer version of the device with a pink-coloured core is said to be slightly more rigid.

Although precoated carriers are convenient, they are relatively expensive and cannot be customized easily for specific canals.

Thermoplastic Delivery Systems. Many injection-type thermoplastic gutta-percha products are available. The devices heat gutta-percha to a molten state for injection into the root canal.[101] Vertical condensation is then required to ensure its adaptation to the canal wall.

The ability of gutta-percha to adapt to the canal walls has been confirmed,[102] and the method produces a seal comparable to lateral condensation,[101] although extrusion of root filling material may occur. With the Obtura III Max (Obtura Spartan, Algonquin, IL, USA) thermoplasticized injected gutta-percha devices, the gutta-percha is heated to 160°C and delivered through the needle tip at approximately 60°C.[103]

Other examples of injection devices include BeeFill Backfill (VDW), the Elements Obturation Unit (SybronEndo) and the BeeFill 2in1 (VDW); cordless versions include the System B Endodontic Cordless Fill (SybronEndo), B&L SuperEndo Beta, (B & L Biotech) and elementsfree cordless (SybronEndo).

The BeeFill 2in1, the Elements Obturation Unit and the elementsfree cordless, combine a gutta-percha extruder and a System B type device. The gutta-percha cartridges heat quickly, and the extruder tips, which may come in different sizes, are easily bent. These high-temperature type devices have been shown to produce clinically acceptable results,[104,105] whereas laboratory studies have demonstrated an apical seal as good as with lateral condensation.[17] Warm injected gutta-percha can also penetrate dentinal tubules to an extent.[60] On the other hand, some studies have reported the apical seal to be less effective[106,107] and the incidence of gutta-percha under, or overextension, to be high.[108]

The enlargement of the foramen needs to be limited[109] and the prepared canal requires a definite stop at the termination of the preparation.[110,111] The use of a sectional injection technique, in which the gutta-percha is deposited and condensed in several increments rather than in one application, has also been found to improve the apical seal as it allows better condensation of the material deposited apically.[112] Improvement of the apical seal has also been reported when a conventional master gutta-percha cone is cemented before injection of the heated gutta-percha.[113] This hybrid technique also offers good length control. Thermoplasticized injected gutta-percha delivery systems are very popular for back-filling the middle and coronal portions after vertical condensation or lateral condensation (Figure 9-13). Concern has been raised regarding shrinkage of

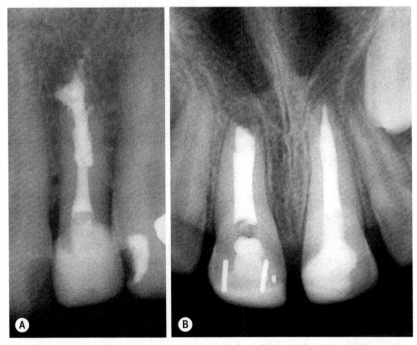

FIGURE 9-13 (A) Maxillary lateral incisor with communicating resorptive defects filled apically with vertically condensed warm gutta-percha and back-filled using an injection delivery system. (B) One-step apexification of maxillary right central incisor using an absorbable collagen matrix and injected thermoplasticized gutta-percha. The left central incisor was filled using lateral condensation. (Part A reproduced courtesy of L Friedlander.)

gutta-percha, which can be quick and extensive. In a study of three injection devices set to 200°C, gutta-percha was provided at between 58°C and 104°C and shrinkage was as high as 2.3% after 10 minutes.[114]

Operator-Coated Carrier-Condenser. The original technique of thermatic condensation of gutta-percha used conventional gutta-percha cones and a rotating condenser to generate heat.[86] Concerns about instrument fracture, its inability to be used effectively in curved canals, excessive heat generation and lack of predictability led to the development of nickel–titanium condensers and a technique in which the condenser is coated with heat-softened gutta-percha (two formulations, one relatively viscous and the other more fluid) before insertion into the canal. A number of methods could be used to obturate canals; one involved sealing a conventional master gutta-percha cone into the canal followed by the immediate use of a condenser coated with heat-softened gutta-percha.[115] Alternatively, the compactor can first be coated with the more viscous material and then with an additional layer of the more fluid material. The concept with the MicroSeal system (SybronEndo) remains as before, but it has been enhanced by the provision of master cones having a different gutta-percha formulation to the one that is warmed and injected onto the condenser. The manufacturer recommends the fitting of a cold master gutta-percha cone before the introduction of the warmed gutta-percha on the condenser.

SOLVENT-SOFTENED GUTTA-PERCHA

Chloroform-softened gutta-percha has a long tradition in endodontics. After drying with alcohol, the root canal is filled with a solution of rosin (colophony) in chloroform into which is seated a master cone. The chloroform softened the surface of the gutta-percha and made it swell, and the rosin acted as a glue to make the mass stick to the canal walls.

The high degree of evaporation and the fluid nature of the rosin solution led to the development of chloro-percha. Primarily a thick suspension of fine shavings of gutta-percha in chloroform, chloro-percha was modified by the addition of zinc oxide and metal salts to act as much as a conventional sealer as merely softening the points. Kloroperka is the best-known

formulation, with studies of its performance reported as favourable.[116]

Chloroform may also be used to customize master gutta-percha cones. This has been popularized as the chloroform dip technique.[117] The apical 2 to 5 mm of the master gutta-percha cone is dipped in chloroform for a few seconds and inserted into the moist canal to the termination of the preparation and then withdrawn and allowed to dry. The chloroform softens the outer layer of the gutta-percha so that when it is seated fully it takes up the shape of the apical portion of the canal. Since the volume of solvent is small and the thickness of gutta-percha affected is minimal, there is potentially little shrinkage after solvent evaporation.[118] The customized cone is then inserted with a conventional sealer, and the remainder of the canal is filled with laterally condensed gutta-percha. The apical seal obtained with this technique is reported to be comparable with traditional cold lateral condensation.[119]

Other Methods of Root Canal Filling

MINERAL TRIOXIDE AGGREGATE

Mineral trioxide aggregate consists of hydrophilic particles that sets in the presence of moisture.[120] Hydration of the powder results in a colloidal gel with a pH of 12.5 that solidifies to a hard structure. Several *in vitro* and *in vivo* studies have shown that MTA has good sealing ability, is biocompatible and promotes tissue regeneration when placed in contact with the periapical tissues.

MTA has application as a root canal filling material without the need for a core material, such as gutta-percha, if the difficulties of placement in the canal can be mastered[121] (Figure 9-14). MTA may be placed with an incremental compaction technique involving pluggers,[121] using a series of K files (Lawaty technique) or with tapered rotary NiTi files used in reverse (Auger technique). Ultrasound, applied indirectly, has been suggested as an aid to MTA condensation; there has been controversy regarding whether it provides a better, void-free result, especially when applied for very short time periods (1 second).[122,123] Manual condensation using increments placed with pluggers also produces a dense fill.[123]

Root fillings of MTA may be also considered for patients seeking 'alternative' filling materials, and for

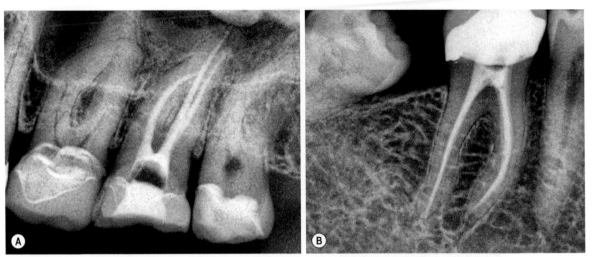

FIGURE 9-14 Root fillings consisting of just Mineral trioxide aggregate (MTA). (A) Maxillary left second molar. (B) Mandibular right first molar. (Reproduced courtesy of I. Lawaty.)

some with a latex allergy who are concerned about the use of gutta-percha.

MTA canal fillings should be considered permanent, as removing it, or any bioceramic materials, from a canal is challenging.[124] The recent discovery of bacterial entombment in dentinal tubules by MTA may be significant[58]; successful root fillings do not need removal, so the requirement for retreatment may be reduced.

The use of MTA as an apical plug for teeth with immature, open apices has proved very successful.[125] The material creates a hard barrier, and the remainder of the canal is then filled with MTA, or the root reinforced by appropriate materials[126] (Figure 9-15). Treatment in one or two appointments avoids the long-term use of calcium hydroxide dressings, which weaken the already thin dentine,[127] while waiting for the formation of a hard tissue barrier. MTA may also be used to root fill the nonvital coronal part of a tooth with a horizontal root fracture, a condition presenting a similar clinical task to an open apex (Figure 9-16).

HYDROPHILIC POLYMERS

The SmartSeal system (SmartSeal DRFP Ltd, Stamford, Peterborough, UK), introduced in 2007, uses a single master cone (SmartPoint) made of materials similar to those used in intraocular and contact lenses. The central cores of the cones are of two polyamide (nylon) polymers covered by a hydrophilic polymer sheath. The coating is designed to swell and to be self-sealing in a 'wet' canal. A resin-based sealer (SmartPaste Bio) is used in conjunction with the SmartPoint cone and contains bioceramics; it too hydrates and swells to fill voids. No special equipment is required and the cones are provided in a variety of tapers and sizes to match preparation instruments. Two points may be used to fill an oval canal. The radiographic appearance differs from gutta-percha, as the polymer sheath is not radiopaque. The system claims to be easier to handle and less technique sensitive than other obturation methods, with cost and time savings in both preparation and obturation. The points have comparable biocompatibility to gutta-percha[128] and have a significant lateral expansion, within 20 minutes when exposed to water.[129] Used with SmartPaste sealer in an *in vitro* study, there was high extension of material into simulated lateral canals and comparable homogeneity of obturation compared with laterally condensed gutta-percha and AH Plus sealer.[130]

MONOBLOCKS

A key disadvantage of gutta-percha is that it does not bond to dentine. A search for simpler methods of filling canals and alternatives to gutta-percha led to the investigation of low viscosity composite resins to seal root canals in the late 1970s.[131] The introduction

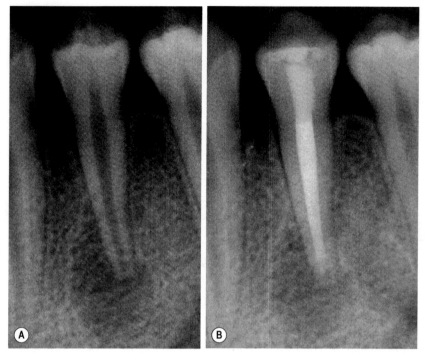

FIGURE 9-15 Mandibular left first premolar with immature apex and periapical lesion a result of pulp exposure of a dens evaginatus tubercle: (A) initial presentation; (B) canal filled with Mineral trioxide aggregate and access cavity sealed with composite resin. (Reproduced courtesy of M. Gordon.)

of fibre posts for restoring root-filled teeth introduced the potential to, simultaneously, fill the root and also reinforce the tooth. The development of a polycaprolactone thermoplastic material (Resilon, Pentron Corp, Wallingford, CT, USA) with bioactive glass, bismuth and barium salts as fillers provided an alternative core material to gutta-percha. With handling characteristics very similar to gutta-percha, it has the potential to bond to suitable sealers.

Together with a UDMA-based sealer (e.g. Epiphany, Pentron Corp; RealSeal or RealSeal SE, SybronEndo), there is the potential to create a form of monoblock,[132] which has a single interface between the dentine of the root canal wall and the filling core. With the smear layer removed, a primer is applied and the dual-cured sealer is coated onto the dentine wall. Cones, or thermoplasticized portions of core material, are then inserted. Tests of these materials indicated less apical leakage[133] and an improvement in the strength of the tooth.[134,135] The work of other researchers has challenged the increase in fracture resistance offered by

these systems,[136] their improved bond strength to dentine,[137-141] and also their sealing ability.[142,143,144] It may be that the initial hopes of increasing the fracture strength of teeth were the result of altered transmission of forces within the canal rather than the direct effect of the material.[145] Many factors are involved in the success or failure of these systems, including the nature of the smear layer (if present), any oxidative layer left by irrigating solutions, dentine tubule permeability, C-factor (the ratio of bonded/nonbonded surface area of the canal space), the thickness of the sealer and its polymerization shrinkage. All self- and dual-cure adhesives have lower bond strengths than the light-activated varieties. In addition to the problem of contraction on setting, no polymer is considered entirely stable over time.

Carrier-type obturators, similar to Thermafil but precoated with Resilon instead of gutta-percha, are available (RealSeal 1, SybronEndo). The other components of the system include verifiers to determine the obturator size required, a conditioning oven and the

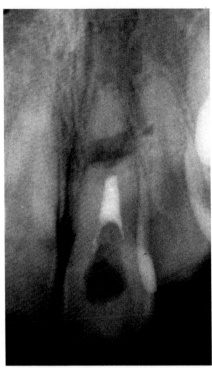

FIGURE 9-16 Maxillary left central incisor with horizontal root fracture. The nonvital coronal part of the canal has been filled with mineral trioxide aggregate (MTA); radiograph to check placement of MTA before restoration.

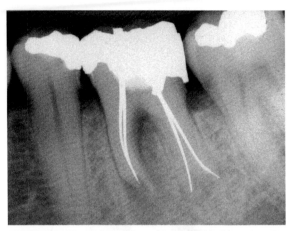

FIGURE 9-17 Mandibular left first molar filled with silver points. The tooth has two distal roots, and inflammatory resorption is evident at the apex of the mesial root.

self-etch resin sealer (RealSeal SE, SybronEndo). Together, the claim is that the obturator is 'warm-bonded' to the canal.

Another family of products designed with the monoblock concept in mind is the Next system (Heraeus Kulzer, Armonk, NY, USA) consisting of Next Post/Obturators, fibreglass carriers tipped with Resilon, for straight canals. Where the subsequent restoration requires an intraradicular post and for curved canals, Next Tapered Obturators, in which the carriers are resin rather than glass fibre can be used. Both types of obturators are bonded to the root dentine using a resin-based (Next) sealer and bonding agents.

Reviews conclude that at this point of development methacrylate-based root canal filling systems have no clear benefits.[146,147]

NONINSTRUMENTATION TECHNOLOGY

A noninstrumentation hydrodynamic method for root canal treatment has been described that allows the cleaning, disinfection and filling of the root canal system without the use of traditional instruments.[148,149] The canals are cleansed by irrigation with sodium hypochlorite under alternating pressure generated by a vacuum pump; the canals are not enlarged, and no smear layer is created. Filling of the canal system is performed using a vacuum pump that produces a negative pressure. When this is achieved, a valve is opened to a reservoir containing freshly mixed sealer and the material is sucked into the root canal system. Laboratory and clinical studies of the technique were promising, and the seal comparable to lateral condensation,[150–152] but it has not materialized into a clinically viable technique.

SILVER POINTS

Silver points were first used in 1931 to fill curved canals.[153] Due to the limitations of early canal preparation instruments, these canals were difficult to enlarge adequately to accept gutta-percha cones. Gutta-percha cones lack rigidity and will bend or deform in narrow, curved canals. Silver points could be forced down narrow canals and provide the appearance of a dense radiopaque filling occupying the full length of the canal (Figure 9-17). Unfortunately, this filling technique encouraged clinicians to pay less attention to thorough cleaning and shaping of the root canal system, often leaving debris and microorganisms present, leading to failure. Silver points have other

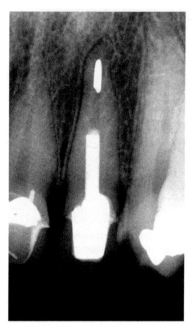

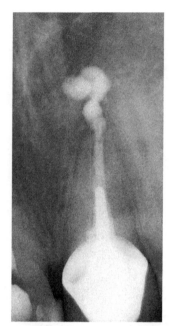

FIGURE 9-18 Maxillary left lateral incisor filled using the sectional silver point technique and restored with a cast post/core and a porcelain jacket crown.

FIGURE 9-19 Maxillary left central incisor filled with paste material; a substantial quantity has been extruded into the periapical region.

disadvantages. They are round in cross-section, and few canals are round, or can be made round, particularly coronally. The seal relies heavily on large volumes of sealer. Silver points are also prone to corrosion when exposed to tissue fluids or saliva.[154] The corrosion products are toxic and may reach the periapical tissues and compound the problems caused by sealer dissolution. In addition, full-length silver points could not be used in teeth where postretained restorations were planned; a sectional technique was devised to overcome this difficulty (Figure 9-18). Finally, the removal of silver points, particularly sectional silver points, for retreatment is also not easy. The use of silver points is not recommended.

PASTE FILLERS

Paste fillers were introduced to speed up root canal treatment[155] and harks back to the dated concept of mummifying pulps. The paste fillers should not be confused with sealers, or cements, designed as luting agents for solid, or semisolid, root canal filling materials.

Paste fillers may contain strong disinfectants (e.g. paraformaldehyde) and antiinflammatory agents (e.g. corticosteroids) and were introduced in the belief that their use could bypass the accepted principles of canal preparation, disinfection and filling. The proponents of paste fillers argued that the medicaments would eliminate microorganisms so that thorough cleaning and shaping were not necessary, and the antiinflammatory agents would reduce the host response. The use of paste fillers is to be condemned as some patients (Figure 9-19) suffered injury as a result of toxic materials being passed into the periapical tissues and beyond.[156,157] Most paste fillers (Endomethasone, Septodont; N2, Indrag-Agsa, Bologna, Italy; SPAD, Quetigny, France) contain paraformaldehyde. If deposited in the periapical tissues this may give rise to severe inflammatory reactions and long-lasting, or permanent injury, particularly to nerve bundles.[157,158] Corticosteroid in paste fillers severely affects the defense responses of the periapical tissues by suppressing phagocytosis, and their use may possibly cause unwanted systemic side effects.[159]

The application of paraformaldehyde to vital tissue will also result in traces of the material, or its components, being spread throughout the body.[160] Individuals may show a hypersensitivity response, and the material may have both mutagenic and carcinogenic potentials.[161] A newer development is Endomethasone N (Septodont), which does not contain paraformaldehyde and claims greatly improved biocompatibility.

Coronal Restoration

A variety of materials are used as provisional restorations between treatment visits.[162] There is overwhelming evidence supporting the concept of coronal leakage[1] and the requirement to restore the root filled tooth with a good quality, permanent coronal restoration[2,163,164]. Root-filled teeth are vulnerable and will not survive unless they are properly restored.[165] A tooth which has lost its provisional, or permanent, restoration may need to have its root canal retreated.[166,167] Provided all the technical requirements of the root canal treatment have been achieved, a permanent coronal restoration should be placed without unnecessary delay, preferably during the canal filling visit.

Follow-Up

It is essential to take a postoperative radiograph straight after completion of root canal filling. Immediately after treatment, teeth may be tender and it is advisable to warn patients of this possibility. Fortunately, the incidence of severe pain after root canal filling is low.[168,169] In most cases, any discomfort is mild and no active intervention is required. If severe pain occurs over an extended period, then further investigation and diagnosis are necessary. In particular, the quality of treatment should be reviewed so that it can be established whether poor technique and/or procedural accidents may have contributed to the problem. Once the cause has been identified, then the correct treatment can be instituted; this may include nonsurgical or surgical retreatment.

Follow-up of root-filled teeth is important to ascertain treatment outcome. Firm guidelines for the timing of recalls are not possible as each case is different, but a clinical and radiographic check after 1 year is advisable.[170]

Treatment Outcome

The outcome of root canal treatment is assessed using a combination of clinical and radiological criteria[170]:
- the tooth should be functional with no signs of swelling or sinus tract;
- the patient should be free from symptoms;
- the radiographic appearance of the periapical tissues should either remain normal or return to normality.

Although the patient's symptoms may improve, and signs such as a swelling, or a draining sinus, may disappear after root canal preparation and dressing, success or failure cannot be declared immediately. Large areas of periapical bone loss may take months, or even years, to heal completely, with extended review necessary especially for retreatment cases.[171]

Learning Outcomes

This chapter should allow the reader to recognise and explain the:
- objectives of filling root canals;
- various materials and the different techniques for root canal filling, with the emphasis on gutta-percha as the core material;
- role and use of different types of root canal sealers;
- newer materials for root canal filling, including MTA, calcium silicates, bioceramics and the 'monoblock' concept;
- shortcomings of older filling techniques and materials, which although no longer recommended or used, may be encountered in clinical practice.

REFERENCES

1. Saunders WP, Saunders EM. Coronal leakage as a cause of failure in root canal therapy: a review. Endodontics and Dental Traumatology 1994;10:105–8.
2. Tronstad L, Asbjørnsen K, Døving L, et al. Influence of coronal restorations on the periapical health of endodontically treated teeth. Endodontics and Dental Traumatology 2000;16: 218–21.
3. Metzger Z, Zary R, Cohen R, et al. The quality of root canal preparation and root canal obturation in canals treated with rotary versus Self-adjusting files: a three-dimensional micro-computed tomographic study. Journal of Endodontics 2010;36:1569–73.

4. Wu M-K, Wesselink PR, Walton RE. Apical terminus location of root canal treatment procedures. Oral Surgery, Oral Medicine, Oral Pathology, Oral Radiology, Endodontics 2000;89: 99–103.

5. Buchanan LS. The standardized-taper root canal preparation. Part I. Concepts for variably tapered shaping instruments. International Endodontic Journal 2000;33:516–29.

6. Byström A, Claesson R, Sundqvist G. The antibacterial effect of camphorated paramonochlorophenol, camphorated phenol and calcium hydroxide in the treatment of infected root canals. Endodontics and Dental Traumatology 1985;1: 170–5.

7. Peters LB, Wesselink PR, Moorer WR. The fate and the role of bacteria left in root canal tubules. International Endodontic Journal 1995;28:95–9.

8. Vera J, Siqueira JF Jr, Ricucci D, et al. One- versus two-visit endodontic treatment of teeth with apical periodontitis: a histobacteriologic study. Journal of Endodontics 2012;38: 1040–52.

9. Xavier ACC, Martinho FC, Chung A, et al. One-visit versus two-visit root canal treatment: effectiveness in removal of endotoxins and cultivable bacteria. Journal of Endodontics 2013;39:959–64.

10. Sjögren U, Figdor D, Persson S, et al. Influence of infection at the time of root filling on the outcome of endodontic treatment of teeth with apical periodontitis. International Endodontic Journal 1997;30:297–306.

11. Trope M, Delano EO, Ørstavik D. Endodontic treatment of teeth with apical periodontitis: single visit vs. multivisit treatment. Journal of Endodontics 1999;25:345–50.

12. Ricucci D, Russo J, Rutberg M, et al. A prospective cohort study of endodontic treatments of 1,369 root canals: results after 5 years. Oral Surgery, Oral Medicine, Oral Pathology, Oral Radiology, Endodontics 2011;112:825–42.

13. Su Y, Wang C, Ye L. Healing rate and post-obturation pain of single- versus multiple- visit endodontic treatment for infected root canals: a systematic review. Journal of Endodontics 2011; 37:125–32.

14. Vela KC, Walton RE, Trope M, et al. Patient preferences regarding 1-visit versus 2-visit root canal therapy. Journal of Endodontics 2012;38:1322–5.

15. Nagas EN, Ozgur Uyanik M, Eymirli A, et al. Dentin moisture conditions affect the adhesion of root canal sealers. Journal of Endodontics 2012;38:240–4.

16. Anbu R, Nandini S, Velmurugan N. Volumetric analysis of root fillings using spiral computed tomography: an *in vitro* study. International Endodontic Journal 2009;43:64–8.

17. Hata G, Kawazoe S, Toda T, et al. Sealing ability of thermoplasticized gutta-percha fill techniques as assessed by a new method of determining apical leakage. Journal of Endodontics 1995;21:167–72.

18. Grossman LI, Oliet S, del Rio CE. Endodontic practice. 11th ed. Philadelphia: Lea and Febiger; 1988. p. 242–70.

19. Spångberg L, Langeland K. Biologic effects of dental materials. I. Toxicity of root canal filling materials on HeLa cells in vitro. Oral Surgery, Oral Medicine, Oral Pathology 1973;35:402–14.

20. Ørstavik D, Mjör IA. Histopathology and X-ray microanalysis of the subcutaneous tissue response to endodontic sealers. Journal of Endodontics 1988;14:13–23.

21. Ørstavik D. Weight loss of endodontic sealers, cements and pastes in water. Scandinavian Journal of Dental Research 1983;91:316–9.

22. Al-Dewani N, Hayes SJ, Dummer PMH. Comparison of laterally condensed and low temperature thermoplasticized gutta-percha root fillings. Journal of Endodontics 2000;26:733–8.

23. Balguerie E, van der Sluis L, Vallaeys K, et al. Sealer penetration and adaptation in the dentinal tubules: a scanning electron microscopic study. Journal of Endodontics 2011;37: 1576–9.

24. Kuçi A, Alaçam T, Yavas Ö, et al. Sealer penetration into dentinal tubules in the presence or absence of smear layer: a confocal laser scanning microscopic study. Journal of Endodontics 2014;40:1627–31.

25. Guimarães BM, Amoroso-Silva PA, Alcalde MP, et al. Influence of ultrasonic activation of four root canal sealers on the filling quality. Journal of Endodontics 2014;40:964–8.

26. Grossman LI. An improved root canal cement. Journal of the American Dental Association 1958;56:381–5.

27. Desai S, Chandler N. Calcium-hydroxide-based root canal sealers: a review. Journal of Endodontics 2009;35:475–80.

28. Jacobsen EL, BeGole EA, Vitkus DD, et al. An evaluation of two newly formulated calcium hydroxide cements: a leakage study. Journal of Endodontics 1987;13:164–9.

29. Barkhordar RA, Nguyen NT. Paresthesia of the mental nerve after overextension with AH26 and gutta-percha: report of a case. Journal of the American Dental Association 1985;110: 202–3.

30. Spångberg LSW, Barbosa SV, Lavigne GD. AH26 releases formaldehyde. Journal of Endodontics 1993;19:596–8.

31. Heling I, Chandler NP. The antimicrobial effect within dentinal tubules of four root canal sealers. Journal of Endodontics 1996;22:257–9.

32. Viapiana R, Guerreiro-Tanomaru JM, Tanomaru-Filho M, et al. Investigation of the effect of sealer use on the heat generated at the external root surface during root canal obturation using warm vertical compaction technique with System B heat source. Journal of Endodontics 2014;40:555–61.

33. Viapana R, Baluci CA, Tanumaro-Filho M, et al. Investigation of chemical changes in sealers during application of the warm vertical compaction technique. International Endodontic Journal 2015;48:16–27.

34. Camilleri J. Sealers and warm gutta-percha obturation techniques. Journal of Endodontics 2015;41:72–8.

35. Zmener O, Pameijer CH. Clinical and radiographic evaluation of a resin-based root canal sealer: 10-year recall data. International Journal of Dentistry 2012;4:ID 763248.

36. Roth KA, Friedman S, Lévesque CM, et al. Microbial biofilm proliferation within sealer-root dentin interfaces is affected by sealer type and aging period. Journal of Endodontics 2012;38: 1253–6.

37. Rahimi M, Jainaen A, Parashos P, et al. Enhancing the bond of a resin-based sealer to root dentine. International Endodontic Journal 2012;45:1141–7.

38. Prado M, Simão RA, Gomes BPFA. Effect of different irrigation protocols on resin sealer bond strength to dentin. Journal of Endodontics 2013;39:689–92.

39. do Prado M, de Assis DF, Gomes BPFA, et al. Adhesion of resin-based sealers to dentine: an atomic force microscopy study. International Endodontic Journal 2014;47:1052–7.

40. Pitt Ford TR. The leakage of root fillings using glass ionomer cement and other materials. British Dental Journal 1979;146: 273–8.

41. Wu M-K, Tigos E, Wesselink PR. An 18-month longitudinal study on a new silicon-based sealer, RSA RoekoSeal: a leakage

study *in vitro*. Oral Surgery, Oral Medicine, Oral Pathology, Oral Radiology, Endodontics 2002;94:499–502.

42. Miletic I, Devcic N, Anic I, et al. The cytotoxicity of RoekoSeal and AH Plus compared during different setting periods. Journal of Endodontics 2005;31:307–9.

43. Zielinski TM, Baumgartner JC, Marshall JG. An evaluation of GuttaFlow and gutta-percha in the filling of lateral grooves and depressions. Journal of Endodontics 2008;34: 295–8.

44. De-Deus G, Brandão MC, Fidel RAS, et al. The sealing ability of GuttaFlow in oval-shaped canals: an *ex vivo* study using a polymicrobial leakage model. International Endodontic Journal 2007;40:794–9.

45. Vasiliadis L, Kodonas K, Economides N, et al. Short- and long-term sealing ability of GuttaFlow and AH-Plus using an *ex vivo* fluid transport model. International Endodontic Journal 2010;43:377–81.

46. Weller RN, Tay KC, Garrett LV, et al. Microscopic appearance and apical seal of root canals filled with gutta-percha and ProRoot Endo Sealer after immersion in a phosphate-containing fluid. International Endodontic Journal 2008;41: 977–86.

47. Camilleri J. Evaluation of selected properties of mineral trioxide aggregate sealer cement. Journal of Endodontics 2009;35:1412–7.

48. Salles LP, Gomes-Cornélio AL, Guimarães FC, et al. Mineral trioxide aggregate-based endodontic sealer stimulates hydroxyapatite nucleation in human osteoblast-like cell culture. Journal of Endodontics 2012;38:971–6.

49. Zhou HM, Du TF, Shen Y, et al. *In vitro* cytotoxicity of calcium silicate-containing endodontic sealers. Journal of Endodontics 2015;41:56–61.

50. Massi S, Tanomaru-Filho M, Silva GF, et al. pH, calcium ion release, and setting time of an experimental mineral trioxide aggregate-based root canal sealer. Journal of Endodontics 2011;37:844–6.

51. Camilleri J, Gandolfi MG, Siboni F, et al. Dynamic sealing ability of MTA root canal sealer. International Endodontic Journal 2011;44:9–20.

52. Candeiro GT, Correia FC, Duarte MA, et al. Evaluation of radiopacity, pH, release of calcium ions, and flow of a bioceramic root canal sealer. Journal of Endodontics 2012;38: 842–5.

53. Gomes-Filho JE, Watanabe S, Bernabé PF, et al. A mineral trioxide aggregate sealer stimulated mineralization. Journal of Endodontics 2009;35:256–60.

54. Huffman BP, Mai S, Pinna L, et al. Dislocation resistance of ProRoot Endo Sealer, a calcium silicate-based root canal sealer, from radicular dentine. International Endodontic Journal 2009;42:34–46.

55. Ersahan S, Aydin C. Dislocation resistance of iRoot SP, a calcium silicate-based sealer, from radicular dentine. Journal of Endodontics 2010;36:2000–2.

56. Sagsen B, Ustün Y, Demirbuga S, et al. Push-out bond strength of two new calcium silicate-based endodontic sealers to root canal dentine. International Endodontic Journal 2011;44: 1088–91.

57. Topçuoglu HS, Tuncay Ö, Karatas E, et al. *In vitro* fracture resistance of roots obturated with epoxy-resin-based, mineral trioxide-based, and bioceramic root canal sealers. Journal of Endodontics 2013;39:1630–3.

58. Yoo JS, Chang S-W, Oh SR, et al. Bacterial entombment by intratubular mineralization following orthograde mineral trioxide aggregate obturation: a scanning electron microscope study. International Journal of Oral Science 2014;6:227–32.

59. Violich R, Chandler NP. The smear layer in endodontics: a review. International Endodontic Journal 2010;43:2–15.

60. Gutmann JL. Adaptation of injected thermoplasticized gutta-percha in the absence of the dentinal smear layer. International Endodontic Journal 1993;26:87–92.

61. Hovland EJ, Dumsha TC. Leakage evaluation in vitro of the root canal sealer cement Sealapex. International Endodontic Journal 1985;18:179–82.

62. Galvan DA, Ciarlone AE, Pashley DH, et al. Effect of smear layer removal on the diffusion permeability of human roots. Journal of Endodontics 1994;20:83–6.

63. Drake DR, Wiemann AH, Rivera EM, et al. Bacterial retention in canal walls *in vitro*: effect of smear layer. Journal of Endodontics 1994;20:78–82.

64. De-Deus G, Brandão MC, Leal F, et al. Lack of correlation between sealer penetration into dentinal tubules and sealability in nonbonded root fillings. International Endodontic Journal 2012;45:642–51.

65. Combe EC, Cohen BD, Cummings K. Alpha- and beta-forms of gutta-percha in products for root canal filling. International Endodontic Journal 2001;34:447–51.

66. Senia ES, Marraro RV, Mitchell JL, et al. Rapid sterilization of gutta-percha cones with 5.25% sodium hypochlorite. Journal of Endodontics 1975;1:136–40.

67. Ingle JI. A standardized endodontic technique utilizing newly designed instruments and filling materials. Oral Surgery, Oral Medicine, Oral Pathology 1961;14:83–91.

68. Beatty RG. The effect of standard or serial preparation on single cone obturation. International Endodontic Journal 1987;20:276–81.

69. Gordon MPJ, Love RM, Chandler NP. An evaluation of .06 tapered gutta-percha cones for filling of .06 taper prepared curved root canals. International Endodontic Journal 2005;38: 87–96.

70. Allison DA, Weber CR, Walton RE. The influence of the method of canal preparation on the quality of apical and coronal obturation. Journal of Endodontics 1979;5:298–304.

71. Van der Sluis LWM, Versluis M, Wu M-K, et al. Passive ultrasonic irrigation of the root canal: a review of the literature. International Endodontic Journal 2007;40:415–26.

72. Blum J-Y, Machtou P, Micallef J-P. Analysis of forces developed during obturations. Wedging effect: Part II. Journal of Endodontics 1998;24:223–8.

73. Wilcox LR, Roskelley C, Sutton T. The relationship of root canal enlargement to finger-spreader induced vertical root fracture. Journal of Endodontics 1997;23:533–4.

74. Madison S, Zakariasen KL. Linear and volumetric analysis of apical leakage in teeth prepared for posts. Journal of Endodontics 1984;10:422–7.

75. Wu M-K, Wesselink PR. A primary observation on the preparation and obturation of oval canals. International Endodontic Journal 2001;34:137–41.

76. Keles A, Alcin H, Kamalak A, et al. Micro-CT evaluation of root filling quality in oval-shaped canals. International Endodontic Journal 2014;47:1177–84.

77. Schilder H. Filling root canals in three dimensions. Dental Clinics of North America 1967;11:723–44.

78. Yared GM, Bou Dagher FE. Apical enlargement: influence on overextensions during *in vitro* vertical compaction. Journal of Endodontics 1994;20:269–71.

79. Wong M, Peters DD, Lorton L. Comparison of gutta-percha filling techniques, compaction (mechanical), vertical (warm), and lateral condensation techniques, part I. Journal of Endodontics 1981;7:551–8.

80. Peng L, Ye L, Tan H, et al. Outcome of root canal obturation by warm gutta-percha versus cold lateral condensation: a meta-analysis. Journal of Endodontics 2007;33:106–9.

81. Khayat A, Lee SJ, Torabinejad M. Human saliva penetration of coronally unsealed obturated root canals. Journal of Endodontics 1993;19:458–61.

82. Hand RE, Huget EF, Tsaknis PJ. Effects of a warm gutta-percha technique on the lateral periodontium. Oral Surgery, Oral Medicine, Oral Pathology 1976;42:395–401.

83. Bailey GC, Cunnington SA, Ng L-Y, et al. Ultrasonic condensation of gutta-percha: the effect of power setting and activation time on temperature rise at the root surface – an *in vitro* study. International Endodontic Journal 2004;37:447–54.

84. Buchanan LS. The Buchanan continuous wave of condensation technique. A convergence of conceptual and procedural advances in obturation. Dentistry Today 1994;13:80–5.

85. Pagavino G, Giachetti L, Nieri M, et al. The percentage of gutta-percha-filled area in simulated curved canals when filled using Endo Twinn, a new heat device source. International Endodontic Journal 2006;39:610–5.

86. McSpadden JT. Self-study course for the thermatic condensation of gutta-percha. York, PA: Dentsply; 1980.

87. Tagger M, Tamse A, Katz A, et al. Evaluation of apical seal produced by a hybrid root canal filling method combining lateral condensation and thermatic compaction. Journal of Endodontics 1984;10:299–303.

88. Johnson WB. A new gutta-percha filling technique. Journal of Endodontics 1978;4:184–8.

89. von Schroeter C. Thermafil obturation technique: an overview from the practitioner's point of view. ENDO (Lond Engl) 2008;2:43–54.

90. Chohayeb AA. Comparison of conventional root canal obturation techniques with Thermafil obturators. Journal of Endodontics 1992;18:10–2.

91. Haddix JE, Jarrell M, Mattison GD, et al. An in vitro investigation of the apical seal produced by a new thermoplasticized gutta-percha obturation technique. Quintessence International 1991;22:159–63.

92. Lares C, ElDeeb ME. The sealing ability of the Thermafil obturation technique. Journal of Endodontics 1990;16:474–9.

93. Ravanshad S, Torabinejad M. Coronal dye penetration of the apical filling materials after post space preparation. Oral Surgery, Oral Medicine, Oral Pathology 1992;74:644–7.

94. Heeren TJ, Levitan ME. Effects of canal preparation on fill length in straight root canals obturated with RealSeal 1 and Thermafil Plus. Journal of Endodontics 2012;38:1380–2.

95. Re D, Augusti D, Cerutti F, et al. A study on undergraduate learning of two obturation techniques: Thermafil versus lateral condensation. ENDO (Lond Engl) 2009;3:227–34.

96. Somma F, Cretella G, Carotenuto M, et al. Quality of thermoplasticized and single point root fillings assessed by micro-computed tomography. International Endodontic Journal 2011;44:362–9.

97. Wilcox LR. Thermafil retreatment with and without chloroform solvent. Journal of Endodontics 1993;19:563–6.

98. Wilcox LR, Juhlin JJ. Endodontic retreatment of Thermafil versus laterally condensed gutta-percha. Journal of Endodontics 1994;20:115–7.

99. Royzenblat A, Goodell GG. Comparison of removal times of Thermafil plastic obturators using ProFile rotary instruments at different rotational speeds in moderately curved canals. Journal of Endodontics 2007;33:256–8.

100. Beasley RT, Williamson AE, Justman BC, et al. Time required to remove GuttaCore, Thermafil Plus and thermoplasticized gutta-percha from moderately curved root canals with ProTaper files. Journal of Endodontics 2013;39:125–8.

101. Yee FS, Marlin J, Krakow AA, et al. Three-dimensional obturation of the root canal using injection-molded, thermoplasticized dental gutta-percha. Journal of Endodontics 1977;3:168–74.

102. Torabinejad M, Skobe Z, Trombly PL, et al. Scanning electron microscopic study of root canal obturation using thermoplasticized gutta-percha. Journal of Endodontics 1978;4:245–50.

103. Glickman GN, Gutmann JL. Contemporary perspectives on canal obturation. Dental Clinics of North America 1992;36:327–41.

104. Marlin J. Injectable standard gutta-percha as a method of filling the root canal system. Journal of Endodontics 1986;12:354–8.

105. Sobarzo-Navarro V. Clinical experience in root canal obturation by an injection thermoplasticized gutta-percha technique. Journal of Endodontics 1991;17:389–91.

106. Bradshaw GB, Hall A, Edmunds DH. The sealing ability of injection-moulded thermoplasticized gutta-percha. International Endodontic Journal 1989;22:17–20.

107. LaCombe JS, Campbell AD, Hicks ML, et al. A comparison of the apical seal produced by two thermoplasticized injectable gutta-percha techniques. Journal of Endodontics 1988;14:445–50.

108. Mann SR, McWalter GM. Evaluation of apical seal and placement control in straight and curved canals obturated by laterally condensed and thermoplasticized gutta-percha. Journal of Endodontics 1987;13:10–7.

109. Richie GM, Anderson DM, Sakumura JS. Apical extrusion of thermoplasticized gutta-percha used as a root canal filling. Journal of Endodontics 1988;14:128–32.

110. Gatot A, Peist M, Mozes M. Endodontic overextension produced by injected thermoplasticized gutta-percha. Journal of Endodontics 1989;15:273–4.

111. George JW, Michanowicz AE, Michanowicz JP. A method of canal preparation to control apical extrusion of low-temperature thermoplasticized gutta-percha. Journal of Endodontics 1987;13:18–23.

112. Veis A, Lambrianidis T, Molyvdas I, et al. Sealing ability of sectional injection thermoplasticized gutta-percha technique with varying distances between needle tip and apical foramen. Endodontics and Dental Traumatology 1992;8:63–6.

113. Olson AK, Hartwell GR, Weller RN. Evaluation of the controlled placement of injected thermoplasticized gutta-percha. Journal of Endodontics 1989;15:306–9.

114. Lottanti S, Tauböck TT, Zehnder M. Shrinkage of backfill gutta-percha on cooling. Journal of Endodontics 2014;40:721–4.

115. Gilhooly RMP, Hayes SJ, Bryant ST, et al. Comparison of lateral condensation and thermomechanically compacted warm α-phase gutta-percha with a single cone for obturating curved root canals. Oral Surgery, Oral Medicine, Oral Pathology, Oral Radiology, Endodontics 2001;91:89–94.

116. Strindberg LZ. The dependence of the results of pulp therapy on certain factors. An analytic study based on radiographic

and clinical follow-up examinations. Acta Odontologica Scandinavica 1956;21(Suppl. 4):1–175.

117. Beatty RG, Zakariasen KL. Apical leakage associated with three obturation techniques in large and small root canals. International Endodontic Journal 1984;17:67–72.

118. Wong M, Peters DD, Lorton L, et al. Comparison of gutta-percha filling techniques: three chloroform-gutta-percha filling techniques. Part II. Journal of Endodontics 1982;8: 4–9.

119. Smith JJ, Montgomery S. A comparison of apical seal: chloroform versus halothane-dipped gutta-percha cones. Journal of Endodontics 1992;18:156–60.

120. Torabinejad M, Hong CU, McDonald F, et al. Physical and chemical properties of a new root-end filling material. Journal of Endodontics 1995;21:349–53.

121. Bogen G, Kuttler S. Mineral trioxide aggregate obturation: a review and case series. Journal of Endodontics 2009;35:777–90.

122. Yeung P, Liewehr FR, Moon PC. A quantitative comparison of the fill density of MTA produced by two placement techniques. Journal of Endodontics 2006;32:456–9.

123. El-Ma'aita AM, Qualtrough AJE, Watts DC. A micro-computed tomography evaluation of mineral trioxide aggregate root canal fillings. Journal of Endodontics 2012;38:670–2.

124. Hess D, Solomon E, Spears R, et al. Retreatability of bioceramic root canal sealing material. Journal of Endodontics 2011; 37:1547–9.

125. Witherspoon DE, Small JC, Regan JD, et al. Retrospective analysis of open apex teeth obturated with mineral trioxide aggregate. Journal of Endodontics 2008;34:1171–6.

126. Desai S, Chandler N. The restoration of permanent immature teeth, root filled using MTA: a review. Journal of Dentistry 2009;37:652–7.

127. Andreasen JO, Farik B, Munksgaard EC. Long-term calcium hydroxide as a root canal dressing may increase risk of root fracture. Dental Traumatology 2002;18:134–7.

128. Eid AA, Nikonov SY, Looney SW, et al. In vitro biocompatibility evaluation of a root canal filling material that expands on water sorption. Journal of Endodontics 2013;39: 883–8.

129. Didato A, Eid AA, Levin MD, et al. Time-based lateral hygroscopic expansion of a water-expandable endodontic obturation point. Journal of Dentistry 2013;41:796–801.

130. Arora S, Hegde V. Comparative evaluation of a novel smart-seal obturating system and its homogeneity of using cone beam computed tomography: In vitro simulated lateral canal study. Journal of Conservative Dentistry 2014;17:364–8.

131. Tidmarsh BG. Acid-cleansed and resin-sealed root canals. Journal of Endodontics 1978;4:117–21.

132. Tay FR, Pashley DH. Monoblocks in root canals: a hypothetical or a tangible goal. Journal of Endodontics 2007;33: 391–8.

133. Shipper G, Ørstavik D, Teixeira FB, et al. An evaluation of microbial leakage in roots filled with a thermoplastic synthetic polymer-based root canal filling material (Resilon). Journal of Endodontics 2004;30:342–7.

134. Teixeira FB, Teixeira ECN, Thompson JY, et al. Fracture resistance of roots endodontically treated with a new resin filling material. Journal of the American Dental Association 2004; 135:646–52.

135. Monteiro J, de Noronha de Ataide I, Chalakkal P, et al. In vitro resistance to fracture of roots obturated with Resilon or gutta-percha. Journal of Endodontics 2011;37:828–31.

136. Stuart CH, Schwartz SA, Beeson TJ. Reinforcement of immature roots with a new resin filling material. Journal of Endodontics 2006;32:350–3.

137. Gesi A, Raffaelli O, Goracci C, et al. Interfacial strength of Resilon and gutta-percha to intraradicular dentin. Journal of Endodontics 2005;31:809–13.

138. Hiraishi N, Papacchini F, Loushine RJ, et al. Shear bond strength of Resilon to a methacrylate-based root canal sealer. International Endodontic Journal 2005;38:753–63.

139. Jainaen A, Palamara JEA, Messer HH. Push-out bond strengths of the dentine-sealer interface with and without a main cone. International Endodontic Journal 2007;40:882–90.

140. Sly MM, Moore BK, Platt JA, et al. Push-out bond strength of a new endodontic obturation system (Resilon/Epiphany). Journal of Endodontics 2007;33:160–2.

141. Üreyen Kaya B, Keçeci AD, Orhan H, et al. Micropush-out bond strengths of gutta-percha versus thermoplastic synthetic polymer-based systems- an ex vivo study. International Endodontic Journal 2008;41:211–8.

142. Paqué F, Sirtes G. Apical sealing ability of Resilon/Epiphany versus gutta-percha/AH Plus: immediate and 16-months leakage. International Endodontic Journal 2007;40:722–9.

143. Saleh IM, Ruyter IE, Haapasalo M, et al. Bacterial penetration along different root canal filling materials in the presence or absence of smear layer. International Endodontic Journal 2008;41:32–40.

144. Shemesh H, van den Bos M, Wu M-K, et al. Glucose penetration and fluid transport through coronal root structure and filled root canals. International Endodontic Journal 2007;40: 866–72.

145. Lertchirakarn V, Poonkaew A, Messer H. Fracture resistance of roots filled with gutta-percha or RealSeal. International Endodontic Journal 2011;44:1005–10.

146. Kim YK, Grandini S, Ames JM, et al. Critical review of methacrylate resin-based root canal sealers. Journal of Endodontics 2010;36:383–99.

147. Shanahan DJ, Duncan HF. Root canal filling with Resilon: a review. British Dental Journal 2011;211:81–8.

148. Lussi A, Messerli L, Hotz P, et al. A new noninstrumental technique for cleaning and filling root canals. International Endodontic Journal 1995;28:1–6.

149. Lussi A, Portmann P, Nussbächer U, et al. Comparison of two devices for root canal cleansing by the noninstrumentation technology. Journal of Endodontics 1999;25:9–13.

150. Lussi A, Imwinkelried S, Hotz P, et al. Long-term obturation quality using noninstrumentation technology. Journal of Endodontics 2000;26:491–3.

151. Portmann P, Lussi A. A comparison between a new vacuum obturation technique and lateral condensation: an in vitro study. Journal of Endodontics 1994;20:292–5.

152. Lussi A, Suter B, Fritzsche A, et al. In vivo performance of the new non-instrumentation technology (NIT) for root canal obturation. International Endodontic Journal 2002;35: 352–8.

153. Jasper EA. Adaptation and tissue tolerance of silver root canal fillings. Journal of Dental Research 1941;20:355–60.

154. Seltzer S, Green DB, Weiner N, et al. A scanning electron microscope examination of silver cones removed from endodontically treated teeth. Journal of Endodontics 2004;30: 463–74.

155. Sargenti A, Richter SL. Rationalized root canal treatment. New York: AGSA; 1965.

156. Alantar A, Tarragano H, Lefevre B. Extrusion of endodontic filling material into the insertions of the mylohyoid muscle: a case report. Oral Surgery, Oral Medicine, Oral Pathology 1994;78:646–9.

157. Allard KUB. Paraesthesia – a consequence of a controversial root-filling material? A case report. International Endodontic Journal 1986;19:2058.

158. Ørstavik D, Brodin P, Aas E. Paraesthesia following endodontic treatment: survey of the literature and report of a case. International Endodontic Journal 1983;16:167–72.

159. Spector RG. Pharmacological properties of the glucocorticoids. International Dental Journal 1981;31:152–5.

160. Block RM, Lewis RD, Hirsch J, et al. Systemic distribution of [^{14}C]-labelled paraformaldehyde incorporated within formocresol following pulpotomies in dogs. Journal of Endodontics 1983;9:176–89.

161. Ørstavik D, Hongslo JK. Mutagenicity of endodontic sealers. Biomaterials 1985;6:129–32.

162. Naoum HA, Chandler NP. Temporization for endodontics. International Endodontic Journal 2002;35:964–78.

163. Kirkevang L-L, Ørstavik D, Hörsted-Bindslev P, et al. Periapical status and quality of root fillings and coronal restorations in a Danish population. International Endodontic Journal 2000;33:509–15.

164. Ray HA, Trope M. Periapical status of endodontically treated teeth in relation to the technical quality of the root filling and the coronal restoration. International Endodontic Journal 1995;28:12–8.

165. Heling I, Gorfil C, Slutzky H, et al. Endodontic failure caused by inadequate restorative procedures: Review and treatment recommendations. Journal of Prosthetic Dentistry 2002;87: 674–8.

166. Ricucci D, Bergenholtz G. Bacterial status in root-filled teeth exposed to the oral environment by loss of restoration and fracture or caries- a histobacteriological study of treated cases. International Endodontic Journal 2003;36:787–802.

167. Keinan D, Moshonov J, Smidt A. Is endodontic re-treatment mandatory for every relatively old temporary restoration? Journal of the American Dental Association 2011;142: 391–6.

168. Harrison JW, Baumgartner JC, Svec TA. Incidence of pain associated with clinical factors during and after root canal therapy. Part II. Postobturation pain. Journal of Endodontics 1983;9:434–8.

169. Yesiloy C, Koren LZ, Morse DR, et al. Post-endodontic obturation pain: a comparative evaluation. Quintessence International 1988;19:431–8.

170. European Society of Endodontology. Quality guidelines for endodontic treatment: concensus report of the European Society of Endodontology. International Endodontic Journal 2006;39:921–30.

171. Fristad I, Molven O, Halse A. Nonsurgically retreated root-filled teeth- radiographic findings after 20–27 years. International Endodontic Journal 2004;37:12–8.

CHAPTER 10

Surgical Endodontics

J. L. Gutmann

Chapter Contents

Summary

Surgical endodontics has been a mainstay for the retention of teeth that cannot be treated with non-surgical endodontic procedures alone. Recent advances in surgical techniques, based on better scientific understanding of the periradicular disease process, and evidence-based principles, have enabled more predictable outcomes when surgery is chosen. Coupled with the introduction of newer instruments and magnification, refined principles of soft and hard tissue management and use of tissue regenerative techniques and materials, surgical endodontics has become a highly predictable procedure when practised by well-trained clinicians. Although there are a variety of surgical endodontic procedures within the scope of this discipline, the primary procedure is periradicular surgery. This chapter will focus on the scientific basis for surgical endodontics, to provide a better understanding of the rationale for their application and to achieve predictable results in clinical practice.

Introduction

The outcome of nonsurgical endodontic therapy is highly favourable, with success rates of 90% or higher being reported in recent decades.[1,2] Despite these impressive statistics, surgery is occasionally indicated to achieve what was not possible with root canal treatment alone or to secure a biopsy for histological examination. The prime determining factors appear to be the inability to manage the complex root canal anatomy and to eradicate bacterial populations and their biofilms from the root canal system.

Recent advances in surgical techniques, based on better scientific understanding of the periradicular disease process, have facilitated greater success rates in surgical endodontic procedures.[3] Empirical decision-making in the past has been replaced by evidence-based principles. Coupled with the introduction of newer instruments and magnification,[4] refined principles of soft and hard tissue management,[5] use of tissue regenerative techniques and materials[6] and enhanced principles of wound closure,[7] surgical endodontics has become a highly predictable procedure when practised by well-trained clinicians. The application of these principles and techniques by the endodontic specialist will ensure the retention of many teeth that may otherwise be considered nonsalvageable.

The most common surgical endodontic procedure is periradicular surgery, which consists of periradicular curettage, root-end resection, root-end preparation and root-end filling. Hence, the use of the terms *apicectomy* and *apicoectomy* appears to be archaic and limiting in scope based on the overall demands of the surgical procedure. Other surgical endodontic procedures include perforation repair, root and tooth resection, crown lengthening, intentional replantation, regenerative techniques, incision and drainage, cortical trephination, marsupialization or decompression and diodontic implants.[8] This chapter will focus primarily on the essentials of periradicular surgery.

Treatment Choices

The clinician must empower the patient to make the best decision based on sound scientific evidence. To provide optimal treatment planning, an accurate assessment of the likely outcome of any potential treatment modality (nonsurgical endodontic treatment, surgical endodontic treatment, or extraction of the tooth followed by implant placement) is required.[9] Failure to fully understand the aetiology of the disease process will result in impaired clinical decision-making detrimental to the overall well-being of the patient.

The best decision can be made when all available evidence is considered. A hierarchy of evidence exists, with randomized, controlled trials at the peak of the evidence pyramid and case reports and personal opinions at the base. The adoption of evidence-based decision-making has greatly advanced clinical treatment planning in dentistry, but the impact of clinician experience should not be ignored.

Indications for Periradicular Surgery

Historically, most texts on surgical endodontics list multiple, 'cookbook'-type indications for surgical intervention.[10,11] These often include instrument separation, apical fracture, inadequate root canal filling and presence of a cyst. Advances in the understanding of the disease process involved in the development of apical periodontitis and in clinical techniques have eliminated most of these indications for surgery. Outcome studies of nonsurgical root canal treatment versus surgical treatment have clearly shown a higher success rate with high-quality nonsurgical root canal treatment procedures using contemporary techniques. Unfortunately, most of the teeth referred to specialists for surgery would more appropriately have been treated nonsurgically.[12] Periradicular tissues usually heal after removal of infection originating from the root canal system combined with the prevention of further contamination.[13,14] The main cause of failure following both nonsurgical and surgical procedures is inadequate enlarging, shaping, cleaning, disinfecting and filling of the root canal system.[15] Therefore, the routine selection of surgery without full case assessment, in particular the status of the root canal system, is unwarranted as is selection of surgery for the convenience of the clinician. Consequently, many of these types of cases would benefit tremendously from specialist assessment and management.

The indications for surgery must always be in the best interest of the patient and within the realm of the clinician's understanding and expertise.[16] These include the following concepts. First, if failure has resulted from nonsurgical root canal treatment and retreatment is impossible or would not achieve a better result, surgery may be indicated (e.g. nonnegotiable canal, perforation or ledge with signs and/or symptoms). Second, if there is a strong possibility of failure with nonsurgical root canal treatment, surgery may be indicated (e.g. calcified canal with concomitant patient signs and/or symptoms). Third, if a biopsy is necessary, then surgery is indicated. Contraindications to surgery are few and far between and are usually limited to patient (psychological and systemic), clinician (experience and expertise) and anatomical factors, or complete lack of surgical access.

Preoperative Assessment

The prognosis after surgery is dependent on careful patient assessment, evidence-based diagnosis and appropriate treatment planning.[17] Contraindications involving the patient's psychological, or systemic conditions must be identified. Patient acceptance of, and cooperation with, the anticipated surgical procedure must be forthcoming. Procedures to minimize stress for patients who are particularly susceptible to pain and anxiety may be required.[5] General systemic factors which usually require medical consultation are listed in Table 10-1. As a general rule, no special precautions need to be taken when surgery is planned, other than those that normally apply to routine dental procedures.[5]

Local factors are related to the management of both soft and hard tissues. These factors include the possible need to remove and revise previous dental restorations that are failing and the need to revise the root filling beforehand as part of the overall management of the case. If the quality of the existing root filling is doubtful, more favourable results have been obtained when the root canal system is retreated before surgical management.[18] The tooth must also be assessed for restorability, and its place in the overall treatment plan should be determined. At times, the need for altering the restorative treatment plan may only become apparent once the gingival tissues have been reflected, and the serious marginal defects in the restorative tooth interface have been identified.

Radiological examination is essential, including assessment of previous radiographs, if available.[17] Radiographs from different angles should be taken, identifying the number, curvature and angle of the roots requiring surgery and the position of the apices relative to adjacent structures. Anatomical structures that may impair surgical or visual access to the surgical site must be identified. These include the mental foramen, zygomatic process, anterior nasal spine and external oblique ridge. The following factors are particularly important in a radiological assessment:

- relation of the apices to the inferior dental canal, mental foramen, the maxillary sinus or adjacent roots;
- number of and access to the roots, including the thickness of the cortical bone;
- approximate length of the roots; this may sometimes be ascertained from the patient's records if nonsurgical endodontic treatment had previously been performed;
- approximate extent of any visible lesion.

Although traditional radiographic techniques provide the clinician with the necessary information needed to assess the surgical site adequately, occasionally, newer techniques such as cone beam computed tomography (CBCT) may be necessary. The three-dimensional images using CBCT are invaluable in allowing the clinician to define the precise extent and location of a lesion that otherwise might be impossible to determine.[19–21]

TABLE 10-1	**General Medical Conditions**
Hypertension	Coronary atherosclerotic disease
Stable angina	Myocardial infarction
	Chronic obstructive pulmonary disease
Anticoagulant therapy	Cerebrovascular accident
Epilepsy	Diabetes
Adrenal insufficiency	Steroid therapy
Organ transplant	Impaired hepatic or renal function

Communication with the patient concerning the need for surgery, outline of the procedure, anticipated difficulties and problems, the prognosis, preoperative medication, or mouth rinses, postoperative care and long-term assessment are all essential.[5] Provision of written information and instructions is beneficial and can help to allay the patient's fears.

The following pretreatment regimens are recommended:

- A periodontal examination must be performed before surgery to assess periodontal pockets and/or sinus tracts. Scaling and/or root planing may be required. The patient's oral hygiene practices should be assessed and good oral hygiene reinforced.
- Patients should be placed on chlorhexidine (0.12–0.2%) rinses in an attempt to reduce the oral microorganisms. These rinses should be performed 1 day before surgery, immediately before surgery and should continue for at least 2 to 3 days afterward.[5]
- Patients can begin taking, if tolerated, nonsteroidal antiinflammatory medication (e.g. ibuprofen) 1 day before surgery or at the latest 1 hour before treatment. The clinician may dictate in the choice, but one of the best antiinflammatory result is obtained using 800 mg of ibuprofen every 6 hours. Alternatively, 400 mg of ibuprofen given along with 500 mg of paracetamol (acetaminophen) can be used every 4 to 6 hours. The same regimen may be used for postoperative pain management.
- Patients should be advised to refrain from smoking.
- If sedation (enteral or parenteral) is to be used, the patient must bring an accompanying person, who will be responsible for escorting the patient home and for compliance with postoperative instructions.

Surgical Kit

A plethora of specialized instruments are available, and the dental industry has formed an effective partnership with clinicians, allowing the development of numerous new instruments. Many of these have been developed specifically for use by clinicians operating with a microscope; these include miniature surgical blades and mirrors, rear-venting surgical handpieces, ultrasonically energized root-end preparation tips in multiple lengths and root-end pluggers (see later). Specific instruments should be chosen that facilitate the procedure according to the individual operator's requirements. Instruments must be sterile, sharp, undamaged and should enable the surgeon to maintain total control of the surgical site. A basic kit should contain the most commonly used instruments and should be readily supplemented with any other instrument considered necessary. Key instruments and their general uses are listed in Table 10-2 and illustrated in Figure 10-1.

MAGNIFICATION AND ILLUMINATION IN SURGICAL ENDODONTICS

Visual aids such as loupes and operating microscopes provide the operator with excellent lighting and magnification.[22] The development of operating microscopes specifically for endodontics greatly enhances the operator's view of the surgical site. However, there is a steep learning curve associated with the operating microscope and proficiency demands regular and continuous use. The enhanced vision facilitates the location of a multitude of anatomical features not easily visible to the naked eye. These include isthmuses, fins and additional or accessory canals. In addition, fractures, perforations and resorptive defects are more easily identified and managed.

Surgical Technique

TISSUE ANAESTHESIA AND HAEMOSTASIS

Profound anaesthesia and tissue haemostasis in the surgical site are essential.[23] Profound anaesthesia will minimize or eliminate patient discomfort during the procedure and for a significant period thereafter, whereas good haemostasis will improve vision at the surgical site, improve root-end cavity preparation and filling, minimize surgical time and reduce surgical blood loss, postsurgical haemorrhage and postsurgical swelling.[5] An anaesthetic solution containing a vasoconstrictor is indicated to achieve these objectives.[24]

The choice of anaesthetic–vasoconstrictor combination is dependent on the health status of the patient and the surgical needs. Lignocaine (lidocaine) with

TABLE 10-2 Surgical Kit

Presurgical Assessment	Root-End Preparation/Placement of Root-End Filling/ Finishing of Resected Root End
Mirror & curved explorer	
Straight & curved periodontal probes	Ultrasonic or sonic unit with appropriate root-end preparation tips
Soft Tissue Incision, Elevation & Reflection	Root-end filling material
Sharp scalpels – Nos. 15, 15c, 11 & 12	Haemostatic agent (avoid bone wax)
Micro scalpels	Miniature material carriers & condensers
Broad-based periosteal elevator	Small ball-ended burnisher
Broad-based periosteal retractor	Paper points or fine aspirator tip
Tissue forceps	Small, fine explorer
Surgical aspirator	**Suturing & Soft Tissue Closure**
Irrigating syringes & needles	Surgical scissors
Periradicular Curettage	Haemostat or fine needle holders
Straight & angled bone curettes	Various suture types & sizes (USP 3–0 to 6–0/metric size 2.0–0.7)
Small endodontic spoon curette	
Periodontal curettes	Sterile gauze for soft tissue compression
Fine, curved mosquito forceps	**Miscellaneous (or Readily Available)**
Small, curved surgical scissors	Adequate aspiration equipment
Bone Removal & Root-End Resection	Additional light source – Magnification
Surgical length round and tapered fissure burs	Root canal filling materials
Straight & angled bone curettes	Anaesthetic syringes, needles & local anaesthetic solution
Rear-venting high-speed handpiece	
Contra-angle slow-speed handpiece	Biopsy bottle containing transport medium

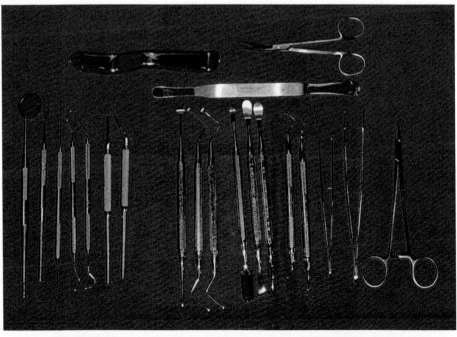

FIGURE 10-1 Basic instruments for periradicular surgery (see Table 10-2 for details).

adrenaline (epinephrine) has long been recognized as an excellent anaesthetic agent for periradicular surgery because of its clinical success in producing profound and prolonged analgesia.[25] Although several studies support the efficacy of 2% lignocaine with 1 : 200 000 to 1 : 100 000 concentrations of adrenaline for profound anaesthesia,[26] clinical evidence suggests that a 1 : 50 000 concentration provides better haemostasis.[27] The prolonged postoperative pain relief is caused by the inhibition of peripheral neuronal discharges, which in turn, helps reduce the subsequent development of central sensitization.[28]

Assessment of the patient's systemic status is essential before the use of 2% lignocaine with adrenaline, especially 1 : 50 000 adrenaline. This is important because lignocaine with adrenaline can elevate systemic plasma levels of the vasoconstrictor,[29] although the haemodynamic response to this increase is still controversial.[30] The potential rise in adrenaline concentration suggests that high-risk patients should be carefully monitored. Great care should be taken during injection to prevent intravascular placement of the solution.[24] When an anaesthetic with 1 : 50 000 adrenaline is unavailable, 1 : 80 000 is clinically acceptable. Whereas 2% lignocaine with 1 : 100 000 adrenaline is recommended for regional nerve blocks before endodontic surgery, this level of vasoconstrictor does not suffice for local haemostasis at the surgical site. Haemostasis must also be established at the surgical site[31] by additional injections supraperiosteally using 2% lignocaine with 1 : 50 000 adrenaline.[23]

In healthy patients, a dose of 2 to 4 mL is recommended. In the maxilla, the achievement of both anaesthesia and haemostasis can be accomplished simultaneously. This requires multiple injections, depositing the solution throughout the entire submucosa superficial to the periosteum at the level of the root apices in the surgical site. The needle, with the bevel toward the bone, is advanced to the target site, and after aspiration, 0.5 mL of solution is deposited slowly (Figure 10-2). The needle may be moved peripherally and similar, small amounts of solution may also be deposited. Additional injections can be made to ensure that the entire surgical field has been covered. Slow, peripheral supraperiosteal infiltration into the submucosa promotes maximum diffusion (Figure 10-3). In the mandible, the anaesthetic–

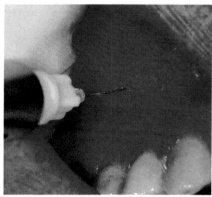

FIGURE 10-2 Placement of anaesthetic solution around the root apex of the tooth to be treated surgically.

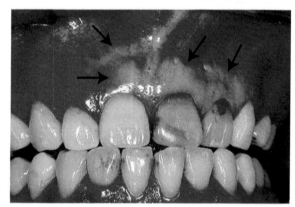

FIGURE 10-3 Slow and careful infiltration of the anaesthetic solution provides widespread and effective tissue haemostasis (delineated by arrows) for treatment of the left maxillary central incisor.

vasoconstrictor solution is injected slowly adjacent to the root apices, along with the block injection of the inferior alveolar nerve. Incisions that are made in alignment with the long axis of the supporting supraperiosteal vasculature coupled with careful elevation and reflection of the tissues will minimize haemorrhage at the surgical site.[5]

The amount of anaesthetic solution containing 1 : 50 000 or 1 : 80 000 adrenaline that is necessary to achieve anaesthesia and haemostasis is dependent on the surgical site, but 2 to 3 mL will usually suffice. The rate of injection can also influence the degree of haemostasis and anaesthesia obtained, with a rate of 1 to 2 mL/min recommended.[32] Injecting at higher rates will lead to localized pooling of solution, delaying and limiting diffusion into the adjacent tissues and resulting in less than optimal anaesthesia and haemostasis. Predictable anaesthesia and haemostasis should be achieved before any incisions are made. Later attempts during surgery to improve anaesthesia and haemostasis are less successful. After administration of the local anaesthetic, sufficient time must elapse before the initial incision (5–10 minutes), to allow proper vascular constriction throughout the surgical site. Other adjunctive agents are available to enhance haemostasis during treatment. These will be discussed later in this chapter.

SOFT TISSUE INCISION AND REFLECTION

Proper surgical access requires predetermined, meticulous tissue flap design followed by the incision and elevation of the soft tissue from the underlying bone. The design is crucial not only to surgical entry and management of the root structure but also to healing of the surgical wound. The design of soft tissue flaps has received wide and varied attention. Contemporarily various flap designs have been advocated based on a biological approach to tissue management and wound healing. The range of contemporary surgical flap designs[5] is outlined in Table 10-3. There are strong biological reasons to consider the use of full mucoperiosteal tissue flaps whenever possible

(see Table 10-3). Figures 10-4 through 10-9 detail diagrammatically each design, while the subsequent text gives a brief description of their application.

Full Mucoperiosteal Tissue Flap

The horizontal incision begins in the gingival sulcus, extending through the gingival fibres to the crestal bone. The scalpel blade is held in a near vertical position (Figure 10-10). In the interdental region, the incision should pass through the midcol area, separating the buccal and lingual papillae and severing the gingival fibres to the depth of the interdental crestal

TABLE 10-3 **Periradicular Surgical Soft Tissue Flap Designs**	
Type of Tissue Flap	**Advantages/Disadvantages**
Full Mucoperiosteal	
Triangular	Maintains intact vertical blood supply
Rectangular	Minimizes haemorrhage
Trapezoidal	Primary wound closure & rapid healing
Horizontal (envelope)	Allows survey of bone and root structure Excellent surgical orientation Minimal postoperative sequelae May have loss of tissue attachment May have loss of crestal bone height Possibility of tissue flap dislodgement Possible loss of interdental papilla integrity
Limited Mucoperiosteal	
Submarginal rectangular (Luebke-Ochsenbein)	Unaltered soft tissue attachment Adequate surgical access – may be compromised in posterior cases or cases with lateral root defects Good healing potential Disruption of blood supply Possibility of tissue shrinkage Delayed secondary healing/scarring Limited orientation to apical region Very limited in posterior surgery
Papilla-base incision	Newer technique & relatively limited data May interrupt blood supply, leading to delayed healing Difficult to perform Good healing potential

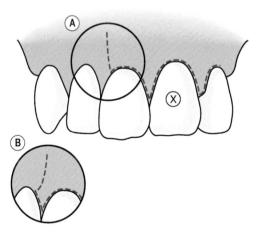

FIGURE 10-4 Triangular tissue flap design with a single vertical releasing incision. The vertical releasing incision can be performed in different ways. Either the incision leaves the interdental papilla intact (A) or (B; insert) the incision includes the interdental papilla. In either case, the incision line should meet the tooth at 90 degrees.

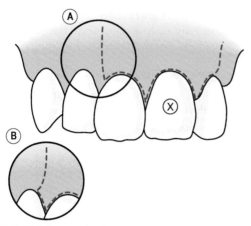

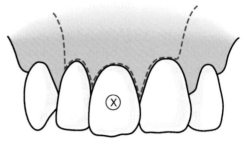

FIGURE 10-6 Trapezoidal tissue flap design. Note that vertical releasing incisions are angled toward the base of the flap.

FIGURE 10-5 Rectangular tissue flap design with double vertical releasing incisions. As with the triangular flap design, variations can be used with vertical incisions (A and B); a description has been included in Figure 10-4.

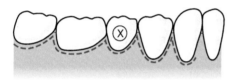

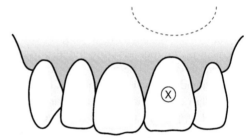

FIGURE 10-8 Semilunar tissue flap design. Note this flap design limits its scope and extension.

FIGURE 10-7 Horizontal tissue flap design. No vertical releasing incisions are used initially, but they can be added later to enhance surgical access if necessary.

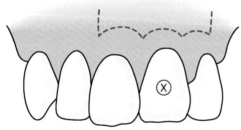

FIGURE 10-9 Luebke-Ochsenbein (submarginal) tissue flap design. This flap may have one or two vertical releasing incisions or may be limited to a horizontal incision, if sufficient surgical and visual access can be obtained.

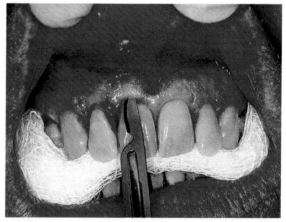

FIGURE 10-10 Intrasulcular incision with a no. 15 scalpel blade. Note the vertical position of the scalpel as it cuts through and releases the crestal fibres.

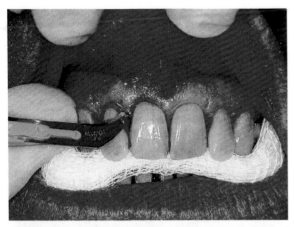

FIGURE 10-11 Use of a no. 12 scalpel blade to release the fibres of the interdental papilla. Note the depth and angulation of the blade.

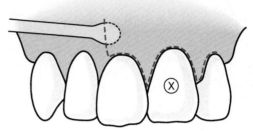

FIGURE 10-12 The periosteum is initially elevated by applying force against the cortical bone in the region of the attached tissues.

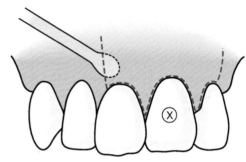

FIGURE 10-13 The periosteal elevator is subsequently moved coronally to elevate the marginal tissues.

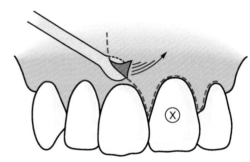

FIGURE 10-14 The entire tissue flap is elevated with minimal force being directed on the marginal and interdental gingival tissues.

bone (Figure 10-11). This is critical to prevent sloughing of the papillae caused by a compromised blood supply. Depending on the shape of the embrasure space, it may be necessary to use a curved scalpel blade, or a miniature surgical blade to follow the interproximal tooth contours (see Figure 10-11).

Vertical (releasing) incisions are used in the triangular and rectangular flap designs (see Figures 10-4 and 10-5) and are oriented by passing between the roots of the adjacent teeth and coursing parallel to the long axes of the roots. The incision should be over intact bone and to the depth of the bone. Vertical incisions should terminate at the mesial or distal line angles of the teeth, and never in the papillae, or in the midroot area. Incisions should be positioned to ensure that the reapposed soft tissue will overlie the solid bone at closure.

The trapezoidal flap design (see Figure 10-6) incorporates angled releasing incisions and is not considered biologically acceptable for periradicular surgery because it cuts across the vertically positioned supraperiosteal vasculature and tissue-supportive collagen fibres. The horizontal or envelope flap design (see Figure 10-7) is often used for maxillary or mandibular molars or as a palatal flap. However, some type of releasing incision is generally incorporated, albeit not as long as that used with triangular or rectangular flaps, and is usually placed between the premolars for molar access.

Tissue reflection always begins in the attached gingiva of the vertical incision. The periosteal elevator is positioned to apply reflective forces in a lateral direction against the cortical bone while elevating the tougher, fibrous-based tissue of the gingiva (Figure 10-12). This also elevates the periosteum and its superficial tissues from the cortical plate. Subsequently, the elevator is directed coronally (Figure 10-13) to elevate the marginal and interdental gingiva with minimal traumatic force (Figure 10-14). All

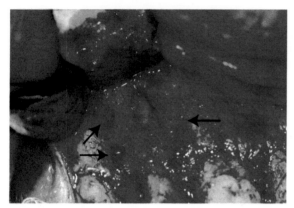

FIGURE 10-15 Tissue tags remain on the cortical bone after flap elevation (*arrowed*).

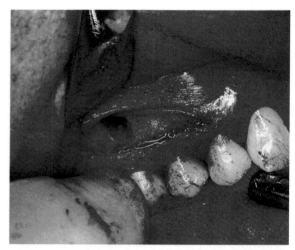

FIGURE 10-16 Pinching of the mucosal tissue with the periosteal retractor should be avoided during surgery.

reflective forces should be applied to the bone and periosteum, with minimal forces on the gingival elements; this is referred to as 'undermining elevation'.[5] After tissue reflection, bleeding tissue tags are often seen on the cortical surface in the crestal region and between root eminences (Figure 10-15). These tissue tags play an important role in healing, so they should not be removed during surgery.

Adequate retraction of the tissue flap is necessary for surgical access to the periradicular tissues. The retractor must always rest on sound bone with light but firm pressure. Pinching of the soft tissue flap with the retractor must be avoided to minimize tissue damage and untoward postsurgical sequelae (Figure 10-16). If this is not possible, the reflected tissue must be elevated further, or the tissue flap extended to release its attachment from the bone.

LIMITED MUCOPERIOSTEAL TISSUE FLAP

Limited mucoperiosteal tissue flaps do not include the marginal and interdental gingiva. The horizontal incision of these flaps should be in the attached gingiva with the vertical incisions involving both the attached gingiva and alveolar mucosa. An absolute minimum of 2 mm (and preferably more) of attached gingiva from the depth of the gingival sulcus must be present before this flap design can be chosen. However, there is a very narrow limit for safe incision between the sulcular depth and mucogingival junction in most patients, especially in the mandible.[33]

The rectangular submarginal flap design, historically referred to as the 'Luebke-Ochsenbein flap', is formed by a scalloped horizontal incision in the attached gingiva and two vertical releasing incisions (see Figure 10-9). Scalloping reflects the contour of the marginal gingivae and provides an adequate distance from the depths of the gingival sulci. Here also, the vasculature and collagen fibres are severed. It may be used in maxillary anterior or posterior teeth in which reflection of marginal and interdental gingival tissue is contraindicated because of tissue inflammation or aesthetic concerns with extensive fixed prostheses. Often, anatomical factors negate the use of a limited mucoperiosteal flap design.

PAPILLA-BASE FLAP

The papilla-base flap has been suggested[34] to prevent recession of the papilla. It consists of two releasing vertical incisions, connected by the papilla-base incision and intrasulcular incision in the cervical area of the tooth. A microsurgical blade that does not exceed 2.5 mm in width should be used, as intricate, minute movement of the surgical blade within the small dimensions of the interproximal space is crucial.

Two different incisions are made at the base of the papilla. An initial shallow incision severs the epithelium and connective tissue to the depth of 1.5 mm from the surface of the gingiva. The path is a curved line, connecting one side of the papilla to the other. The incision begins and ends perpendicular to the gingival margin. In the second step, the scalpel retraces the base of the previously created incision while inclined vertically, toward the crestal bone margin. The second incision results in a split-thickness flap in the apical third of the base of the papilla. From this point on, moving apically, a full-thickness mucoperiosteal flap is elevated. Although the papilla-base flap can result in predictable healing results, this technique is challenging to perform. Atraumatic handling of the soft tissues is of utmost importance to obtain rapid healing through primary intention. The epithelium of the partial-thickness flap has to be supported by underlying connective tissue; otherwise, it will necrose and lead to scar formation. On the other hand, excessive thickness of the connective tissue layer of the split flap portion could compromise the survival of the buccal papilla left in place.[7]

Patients should be informed about the possible changes in the relationship of the gingival tissues to teeth (recession and loss of attachment) that may occur over time after periradicular surgery. Some changes may be caused by the surgery itself, but patient- and healing-related factors may further affect the tissue architecture over time.[35]

OSSEOUS ENTRY AND ROOT IDENTIFICATION

Before root-end resection and removal of any diseased soft tissue surrounding the root, bone may need to be removed to gain visual access to the surgical site. Removal of the bone is usually accomplished with a large round bur (ISO size 018 or 024), using a low- or high-speed handpiece. However, the use of piezoelectric devices and piezosurgical concepts have recently been introduced into endodontics.[8]

When using a bur, the bone is removed in a brush-stroke fashion with copious irrigation, creating a window over the root apex. Ideally, this window should be as small as possible in a mesial-distal dimension to encourage rapid and thorough osseous healing.[36] Adherence to this technique will reduce the heat produced during the osteotomy procedure, thereby minimizing the potential for damage to the living bone tissue. In many cases, the osteotomy may need to be started from a coronal position, moving apically once the root structure has been identified. Care should be taken to avoid removing cementum from the root surface in order to prevent resorption at a later time. Entry as close to the apex, however, is recommended, with the angle of entry facilitating visibility and surgical access. Measuring the approximate

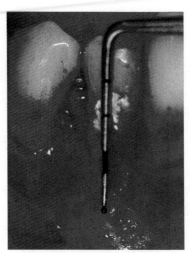

FIGURE 10-17 Placement of a calibrated periodontal probe to determine the approximate position of the root apex.

length of the root on the bone, as estimated from the preoperative radiological assessment, facilitates location of the root apex (Figure 10-17).

The apex may also be identified during osseous palpation after soft tissue reflection. Where the bone is thin or the root apex is prominent, a straight bone curette can be used in a rotating motion to penetrate the cortical plate and identify the root structure (Figure 10-18). In cases with large periradicular lesions, the loss of the cortical plate of bone may directly expose the root apex. Once exposed, the bur can be used to create a larger window to outline the root apex. In those cases in which the bone is thick and location of the apex is difficult, the same type of initial osseous penetration can be made and a sterile radiopaque object placed in the hole. A radiograph can then provide additional information on the location of the root apex.

Root structure can be differentiated from surrounding bone by texture (smooth and hard), lack of bleeding on probing, outline (presence of periodontal ligament) and colour (yellowish). The perimeter of the root and its periodontal ligament may also be identified by painting 1% methylene blue dye on the surface.[37]

REMOVAL OF DISEASED SOFT TISSUE (PERIRADICULAR CURETTAGE)

This procedure can often be performed before or in conjunction with root-end resection. The purpose is

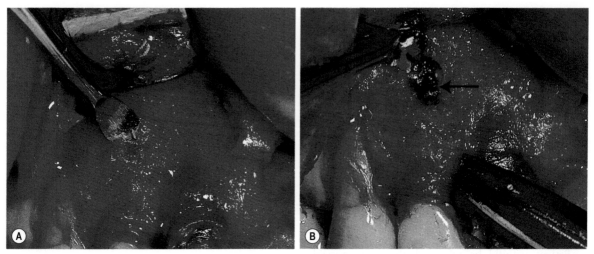

FIGURE 10-18 (A) Use of a straight curette to peel away the surface cortical bone. (B) Penetration through the bone with a curette alone to expose the root (*arrowed*). Note bone chips on the curette.

to remove the reactive tissue.[38] Contrary to previous belief, every remnant of this soft reactive tissue need not be removed to avoid failure as the tissue elements in the periphery of these lesions usually contain fibroblasts, vascular buds, new collagen and bone matrix. In cases where the soft tissue mass is exposed on flap reflection, or initial bone removal, curettage can proceed before root-end resection. In other cases, resection is necessary to gain access to most of the tissue.

Curettage is performed with straight or angled surgical bone curettes and periodontal curettes (Figure 10-19). Initially, the bone curettes are used to peel the soft tissue from the lateral borders of the bony crypt. This is achieved using the concave surface of the curette facing the bony wall, applying pressure only against the bone (Figure 10-20).[39] The clinician should avoid penetration of the soft tissue as this may sever the vascular network and increase local haemorrhage. Once the tissue is freed along the lateral margins, the bone curettes can be turned round and used in a scraping fashion along the deep walls of the crypt. This will detach the soft tissue from its lingual or palatal base. Once the tissue is loosened, tissue forceps are used to grasp the tissue gently as it is teased from its position with a bone curette. The tissue sample is placed directly into a bottle of neutral buffered formalin or transport medium for biopsy. In cases requiring root-end

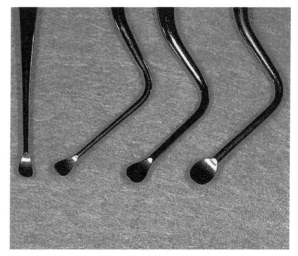

FIGURE 10-19 Straight and angled bone curettes are useful to manage the wide variety of challenges encountered in bone and soft tissue removal.

resection before curettage, the root structure must be exposed sufficiently to minimize shredding of the soft tissues during resection. Despite profound anaesthesia at the surgical site as a whole, it is often found that the centre of the periradicular lesion remains sensitive. This is explained by the proliferation of neural endings stimulated by inflammatory mediators.[40] Infiltration of local anaesthetic into the reactive tissue will invariably eliminate any residual sensation.

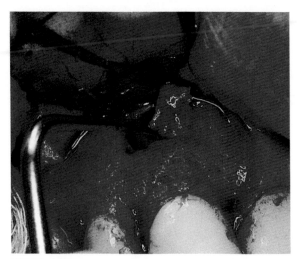

FIGURE 10-20 Use of the bone curette to peel the soft tissue lesion from the bone cavity.

In the presence of large lesions, care must be exercised during curettage of the lateral surfaces of the bony crypt to avoid damage to adjacent roots and their pulpal vasculature. Presurgical radiographs should warn of this possibility, and the tissue in these areas may need to be left in position. Caution is necessary to prevent damage to vital structures when operating close to the maxillary antrum, mental foramen or mandibular canal. When soft tissue is adherent, either lingually to the root or in the furcation region, periodontal curettes facilitate its removal. Periradicular curettage is normally performed in conjunction with the resection of the root end.[41]

BIOPSY

The vast majority of periradicular lesions that are biopsied are granulomas. However, a small percentage (0.7–5.0%) are reported to be different based on histological examination.[42] These 'other' lesions include odontogenic cysts (odontogenic keratocyst, dentigerous cysts), nonodontogenic cysts (globulomaxillary cyst, nasopalatine cyst), ossifying fibroma, Pindborg tumour, Langerhans cell disease, or osteoblastoma, among others. More seriously, however, are lesions that might be neoplastic. Many reports exist in the literature documenting cases of misdiagnosis.[43–45] Considering the potential gravity of this situation, it is widely agreed that tissue excised during surgical endodontic procedures should be sent for histological examination.[46]

ROOT-END RESECTION

The term *root-end resection* refers specifically to the removal of the apical portion of the root. There are many indications for resection of the root end during periradicular surgery, each designed to eliminate aetiological factors.

Historically, the technique of root-end resection involved the creation of a bevel on the root face to improve surgical access and visibility.[41,47–49] The angle of resection was determined by the root inclination and curvature, number of roots, thickness of bone and position of the root in the bone. Current evidence indicates that reducing the angle of the bevel will reduce dentinal tubule exposure.[50] Based on the number of dentinal tubules communicating between the root canal and resected root face, the angle of the bevel should be kept to a minimum.[50] A significant increase in leakage from the root canal system has been demonstrated as the bevel increased.[51] Ultrasonic instruments have been developed that greatly facilitate preparation along the long axis of the root, and, therefore, eliminated the need for extensive bevelling of the root face.

The root end can be resected in one of two ways. First, after the root end has been exposed, the bur (narrow straight fissure) is positioned at the desired angle and the root is shaved away, beginning from the apex, cutting coronally (Figure 10-21). The bur is moved from mesial to distal, shaving the root to a smooth and flat finish until the entire canal system and root outline is exposed. As mentioned earlier, the root outline can be more easily visualized by staining the periodontal ligament with 1% methylene blue dye.[47] This approach allows for continual observation of the root end during cutting. The second technique of resection is to predetermine the amount of root end to be resected. The bur and handpiece are positioned, and the apex is resected by cutting through the root from mesial to distal (see Figure 10-21). Once the apex is removed, the root face is gently shaved with the bur to smooth the surface and ensure complete resection and visibility of the root face. This technique works well when an apical biopsy is desired or to gain access to significant amounts of soft tissue located

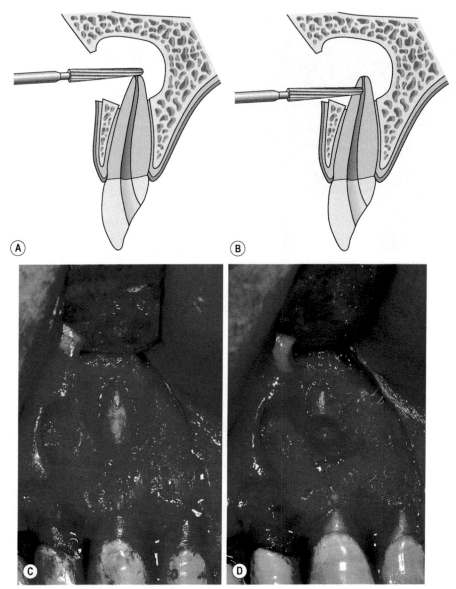

FIGURE 10-21 Diagrammatic representation of (A) the root-end resection from the apex to coronal; (B) the root-end resection when the amount of root to be resected has been determined. (C) Clinical case of the root-end resection in which the amount of the root to be resected has been predetermined. (D) Resection of the root apex.

lingual to the root. It is also the technique of choice in cases in which the root end is located in close proximity to structures such as the mental foramen, or inferior alveolar canal. The disadvantage, however, is that this approach may remove more root structure than necessary.

The appearance of the root face after root-end resection will vary depending on the type of bur used, external root anatomy, anatomy of the canal system exposed at the particular angle of resection and nature and density of the root canal filling material. Various types of burs have been recommended for root-end

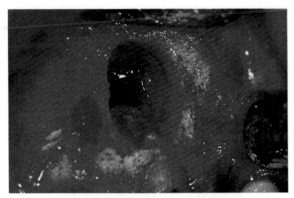

FIGURE 10-22 Severely angled resections, often coupled with large periradicular lesions, compromise the amount of remaining crestal bone.

resection[5]; each will leave a characteristic imprint on the root face, from rough grooved and gouged to smooth.[52] To date, no study has determined the advantages of one type of bur over another, although for years, clinical practice has favoured a smooth, flat root surface.[53]

The level to which the root end should be resected will be dictated by the following factors[5]:

- access and visibility to the surgical site;
- position and anatomy of the root within the alveolar bone;
- presence and position of additional roots (e.g. an additional palatal or lingual root)
- anatomy of the cut root surface relative to the number of canals and their configuration;
- need to place a root-end filling;
- presence and location of a perforation;
- presence of an intraalveolar root fracture;
- anatomical considerations (e.g. proximity of adjacent teeth, mental foramen, or inferior dental canal, level of remaining crestal bone);
- presence of significant accessory canals, which may dictate a more extensive resection.

Regardless of the rationale for the extent of root-end removal, there is no reason to resect the root to the base of a large periradicular lesion as was previously advised. Likewise, resection to the point where little (<1 mm) or no crestal bone remains covering the buccal aspect of the root may very well doom the tooth to failure (Figure 10-22). On the other hand, omitting to remove sufficient root structure to be able to inspect

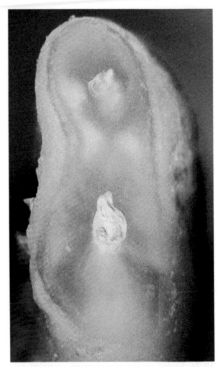

FIGURE 10-23 Resected root outline. Note the kidney bean shape along with the position of the canals. No canal anastomosis is visible.

the resected root face and place a root-end filling may also contribute to failure. Root canals or anastomoses may be missed or may be improperly managed in confined spaces.

The complete root face must be identified and examined after resection. This is inspected, preferably under high magnification, such as a microscope or endoscope,[54] and good illumination with a fine, sharp probe guided around the periphery of the root and root canal. The external root anatomy will determine the ultimate shape of the cut root end, such as oval, round, dumbbell shaped, kidney bean shaped or teardrop shaped (Figure 10-23). The outline of the resected root end will vary depending on the tooth, angle of any bevel and position of the cut on the root. However, the entire surface must be visible. If visibility is impaired or the root has an unusual cross-section, 1% methylene blue dye can be placed on the root face for 5 to 10 seconds using a sterile sponge applicator and rinsed off with a stream of sterile water or saline. Cotton pellets should not be used as the remnants of cotton fibres left

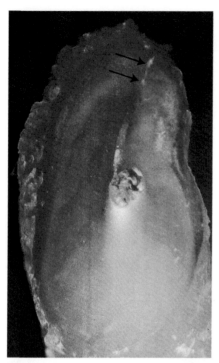

FIGURE 10-24 Angled resection reveals an extended canal space. Removal of additional root palatally will be necessary to manage the uppermost part of the canal system (*arrowed*).

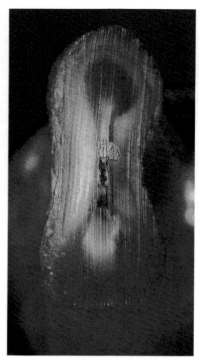

FIGURE 10-25 Root-end resection reveals a poorly compacted gutta-percha filling. Voids filled with sealer are present between the gutta-percha cones, and an anastomosis is present that is filled with tissue remnants (bluish colour).

in the surgical site have been shown to induce a foreign-body reaction in healing tissues.[5] The dye will stain the periodontal ligament dark blue, highlighting the root outline.[47] The shape of the exposed canal system will vary depending on the angle of the bevel and canal anatomy at that level. Canal systems will generally assume a more elongated and accentuated shape with increasing angles of bevel[55] (Figure 10-24).

Also visible on most resected root end is the presence of root canal filling material and the interface between the filling material and root dentine. Variations in the quality of the filling will be seen in both the type of filling material and nature of the filling technique (Figure 10-25). Furthermore, the different burs used for resection will create discrepancies in the surface of the filling material and its adaptation to the canal walls. For example, coarse diamond burs will tend to rip and tear at the gutta-percha root canal filling, spreading the gutta-percha over the edge of the canal aperture and onto the resected root face (Figure 10-26). Surface finishing with an ultrafine diamond is

recommended (Figure 10-27; Ultrafine no. 862–012 diamond bur, Brasseler, Savannah, GA, USA).

The presence of additional canals, anastomoses, fracture lines and the quality of the apical adaptation of the root canal filling must be checked on the resected root surface[54] (Figure 10-28). If methylene blue dye has been used, it will also stain the periphery of the canal system and highlight fracture lines.[47,55] A fibre optic light can be aimed at or behind the root end to enhance visibility.[10] Occasionally, it may be necessary to remove additional root structures to identify the canal system or in the case of a fracture line, to observe its direction and extent.

A major area of concern after root-end resection and dentinal tubule exposure is the possibility that these tubules serve as a direct source of contamination from the uncleaned root canal system into the periradicular tissues. Root ends resected from 45 degrees to 60 degrees have as many as 28 000 tubules/mm^2 immediately adjacent to the canal.[50] At the

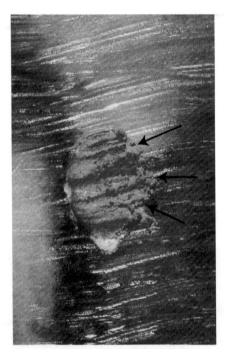

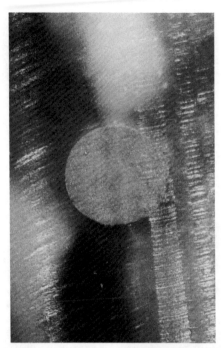

FIGURE 10-26 Rough surface of resected root after being cut with a coarse diamond. Note the gutta-percha has been dragged across the surface of the root (*arrowed*).

FIGURE 10-27 Smooth surface of resected root and root filling created with an ultrafine diamond and water spray. Note the adaptation of the root filling material to the outline of the canal.

dentino-cemental junction, areas that may communicate with the root canal even in the presence of a root-end filling with 13 000 tubules/mm² are found. Likewise, angular changes in the tubules at the apex can cause patent communication with the main canal if the depth of the root-end preparation in the buccal aspect of the cavity is insufficient.[56,57] Root-end resections in older teeth have shown less leakage than that seen in teeth from younger patients[58]; this corroborates with the findings of sclerosis and reduced patency in apical dentinal tubules.[59]

Another concern after root-end resection is performed is the formation of a contaminated smear layer over the resected root end (Figure 10-29). This may serve as a source of irritation to the periradicular tissues, primarily preventing the intimate reformation of a layer of cementum against the resected tubules. A thicker smear layer is usually created when cutting without water spray[60] or when using coarse diamond burs rather than tungsten carbide burs.[61] Therefore, it is recommended that root-end resection be performed under constant irrigation, which minimizes

the dentinal smear layer. If diamond burs are used to resect the root, a medium grit is preferred, followed by a fine or ultrafine grit diamond.

ROOT-END CAVITY PREPARATION

In order to seal the potential avenues of communication from the resected root end to the canal system adequately, a root-end preparation should be made into the root to the coronal extent of the resected apical tubules.[51] A depth of 2 to 4 mm is generally sufficient[49,62] depending on the angle of the resection. Increasing the depth of the root-end filling significantly decreases apical leakage,[51] and to this end, ultrasonic tips measuring 3, 6 and 9 mm in length have been developed (Acteon, Mount Laurel, NJ, USA). The minimum depths for a root-end cavity, measured from the buccal aspect of the cavity, are 1.0, 2.1 and 2.5 mm for a 90-, 30- and 45-degree angle of resection, respectively.[51] Ideally, this preparation is made in the long axis of the root, parallel to the anatomical outline of the root, possesses adequate retention form and encompasses all exposed orifices

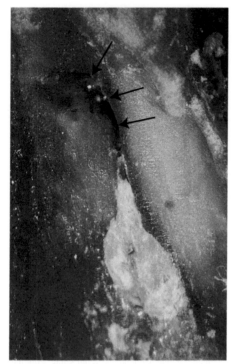

FIGURE 10-28 Resected root end. The main canal has been filled, but the canal extension contains necrotic debris (*arrowed*). A root-end preparation and filling must be performed.

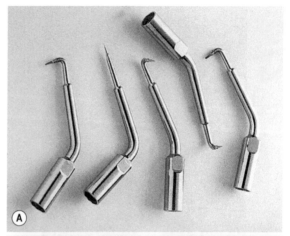

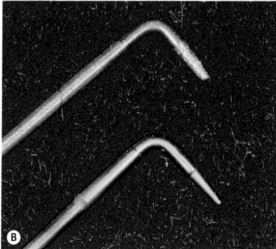

FIGURE 10-30 (A) Variously shaped and angled ultrasonic tips for preparing a root-end cavity. (B) Top, Berutti ultrasonic tip (EMS, Nyon, Switzerland); bottom, RE-2 tip (EMS).

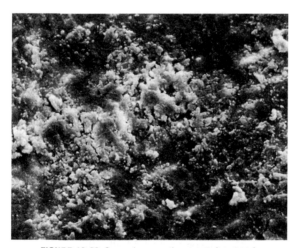

FIGURE 10-29 Smear layer on the resected root end.

of the root canal system. If this is the case, then the depths indicated will be sufficient in all aspects of the preparation.

The final outline of the preparation will depend mainly on the anatomy of the exposed canal space and in some cases, the nature of the root outline. For example, in maxillary central incisors, the shape of the root-end preparation will generally be round to oval. In premolars or molars, it may be very elongated and narrow in conjunction with oval or round shapes.

Root-end preparations are best created with specially designed, ultrasonically energized instruments (Figure 10-30). These ultrasonic tips eliminate many

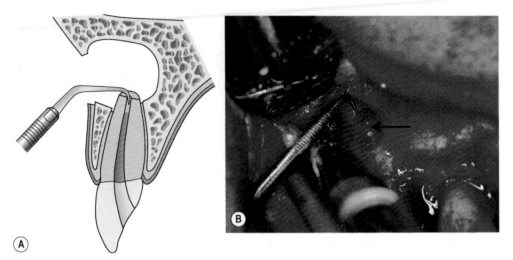

FIGURE 10-31 (A) Diagrammatic representation of root-end cavity preparation along the root axis using an ultrasonic tip. (B) An ultrasonic tip near the resected root end. Note good access and two canals (identified by gutta-percha) united by a thin white line of the anastomosis (*arrowed*). Preparation of the anastomosis is essential.

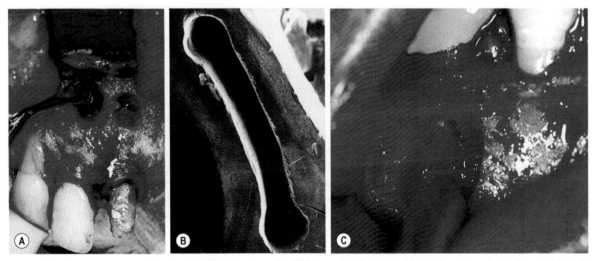

FIGURE 10-32 (A) Preparing a root-end cavity with an ultrasonic tip. (B) Root-end cavity prepared in a molar root uniting the two mesial canals through the anastomosis (SEM). (C) Ultrasonic root-end preparation in the mesial root of a mandibular molar.

of the difficulties associated with root-end preparation with burs. The small, angled tips allow for ultrasonic shaping of apical preparations parallel to the long axis of the root after minimal root-end resection and minimal bevelling of the root face (Figure 10-31). They are effective in the debridement and enlargement of canal anastomoses and irregularities commonly found in molar roots (Figure 10-32)[63]; the ability of this technique to achieve better-shaped and cleaner

root-end preparations as opposed to bur preparations has been highlighted.[64–66] The creation of clean, good quality root-end preparations can also been achieved with the use of sonic tips,[67,68] and clinical experience would support the routine use of either of these techniques. However, a note of caution has been sounded by some authors,[69,70] who have demonstrated cracks in the root surface after use of ultrasonic root-end preparation instruments. An assessment of the

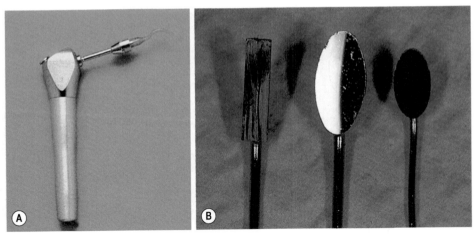

FIGURE 10-33 (A) Stropko irrigator. (B) Miniature mirrors.

root-end preparations using ultrasonic tips indicated that the shortest preparation time that may minimize both the potential for cracks and cavities that may leak after restoration was obtained with diamond-coated tips used on a high-power setting.[71]

After root-end preparation, the cavity should be irrigated with sterile saline or water. Small suction tips, made from 20- or 18-gauge needles that can be bent and adapted to a high-speed suction device, are used to remove fluid and debris from the cavity. Some clinicians prefer to use paper points to dry the preparation. The Stropko irrigator/dryer device (SybronEndo, West Collins, Orange, CA, USA) is a simple and effective means of drying the root-end preparation (Figure 10-33A).[55] Although rinsing the cavity with citric acid has been recommended to remove the smear layer,[63] studies have indicated that this may actually enhance the amount of leakage after root-end filling.[70,72] Despite creating cleaner root-end cavity walls and assisting in debris removal, the routine use of citric acid is questionable. After drying, the cavity must be inspected to ensure that it is clean and that it encompasses all of the canal extensions. Small mirrors have been designed specifically for this purpose (Figure 10-33B).

ROOT-END CAVITY FILLING

Irrespective of whether a root-end filling is placed or not, it is important that the canal system is cleaned and sealed as well as possible. In many cases, this may necessitate that the old root canal filling should be revised before surgery. Under these circumstances, many cases may be successful without the need for a root-end filling.

In some cases, in which time is a factor, or cases in which there are persistent exacerbations between visits, root canal retreatment can be performed at the same time as surgery. The elevated tissue is reflected, and the root apex is exposed and resected. The canal preparation is carried out with the file tips protruding through the resected root end (Figure 10-34A). Small aspirators can be placed next to the apical opening to prevent root canal irrigant entering the bony cavity. After adequate preparation, the canal is dried with paper points. Filling should follow with a suitable material, and any excess removed (Figure 10-34B). An ultrafine diamond bur, or composite finishing bur can be run over the root surface with sterile water, or saline spray (Figure 10-34C). If the canal is filled properly, the result will be a very smooth, well-adapted root canal filling.

Before filling, the root-end cavity must be isolated to ensure moisture control. The appropriate use of vasoconstrictors will greatly reduce the blood flow in the surgical site, but other supplementary agents are frequently used. In recent years, more biocompatible and biodegradable products have been developed; these include collagen-based products such as Hemocollagene (Septodont, Saint-Maur-des-Fossés Cedex, France), CollaPlug (Integra, Plainsboro, NJ, USA),

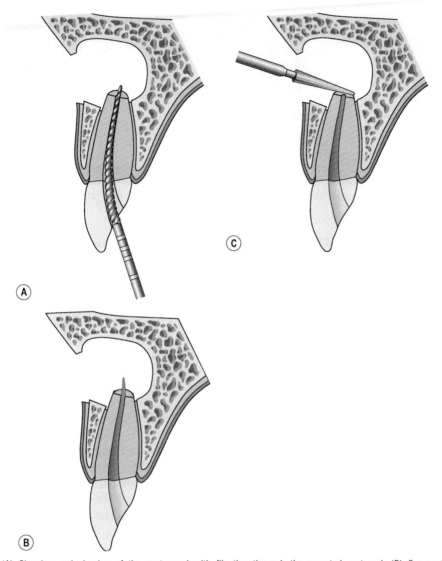

FIGURE 10-34 (A) Cleaning and shaping of the root canal with file tips through the resected root end. (B) Compaction of the gutta-percha filling with the tip through the root end. (C) Removal of excess root filling material and finishing of the root surface with an ultrafine diamond bur.

CollaCote (Integra), Avitene (Davol Inc., Cranston, RI, USA), or Superstat (DPO Medical, Henderson, NV, USA) that can remain in the osseous cavity, or be removed before closure (Figure 10-35).[5] Noncollagen products include Surgicel (Johnson & Johnson, Piscataway, NJ, USA), Oxycel (Becton Dickinson, Sandy, UT, USA) and Gelfoam (Pfizer, New York, NY, USA). These products can exert their influence on haemostasis by stimulating the intrinsic clotting pathway and physically by creating a tamponading effect when packed into the crypt. The use of aluminium chloride paste (Expasyl, Kerr Corporation, West Collins, Orange, CA, USA) has also been shown to be effective, even more so than the use of products impregnated with vasoconstrictors.[73] Other less bio-compatible products include Astringedent (Ultradent,

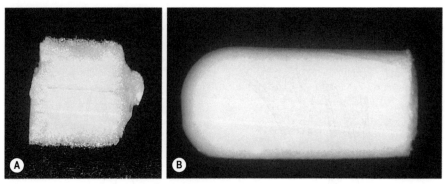

FIGURE 10-35 Collagen sponge materials for haemorrhage control in the apical bony cavity: (A) Hemocollagene; (B) CollaPlug.

TABLE 10-4 **Current Materials Recommended for Root-End Filling**
Super ethoxybenzoic acid (Super EBA)
Intermediate restorative material (IRM)
Glass ionomer
Composite resin (dentine bonded)
Mineral trioxide aggregate (MTA) – ProRoot (regular and white)

South Jordan, UT, USA), Cut-Trol (Kisco, Wichita, KS, USA) and ViscoStat (Ultradent); these are solutions of ferric sulphate which must be removed from the bone cavity before tissue closure.[74,75] Haemostasis in periradicular surgery has been reviewed.[76]

ROOT-END FILLING MATERIALS

The purpose of the root-end filling is to seal the canal system apically and prevent the egress of bacteria and bacterial products into the periradicular tissues. Presently, there are no commercially available materials that provide a perfect seal; therefore, the materials that are used must be prepared and placed carefully to ensure the best possible adaptation to the root-end cavity walls. When using modern materials as root-end fillings, adherence to manufacturers' recommendations during preparation, manipulation and placement is important. Table 10-4 lists current materials that have been recommended for root-end filling. Amalgam has previously been the most widely used root-end

filling material and has been associated with a reasonable level of success. However, problems have existed with corrosion and tissue argyria, persistence of apical inflammation and long-term failure.[77] Coupled with concerns over the mercury component, it is recommended that more biocompatible materials be used; several clinical studies also support the use of alternative materials.[78–84]

Root-end filling materials commonly in use, or used in recent years, include amalgam, intermediate restorative material (IRM; Dentsply, Milford, DE, USA), Super ethoxybenzoic acid (Super EBA), glass ionomer cement, dentine-bonded composite resin, polyketone-based sealer (Diaket) and Mineral trioxide aggregate (MTA). Discussion will be restricted to those materials associated with the highest levels of success, both clinically and histologically. Evidence-based data from randomized clinical trials appears to indicate that two root-end filling materials, when used properly, will result in a high level of predictable clinical and radiographic healing.[85,86] IRM and MTA are discussed in the following section.

Intermediate Restorative Material

Intermediate restorative material is a resin-reinforced zinc oxide-eugenol cement that has been shown to provide a better seal than amalgam, especially against the passage of microorganisms.[87] Healing of the periradicular tissues in the presence of IRM root-end fillings has been quite favourable.[87] Likewise, clinical studies have shown enhanced success with IRM root-end fillings (91%) compared with amalgam (75%) over long periods.[78] When using this material as a root-end filling, a higher powder-to-liquid ratio has been recommended to enhance placement, decrease setting time, reduce toxicity and reduce dissolution in tissue fluids.[88] Therefore, the use of IRM as a root-end filling material is recommended when mixed at a higher powder-to-liquid ratio.

Mineral Trioxide Aggregate

Mineral trioxide aggregate is a newer material.[81,89–91] A series of studies have illustrated the useful properties of MTA as a root-end filling material, including its biocompatibility, sealing properties and ability to promote tissue regeneration.[6,81,89,90] Additional studies have demonstrated the superior sealing properties of MTA over other root-end filling materials with either dye leakage, electrochemical testing,[92] or endotoxin tracer tests.[93] The properties of this material have been shown to be relatively unaffected by blood contamination.[91] Complete regeneration of the periodontal apparatus has been demonstrated but not in all cases.[80]

The cellular response to MTA has been shown to be more favourable than the response to IRM or amalgam. MTA promotes regeneration of the periradicular architecture.[94] However, the physical handling characteristics of MTA leave much to be desired. It is very difficult to deliver the material to the root-end cavity and to adequately compact it to the full length of the preparation. Although moisture, such as bleeding, does not affect the setting ability of the material, it compounds the handling difficulties. A number of instruments have been devised to facilitate the placement of the material, such as the MAP system (Produits Dentaires, Vevey, Switzerland; Figure 10-36), Dovgan MTA carriers and the Lee MTA pellet forming block (Hartzell, Concord, CA, USA; see Chapter 6). The usage of this material is greatly helped by ensuring that the powder/water ratio is correct. After placement into the root-end cavity, the material can be effectively compacted using root-end pluggers and ultrasound transmitted by applying an ultrasonic instrument to the nonworking part of the metal plugger. It is prudent to take a radiograph at this stage to confirm adequate placement of the material. MTA has a working time of approximately 3 to 4 hours and requires the presence of moisture for its final set; however, some newer products on the market have decreased setting times and enhanced handling properties.

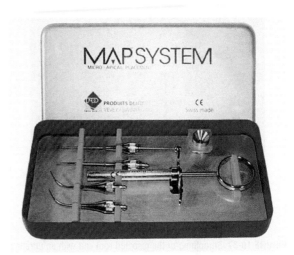

FIGURE 10-36 Miniature carriers, such as the MAP System, are used to carry small increments of root-end filling material.

TREATMENT OF THE ROOT FACE

Removal of the smear layer and exposure of the apical collagen fibres is recommended after root-end resection, primarily to remove potentially contaminated debris and to enhance the healing environment for cemental deposition. Various agents have been recommended including phosphoric acid,[60,95] ethylenediaminetetraacetic acid (EDTA),[96] hydrochloric acid[97,98] and citric acid.[99] The optimal exposure of collagen and demineralization occurs with a burnishing application of citric acid (pH 1.0) for 3 minutes.[100] Longer applications result in collagen denaturation. The peak activity pH of citric acid is 1.42.[101] Demineralization of resected root ends with a 2-minute burnishing of 50% citric acid at pH 1.0 resulted in a rapid and predictable layering of a cementoid type of material on the resected surface of dogs' teeth after 45 days.[102] No direct application to human teeth, under similar circumstances, has been studied, although the omission of an acid cleaner does not preclude the formation of a viable cementum layer.[103]

Studies have identified the use of the ferric ion, as an aqueous solution of 10% citric acid and 3% ferric chloride (10:3), to stabilize dentine collagen during the demineralization process[104,105]; however, applications lasted less than 30 seconds, as longer exposure increased demineralization and denaturation of the collagen. This approach has enhanced the bonding

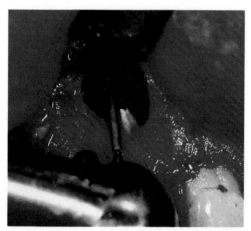

FIGURE 10-37 Smoothing of the resected root end with an ultrafine diamond.

that occurs with restorative materials, and may also stimulate adhesion of the exposed, intact collagen with fibrin and fibronectin[106] and the splicing of collagen with newly formed collagen fibrils[107] during the wound healing process. Further work on its use on the resected root end is warranted.

The following treatment steps are indicated for the resected root face after placement of a root-end filling or root-end resection in which a well-condensed gutta-percha root filling is in place:

1. Finish the surface with an ultrafine diamond or 30-flute tungsten carbide composite-resin finishing bur[63,106] (Figure 10-37).
2. Burnish the surface gently with a weak acid cleaner (10%) for a short period (30 seconds).[106]

These procedures achieve the desired result of a smooth root face devoid of smear layer, regardless of the root or canal configuration type (Figure 10-38). However, when using MTA as a root-end filling, such treatment of the root face is inappropriate. In these cases, the gross excess of MTA is removed with suction, or spoon excavators and a saline-moistened sponge is used to clean the root face.

CLOSURE OF THE SURGICAL SITE

Before repositioning the tissue flap, the underside of the reflected tissue, the surrounding bone and the periradicular bone cavity should be inspected for debris. The surgical site is carefully flushed with saline, except where MTA has been used as the root-end filling. A radiograph is taken to ensure that all debris has been removed and that the goals of the surgical procedure have been accomplished. Final irrigation with saline is often warranted followed by tissue repositioning to the wound edges to ensure primary closure.

When surgery has been performed and there is a stable buccal cortical plate of bone to protect the root structure and no evidence of marginal periodontitis, tissue closure is straightforward. Intimate approximation of the healthy soft tissues and bone with sutures will suffice, and healing will occur uneventfully. Ideally, bony dehiscences or large fenestrations should be detected before surgery so that adjunct procedures such as guided-tissue regeneration can be planned (Figure 10-39).[6,107–109] When there has been loss of the cortical bone, especially in the crestal region, or the presence of marginal periodontitis, the chances for long-term success are highly guarded.[110,111] Persistent periradicular inflammation after root-end surgery has been associated with marginal periodontitis at the time of surgery.[49]

Many clinicians will also apply gentle pressure to the repositioned tissue at this time to remove residual blood and to begin the intimate reattachment process. Gentle pressure can be applied using saline-soaked gauze squares. Suturing will be necessary in most cases. A variety of suturing techniques are frequently used and include interrupted, mattress, continuous or sling sutures. The suture is first placed in the flap and is then carried into the attached tissues. While there is no one formula for the number of sutures and their position, the clinician must exercise judgement in their placement to ensure adequate and stable positioning, especially in the crestal region. Vertical incisions may require several sutures depending on the length and nature of the tissue (Figure 10-40). Avoidance of postoperative gingival recession and delayed healing is dependent on correct suturing techniques and tissue handling.

A variety of suture materials are available, each demonstrating advantages and disadvantages.[105] Suture materials are either absorbable or nonabsorbable. They can also be either monofilament or braided; the latter have a tendency to facilitate the movement of saliva and bacteria along the suture into the tissues. This property, called 'wicking', contributes to irritation

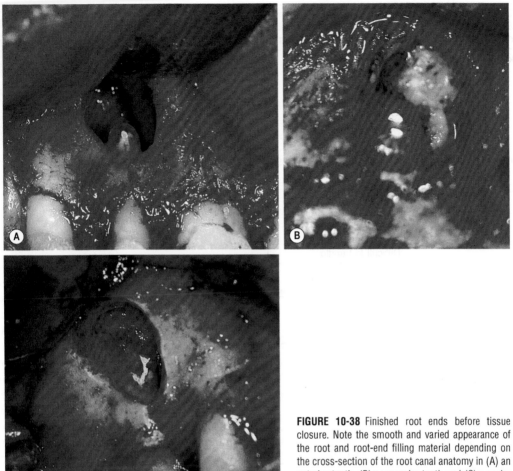

FIGURE 10-38 Finished root ends before tissue closure. Note the smooth and varied appearance of the root and root-end filling material depending on the cross-section of the root canal anatomy in (A) an anterior tooth, (B) a premolar tooth and (C) a molar tooth.

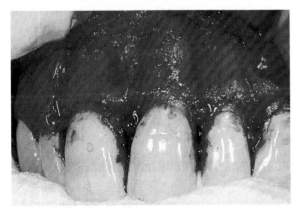

FIGURE 10-39 Loss of buccal cortical bone over the root of a left maxillary central incisor with a periradicular lesion. Correct treatment planning should be able to determine or at least anticipate the presence of these defects before surgical entry.

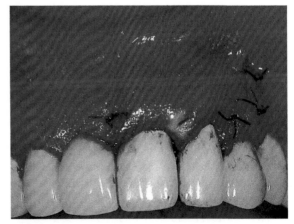

FIGURE 10-40 Close tissue flap approximation with minimal suturing and tissue damage.

TABLE 10-5	**Suture Materials**
Material	**Advantages/Disadvantages**
Black silk	Nonabsorbable Historically the most commonly used Good handling characteristics Braided; wicking effect delays healing
Surgical gut (collagen) Chromic acid treated surgical gut	Absorbable; manufacturing process determines longevity of catgut sutures Treatment with chromic acid prolongs retention in tissues Difficult to handle
Nylon	Nonabsorbable Monofilament
Polyglycolic acid (PGA)	Absorbable May be braided or monofilament
Expanded polytetrafluoroethylene (PTFE; GORE-TEX)	Single filament; smooth, strong Nonporous surface; nonabsorbable Provokes little tissue reaction
PTFE-coated polyester (Tevdek)	Nonabsorbable Usually braided
Polyamide	Nonabsorbable Strong Smooth, nonporous

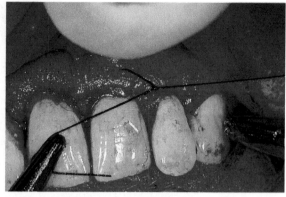

FIGURE 10-41 Suture knots must be kept away from the incision line to minimize infection of the wound.

of the tissues and may delay healing. A list of suitable suture materials is shown in Table 10-5.

For years, silk sutures have been most widely used in the procedure; their main disadvantage is bacterial colonization, which will delay healing. However, with proper suture placement, adequate cleaning of the surgical site by the patient, and timely suture removal in 48 to 72 hours, this problem can be minimized. Gut sutures can also be used, but their handling characteristics can be a challenge. A number of new synthetic suture materials are now available and may have relegated the silk suture to history. Materials such as polyglactin, polypropylene, polyethylene and Teflon (PTFE) cause minimal tissue reaction. With these newer monofilament synthetic materials, the preferred suture size for wound closure in periradicular surgery is either USP 5-0 (metric size 1.0) or USP 6-0 (metric size 0.7). Smaller USP 7-0 (metric size 0.5) or even USP 8-0 (metric size 0.4) sutures are advocated by some operators, particularly in situations such as the papilla-based incision.[34] Different needle sizes and shapes are often necessary as a result of osseous contours and tissue thickness.[112] No single needle shape or radius is ideal for every situation. Thin tissue is often found along the vertical releasing incision and requires a small radius needle. Larger radius needles are generally used in the horizontal incision to facilitate passage interproximally.

Suture knots should always be placed away from the incision line to minimize microbial colonization in that area (Figure 10-41). Sutured tissue should be cleaned routinely by the patient with chlorhexidine or warm saline rinses. Immediately after suturing, the tissue must be compressed with firm finger pressure for 3 to 5 minutes to ensure correct tissue position with a minimal blood clot between the bone and tissue flap (Figure 10-42). During this time, the patient can be given postoperative instructions. All sutures should ideally be removed in 48 to 72 hours.

POSTOPERATIVE RADIOLOGICAL ASSESSMENT

As previously indicated, a postoperative radiograph should be taken before closure of the surgical site; mistakes or deficiencies in techniques can be rectified easily at this point. In some cases, especially posterior

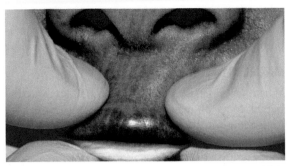

FIGURE 10-42 Compression of the tissue flap with gauze and light pressure is essential to minimize blood clot between tissue and cortical bone.

teeth, angled radiographs should be considered. Radiographs taken with a film-holding device are preferred. When review examination radiographs are taken with the same device, healing can be assessed more accurately. Some points for the clinician to consider are:

- Is there any remaining unresected root structure, or have the wrong roots been inadvertently resected or damaged?
- Has any resected root tissue been left in the surgical site?
- Are the correct root ends surgically filled?
- Do the root-end fillings appear adequate in depth and adaptation and appear well compacted?
- Is there scattered radiopaque material within the surgical site?
- Has root-end filling material been pushed into the maxillary sinus or mandibular canal?
- Is there evidence of a fracture that was not seen clinically?

POSTOPERATIVE PATIENT INSTRUCTIONS

When the soft tissues are managed properly and surgical time is minimized, healing is generally uneventful. Careful attention to postoperative instructions is essential for patient comfort and tissue healing during the next few days. The following postoperative instructions should be given verbally and supported in writing for the patient's reference[113]:

- Strenuous activity should be avoided, along with drinking alcohol and smoking.
- An adequate diet consisting of fruit juices, soups, soft foods and liquid food supplements should be consumed after the effects of the local anaesthesia have worn off. Avoid hard, sticky or chewy foods.
- Do not pull on, or unnecessarily lift, the facial tissues.
- Oozing of blood from the surgical site is normal for the first 24 hours. Bleeding is managed by applying a gauze pack to the site. Slight and transient facial swelling and bruising may be experienced.
- Postsurgical discomfort is minimal, but the surgical site will be tender and sore. The use of analgesics for 24 to 48 hours will help to alleviate this occurrence. Normally, continue with the analgesics given presurgically.
- For the first day, place ice packs with firm pressure directly on the face over the surgical site for 20 minutes and then remove for 20 minutes. Repeat as necessary until retiring that evening.
- Chlorhexidine rinses should be used twice daily. On the day after surgery and for the next 3 to 4 days, warm hypertonic saltwater rinses can be used every 1 to 2 hours if possible (half a teaspoon of salt in a glass of warm water).
- Sutures will be removed in 48 to 72 hours.
- Brushing of the surgical site is not recommended until the sutures are removed. Before that, the surgical area can be cleaned using a large cotton puff or ball saturated with warm salt solution.
- Telephone numbers are provided for your convenience should complications arise.

POSTOPERATIVE EXAMINATION AND REVIEW

Review of the patient, both clinically and radiologically, is normally scheduled at 1 year. In most cases, osseous repair is virtually complete at this time; evidence of this, as well as clinical healing, has been considered as a valid criterion for success. Therefore, no additional follow-up may be necessary.[79,114,115] Failure to observe complete repair, or delayed healing should warrant additional evaluation for as long as 4 years[116] until repair is evident or signs and symptoms indicate failure.

Radiological interpretation is highly variable and can easily be influenced by the quality and angulation of the film and processing irregularities. Therefore, the clinician should use a film-holding device for all follow-up radiographs. Likewise, familiarity with radiological classifications of healing (success/failure) is essential.[5,15,49] This will enable case outcome assessment to be based on a sound, logical and consistent decision-making process.[39]

Periradicular Surgery of Particular Teeth

MAXILLARY ANTERIOR TEETH

Surgical access to maxillary anterior teeth is relatively straightforward because of the root position in relation to the labial cortical bone. The lateral incisor may pose more of a challenge because of its common distopalatal root inclination and curvature. Deeper osseous penetration is often necessary, and the root apex may impinge on the palatal cortical plate of bone. Common also in this region is the excessively long canine that requires extensive soft tissue elevation for access to the root end. Anatomical cross-sections after root-end resection usually reveal a round, oval or slightly oblong root outline with canals placed centrally on the root surface. As the apex of the lateral incisor is commonly positioned more toward the palatal, both the buccal and palatal cortical plates of bone may be destroyed from advancing periradicular disease or surgical intervention. This usually leads to a greater frequency of scar tissue (incomplete healing) as opposed to complete bony repair.

MAXILLARY PREMOLARS

Surgical access to single-rooted premolars is also straightforward, with a minimal thickness of cortical plate covering the root apex. Complications generally occur when multiple roots are present, widely divergent in a buccopalatal dimension and/or when the position of the maxillary sinus is such that penetration into the sinus cannot be avoided. Often, these teeth have buccal apices that have fenestrated the buccal cortex, and access is relatively simple.

The resected root outlines of single-rooted premolars are oval, oblong, dumbbell shaped, or round. In multirooted premolars, canals are centrally placed and generally oval or circular on the resected root surface. In a two-canal, single-rooted premolar, two oval or round canals can be expected with an anastomosis. In this situation, the root-end cavity must encompass not only the canal openings but also the anastomosis for which ultrasonic, or sonic, root-end preparation is particularly helpful.

MAXILLARY MOLARS

When buccal fenestrations exist, surgical access to the buccal roots of maxillary molars is relatively easy. Depending on the position of the inferior border of the zygomatic process, extensive removal of bone may be necessary. Root outlines, after resection, are usually oval or circular for the distobuccal root and oblong, teardrop shaped, figure-of-eight shaped, or narrow and curved for the mesial buccal root. This root has a high incidence of two canals with an anastomosis, and therefore, all orifices on the resected root face must be identified.

In palatal root surgery, soft tissue management is more difficult during reflection and retraction as a result of the thickness of the palatal flap and an irregular surface of the underlying cortical plate. Palatal roots have a tendency to curve toward the buccal, and the root seldom fenestrates the bone at the apex. This often implies that large amounts of bone must be removed in a site that has restricted access and visibility. Penetration into the sinus is not uncommon. The greater palatine nerve and vessels will invariably be encountered with the palatal root of a second molar. Resected root outlines are generally oval, round or oblong, with the canal placed centrally on the root surface.

MANDIBULAR ANTERIOR TEETH

Surgical access to the root apices of the mandibular anterior teeth is often difficult because of lingual tooth inclination, wide buccolingual roots, thick cortical bone apically with increased amounts of cancellous bone between the cortex and root and root dehiscences in the coronal half of the root. It is common for the root apices of mandibular incisors to be in close proximity, which may pose problems in root-end management. Resected root outlines are narrow, oblong or figure-of-eight shaped, with canal space on the resected root that is usually narrow mesiodistally and wide buccolingually. The incidence of two canals, or joining canals on the root surface is high after root-end resection.

When considering surgery on mandibular anterior teeth, make sure that any history of orthodontic tooth movement has been elicited from the patient. Often during tooth movement, the roots are moved facially outside the bone. Palpation of this area is essential, or a CBCT scan may be necessary, as once the tissue has been reflected, the roots may be completely denuded of any coverage, bone and soft tissue alike. This finding will impact significantly on the surgical outcomes.

MANDIBULAR PREMOLARS

Surgical access to the mandibular premolars is usually direct, except for the occasional presence of significant muscle attachments in the soft tissues and the mental foramen in the bone. Surgical entry is often from a superior direction to avoid the foramen, which is most commonly close to the second premolar. The thickness of the cortical bone overlying the root apices is variable depending on tooth inclination in the arch. Root outlines are generally oval to oblong in a buccolingual dimension, with a small incidence of multiple canals exiting on the resected root surface; preoperative radiographs should warn of this possibility.

MANDIBULAR MOLARS

Surgical entry through the cortical plate to mandibular molars can be straightforward but is more often complicated by limited access, shallow vestibule, thick cortical plate, the external oblique ridge, root length,

position and inclination. Although the apices of molar roots are inclined buccally,[10] the roots are often housed within a thick cortical plate of bone. Additionally, individual root variations and curvatures often place the apices in difficult-to-reach positions. Therefore, these anatomical problems must be considered during treatment planning. Radiological assessment is essential; the location of the mandibular canal must be identified through use of angled films in a superior or inferior direction. Likewise, proximally angled films will provide information about the number and curvature of roots. This information may also be gleaned from a CBCT scan.

Root outlines after resection are oval, dumbbell shaped, oblong and wide in a buccolingual dimension. Canals often have anastomoses in both mesial and distal roots. The use of staining is strongly advised to improve visual definition. Root-end cavities, by necessity, are oblong encompassing the entire canal system as it exits on the resected root surface (see Figure 10-32).

GENERAL ANATOMICAL CONSIDERATIONS

It is uncommon to penetrate the maxillary sinus during periradicular surgery. If this occurs, however, the opening must be protected to prevent debris entering the sinus during the management of the root end (Figure 10-43). This can be done with collagen-based

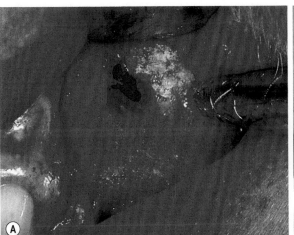
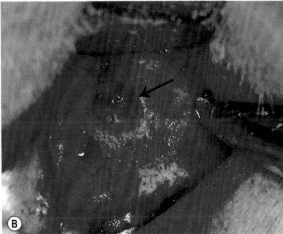

FIGURE 10-43 (A) Penetration into the maxillary sinus apical and distal to a premolar. (B) Blocking of the sinus perforation with a collagen sponge (*arrowed*). Note root-end preparation has been made with good haemorrhage control around the resected apex. Collagen was left in place to serve as a matrix for the closure of the sinus perforation.

haemostatic agents, as previously mentioned. Bone wax should not be used because it can be pushed into the sinus and evoke a significant foreign-body giant cell reaction along with delayed healing.[117] The post-surgical need for antibiotics or antihistamines has not been established.[39] Since primary closure can be achieved with soft tissue repositioning and suturing, an effective seal is obtained, avoiding the need for drug therapy.

The mental foramen also poses a challenge for many clinicians. Discussion with the patient at the treatment planning stage is essential to disclose the nature of the problem, the methods used to manage it and the potential for untoward postoperative seque-lae. The best way to manage this entity is to:

- identify its position; a CBCT scan may be necessary;
- plan surgical entry away from it;
- use the periosteal retractor to protect the foramen and its contents during surgery;
- avoid pinching the soft tissues with the retractor.

An additional concern with all periradicular surgery is the presence of fenestrations and dehiscences, along with large penetrating periradicular lesions, which have destroyed buccal and lingual cortical plates of bone.[108,109,118] Previous studies have identified less than favourable results when the surrounding bone has been compromised.[110,111,115] Management of these osseous defects often requires a guided tissue/bone regenerative procedure, which is becoming more widespread. These situations should be diagnosed and treatment planned carefully; when appropriate, it is prudent to consider help from experienced specialists.

Repair of Perforation

A root perforation is a mechanical, or pathological, communication formed between the supporting peri-odontal apparatus of the tooth and the root canal system. Nonsurgical repair of root perforations is rea-sonably successful,[119–122] but when it fails or is impractical, surgery may be necessary. The surgical repair of root perforations is generally more difficult than root-end procedures. Perforations pose greater radiological difficulties in identification, diagnosis

and postsurgical assessment.[123] Surgical management of perforated roots depends on access to the defect and the relationship of the perforation to crestal bone and the epithelial attachment. Perforations have been classified according to their relationship to the epi-thelial attachment and the crestal bone – the 'critical crestal zone'.[124,125]

Perforations occurring in the apical third pose the least problem in surgical management and are gener-ally amenable to root-end resection.[125–128] Midroot perforations present a different set of challenges. Typi-cally, they are not in line with the coronal aspect of the canal and may only be identified by radiographs taken from different angles. Once identified, surgically, they can be managed like any root end (Figures 10-44 and 10-45). Access to the defect margins, however, is more difficult when the perforation is located on the proximal surface of the root, and it is necessary to ensure complete marginal adaptation of the sealant material while preventing its placement into the sur-rounding bone (see Figure 10-45). Access to lingual perforations is almost impossible on most teeth, so other treatment options must be considered.

A common cause of perforation is caused by post space preparation and placement (Figure 10-46).[125,129] Often the post must be removed before root repair and a shorter post is placed. In some cases, the post may be ground down so that it lies inside the root, and a filling material is placed to seal the perforation.

The prognosis for surgically repaired root perfora-tions is based on a number of factors, similar to those for nonsurgical repair of root perforations. Success is highly dependent on the following factors:

- Proximity of the perforation to the critical crestal zone. The prognosis for furcation perforations is very poor because of the potential for microbial contamination.
- Extent of microbial contamination of the perforation.
- Timely management of the perforation; the shorter the time interval between occurrence of the perforation and repair, the better the prognosis.
- Use of a biocompatible repair material. Any material that is cytotoxic will significantly reduce the prognosis. For example, the placement of phenolic compounds in the root canal after a

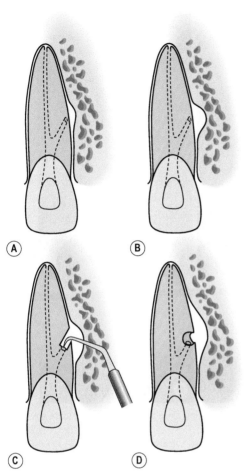

FIGURE 10-44 Access to a midroot proximal perforation. (A) Perforation; (B) access improved by careful removal of overlying bone; (C) creation of a cavity with an ultrasonic tip; (D) if necessary, additional bone can be removed to enhance access to the defect.

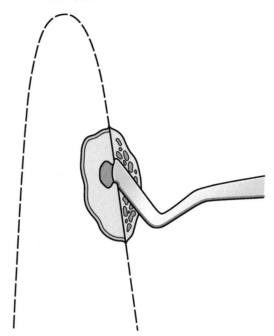

FIGURE 10-45 Repair of perforation. A flat, plastic instrument or the convex side of a small curette is used to apply the filling material to the prepared cavity; it may also serve as a matrix, against which the filling material is compacted with pluggers.

Replantation/Transplantation

Replantation is defined as replacing a tooth in its socket after deliberate, or traumatic, avulsion. In the case of surgical, or deliberate removal of a tooth and its replacement, it is defined as intentional replantation.[130] Transplantation involves the transfer of a tooth from one alveolar socket to another either in the same or another person.[130]

Few true indications exist for choosing intentional replantation as a primary method of treatment.[5] The presence of calcified canals, separated instruments, nonnegotiable root canals, perforations, or anatomical closeness of, e.g. the mandibular canal, are not valid indications for choosing intentional replantation. The patient's symptoms and signs, the strategic value of the tooth and the overall dental condition, including arch continuity, occlusion, function, tooth restorability and periodontal status must be considered along with the patient's understanding and cooperation. Finally, awareness of the potential for adverse

perforation has occurred, and before surgical repair, will cause irreparable damage to the periodontium at the perforation site. Likewise, the use of a cytotoxic material to seal the perforation will cause tissue damage.

- Sealing of the defect with minimal to no excess material in the surgical site that may cause persistent inflammation and possibly stimulate root resorption.
- Maintenance of optimal oral hygiene in the area of any perforation repair.

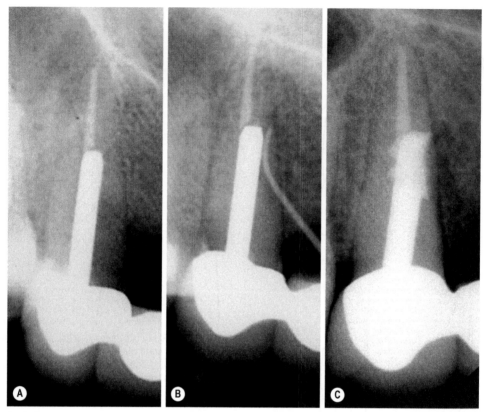

FIGURE 10-46 (A) Maxillary canine with postcore crown. (B) Patient presented with a draining sinus tract that was traced to the apical position of the post midroot. (C) Repair of post perforation with MTA.

sequelae such as bone loss, tooth resorption and tooth fractures during extraction must be considered. When viewed from this perspective, the only true indication for intentional replantation is when there is absolutely no other treatment available to maintain a strategic tooth.[131–133] Even then it is essential that all phases of this planned procedure be communicated to the patient, in addition to providing a realistic appraisal of the treatment plan, sequelae, prognosis and alternatives.

Once a decision has been reached to perform intentional replantation, all efforts should be taken to ensure removal of all tissue debris within the tooth. Root canals must be as clean as possible, canals filled as far as possible and the access opening closed with a permanent restoration. Occlusal adjustments and teeth cleaning should also be performed. Ideally, a two-person team should perform the procedure, one

to remove the tooth and the other to assess and fulfill the endodontic needs of the tooth. The surrounding tissue is disinfected with an antiseptic solution. Elevators should be used to carefully loosen the tooth, minimizing injuries to the soft tissue, bone and root. If necessary, the extraction forceps can be wrapped with gauze to minimize damage to the root. Once removed the crown of the tooth is grasped with gauze sponges soaked in sterile saline. The socket is gently curetted to remove foreign debris. Care is exercised to avoid damage to the socket-retained periodontal fibres; gauze or cotton products should not be placed into the socket.

The extracted tooth is examined for fractures, extra roots or foramina, or any unusual anatomical configurations. Root ends are easily resected with a high-speed fine diamond bur under sterile saline spray. The nature of the canal system and its orifices are examined and apically prepared with ultrasonics and filled if necessary. Time is of the essence with these procedures, and all members of the team must be fully aware of their responsibilities and be skilled in their execution.

When the tooth is ready to be replaced in its socket, the walls should be gently rinsed with saline to remove the blood clot. Additionally, the tooth is rinsed to remove any residual cotton fibres, or debris from the root-end filling material. The tooth is teased carefully and slowly into its original position in the socket, allowing for the slow escape of the blood that has built up in the socket. Slight pressure is applied to the buccal and lingual cortical plates to ensure adaptation. The occlusion is rechecked, and a splint is placed if necessary. Often only a periodontal pack is necessary. If a splint is used, the tooth must be in physiological function. Convenient splints can be made from soft, clear resin, or nylon line that is acid-etched and cemented to the buccal surface. Splints are removed after 5 to 7 days.

The prognosis for intentionally replanted teeth is primarily dictated by the presence, or absence, of inflammatory and replacement resorption. Long-term studies provide mixed results with this technique, with 50% to 60% success over a 5- to 10-year period.[5,134]

Regenerative Procedures

A major factor influencing the prognosis of endodontic surgery is the complete loss of cortical bone overlying the root.[110,111] If the buccal or lingual cortical bone is lost, or a naturally occurring dehiscence is revealed upon entry to the periradicular surgical site, the success rate is reduced.[18,110,111,115,135,136] When there is loss of the cortical plates both buccally and lingually, the success rate is reduced even further. In an attempt to improve the chance of success, regenerative procedures have been advocated as a means of encouraging formation of bone. Regenerative procedures have been used widely in periodontal surgery. Regeneration of the periradicular tissues subsequent to surgery, or due to the ravages of disease processes implies replacement of the various components of the tissues in their appropriate locations, amounts and relationships to each other.[137] There are a number of clinical situations

in endodontic surgery where regenerative procedures might be suitable.[6] These include:

- apical periodontitis without communication to the alveolar crest;
- apical periodontitis with communication to the alveolar crest;
- dehiscence;
- proximal bone loss;
- developmental grooves;
- root or furcation bone loss caused by perforations;
- cervical root resorption;
- oblique root fracture;
- ridge augmentation.

At present, the prognosis for regenerative procedures in endodontic surgery in patients is inconclusive. However, animal studies,[138–141] case reports[107,142–145] and empirical data would suggest that more favourable healing is likely when regenerative procedures are used. Unfortunately, successful regeneration can only be demonstrated histologically. Clinically, measurements such as gain in probing attachment level, decrease in probing depth and increased filling of the osseous defect have been used to measure and compare results.

Clinical Techniques in Regenerative Procedures

In guided-tissue regeneration, the type of healing that occurs after surgery is considered to be determined by the cells that first repopulate the root surface[146]; this has been supported by experimental work.[147–149] Membrane therapy has resulted in predictable formation of new attachments by preventing gingival connective tissue and gingival epithelium from contacting the root surface.[150] Regenerative membrane procedures aim to delay the advance of rapidly growing epithelial cells in order to allow the more slowly growing progenitor cells from the bone and periodontal ligament to repopulate the root surface and produce a new connective tissue attachment. The objectives of membrane application in endodontic surgery are as follows[151]:

- to facilitate tissue regeneration by creating an optimal environment (stable and protected wound);

- to exclude undesirable, fast-proliferating cells that interfere with desired tissue regeneration.

A classification for guided-tissue regeneration (GTR) application in endodontic surgery based on the location, extent and nature of the lesion has been proposed:

- Class I – bony defects located at the apex;
- Class II – apical lesions with concomitant marginal lesions;
- Class III – lateral or furcation lesions with or without a marginal lesion.

Two main types of membrane have been used, absorbable and nonabsorbable. The first commercially available membrane was an expanded polytetrafluoroethylene (ePTFE) nonabsorbable membrane (GORE-TEX, W.L. Gore & Associates, Flagstaff, AZ, USA). The use of GORE-TEX membrane necessitated a second surgical procedure to remove it. With the development of absorbable membranes, single-visit surgical procedures became possible. Studies have subsequently shown that there is no significant difference in the healing with either type of membrane.[152]

The absorbable membranes can be either natural materials such as collagen (BioMend, Zimmer Dental, Carlsbad, CA, USA, or Bio-Gide, Geistlich, Wolhusen, Germany), or synthetic polymers such as polyglactin. The natural materials are absorbed by enzymatic action, whereas the synthetic materials are absorbed by hydrolysis. The use of an absorbable membrane (Bio-Gide) in combination with a bone substitute material (Bio-Oss, Geistlich) has been shown to stimulate substantial new bone and cementum formation with Sharpey's fibre attachment.[153] Histological evaluation suggests that the combined approach compares favourably with other regenerative treatments.

Treatment Outcome – Aetiology and Evaluation

Although many studies have attempted to determine success–failure rates for periradicular surgery, none have been able to integrate fully all parameters of evaluation with techniques performed, materials used, patient compliance, clinician expertise, variability and interpretative skills. Attempts at multivariate analysis

have provided some trends and correlations, but even these findings may only be applicable to specifically controlled cases.[115,154]

Success (complete healing) with periradicular surgery has been reported to range from very low levels to levels as high as 96.8%[154] using mixed populations, at frequently less than ideal percentages of review examinations and short follow-up periods. With longer follow-up periods of up to 8 years, a success rate of 91.5% has been achieved,[3] which correlates closely with other long-term prospective studies (91.2%).[155] Although significant variability in results makes comparisons of studies questionable, the identification of factors that have contributed to the success or failure of periradicular surgery is essential, and these should be integrated into all phases of case assessment and treatment.[156] Often the aetiology of failure may be difficult to identify and may encompass a multitude of factors. For periradicular surgery, most failures can be attributed to specific causes. At the same time, when failure cannot be explained, uncertain aetiological factors and treatment may be speculated. Table 10-6 lists the aetiological factors often cited as valid or uncertain in the failure of periradicular surgery.

Evaluation of success or failure after root-end surgery is limited to clinical and radiological examinations. Clinical criteria for success or failure are used most commonly and in conjunction with the radiological findings. The clinical outcome is classified into one of three categories at the time of review (Table 10-7). Patient assessment, however, must be made in conjunction with both clinical and radiological parameters of evaluation (Table 10-8). If the only goal of periradicular surgery is to retain the tooth in adequate clinical function, then many cases can be classified as successful. Many factors, however, such as case selection, evaluator bias and patient factors, can skew levels of success or failure. Likewise, many clinically symptom-free teeth may have histopathological changes at the root apices, along with minimal or extensive radiological changes. Even in the presence of an apparently normal radiological appearance, a clinically symptom-free tooth may exhibit histopathological changes in the periradicular tissues. This is especially true adjacent to resected root surfaces, which are difficult to assess radiologically.

TABLE 10-6 Factors Influencing Success or Failure of Periradicular Surgery
Valid Causes for Surgical Failure
Failure to debride the root canal space thoroughly.
Failure to seal the root canal space adequately.
Tissue irritation from toxic root canal or root-end fillings.
Failure to manage root canal or root-end materials properly.
Superimposition of periodontal disease.
Longitudinal root fracture.
Recurrent cystic lesion.
Improper management of the supporting periodontium.
Uncertain Causes for Surgical Failure
Infected dentinal tubules.
Infected periradicular lesion.
Failure to use antibiotics when indicated.
Accessory or lateral canals.
Loss of alveolar bone.
Root resorption.
Timing of root canal filling (before or during surgery).
Type of root-end filling.

TABLE 10-7 Clinical Evaluation of Success and Failure
Clinical Success
No tenderness to percussion or palpation.
Normal mobility and function.
No sinusitis or paraesthesia.
No sinus tract or periodontal pocket.
No infection or swelling.
Adjacent teeth respond as expected to stimuli.
Minimal to no scarring or discolouration.
No subjective discomfort.
Clinical Uncertainty
Sporadic, vague symptoms.
Pressure sensation or feeling of fullness.
Low-grade discomfort on percussion, palpation or chewing.
Discomfort with tongue pressure.
Superimposed sinusitis focused on treated tooth.
Occasional need to use analgesics.
Clinical Failure
Persistent subjective symptoms.
Discomfort to percussion and/or palpation.
Recurrent sinus tract or swelling.
Evidence or irreparable tooth fracture.
Excessive mobility or progressive periodontal breakdown.
Inability to chew on the tooth.

Retreatment of Surgical Procedures

Not all surgery is successful, but when a case has been identified as failing, it is necessary to use all tests and information available to determine the cause before further surgery. Table 10-9 lists some of the more common unsuspected, anatomical and technical causes for failure. Not all of these causes are amenable to further surgery, and a tooth may require extraction and prosthetic replacement.

Very few studies have evaluated the results of periradicular surgery that was performed subsequent to previous surgical failure.[49,157] The success rates of repeat surgery were 50% or less with little subsequent alteration in healing after 1 year, but these figures relate to discontinued surgical techniques. In a recent, systematic review and meta-analysis of the outcomes of resurgery,[15,72,115] there was a near equal distribution of the cases between the three outcome groups: 35.7%

healed successfully, 26.3% healed with uncertain results and 38% did not heal.

The primary reason for failure after periradicular surgery is the presence of infected debris in uncleaned and poorly filled canal spaces.[15,115] The primary cause of failure with root canal treatment has been identified as coronal leakage caused by poor quality of the coronal restoration.[94,158] Therefore, it is essential to access, clean and fill as much of the canal space as possible and to seal thoroughly the coronal aspects of the root canal system before resorting to surgical

TABLE 10-8 **Radiological Evaluation of Success and Failure**
Radiological Success
Normal periodontal ligament width or slight increase.
Normal lamina dura or elimination of radiolucency.
Normal to fine-meshed osseous trabeculae.
No resorption evident.
Radiological Uncertainty
Slight increase in periodontal ligament width.
Slight increase in width of lamina dura.
Size of radiolucency static or slight evidence of repair.
Radiolucency is circular or asymmetric.
Extension of the periodontal ligament into radiolucency.
Evidence of resorption.
Radiological Failure
Increased width of the periodontal ligament and lamina dura.
Circular radiolucency with limited osseous trabeculae.
Symmetric radiolucency with funnel-shaped borders.
Evidence of resorption.

TABLE 10-9 **Causes of Surgical Failure**
Unsuspected
Root fracture not readily visible.
Posthole perforation, especially on the buccal or lingual surface.
Instrument perforation coronal to the resected root end.
Persistent infection in the apically resected tubules.
Corrosion of previously placed amalgam root-end filling.
Anatomical
Fenestrations or dehiscences – loss of marginal bone.
Aberrant root anatomy or canal space.
Proximity of root of adjacent teeth.
Proximity of maxillary sinus.
Technical
Poor canal cleaning and filling.
Inadequate root-end resection.
Inadequate root-end preparation and filling.
Toxicity of root-end filling material.
Improper soft tissue management.

intervention. Failing to adhere to this will inevitably result in failure.

Learning Outcomes

Upon completion of this chapter, the reader should be able to describe and discuss the:

- indications for periradicular surgery and the preoperative assessment process;
- key instruments and their usage in surgical endodontics;
- importance of tissue anaesthesia and haemostasis;
- management of the soft tissue, including tissue flap design, tissue incision, elevation and reflection;
- procedures for osseous entry and root identification in the various tooth groups;
- rationale, techniques and instruments for removal of soft tissue lesions and tissue biopsy;
- root-end filling materials available and the choice of material;
- techniques for primary closure of the surgical site to minimize postoperative sequelae;
- importance of the postoperative examination and case review, including radiographic assessment;
- implications and anatomical concerns when considering periradicular surgery of particular teeth;
- repair of tooth/root perforations and the rationale for tooth replantation, or transplantation;
- rationale for, and clinical techniques of, regenerative procedures that may be used in conjunction with periradicular surgery;
- importance of assessing treatment outcome, including identification of adverse aetiological factors that may require the revision of previous surgical procedures.

REFERENCES

1. Naito T. Single or multiple visits for endodontic treatment? Evidence-based Dentistry 2008;9:24.
2. Suchina JA, Levine D, Flaitz CM, et al. Retrospective clinical and radiologic evaluation of nonsurgical endodontic treatment in human immunodeficiency virus (HIV) infection. Journal of Contemporary Dental Practice 2006;7:1–8.
3. Rubinstein RA, Kim S. Long-term follow-up of cases considered healed one year after apical microsurgery. Journal of Endodontics 2002;28:378–83.
4. Rubinstein R, Torabinejad M. Contemporary endodontic surgery. Journal of the Californian Dental Association 2004; 32:485–92.
5. Gutmann J, Harrison JW. Surgical endodontics. St. Louis, MO: Ishiyaku EuroAmerica; 1994.
6. Rankow HJ, Krasner PR. Endodontic applications of guided tissue regeneration in endodontic surgery. Oral Health 1996;86:33–5, 7–40, 33–5.
7. Velvart P, Peters CI. Soft tissue management in endodontic surgery. Journal of Endodontics 2005;31:4–16.
8. Gutmann JL. Surgical endodontics: past, present, and future. Endodontic Topics 2014;30:29–43.
9. Doyle SL, Hodges JS, Pesun IJ, et al. Retrospective cross sectional comparison of initial nonsurgical endodontic treatment and single-tooth implants. Compendium of Continuing Education in Dentistry 2007;28:296–301.
10. Arens D, Adams WR, DeCastro RA. Endodontic surgery. Hagerstown, MD: Harper & Row; 1981.
11. Ingle JI, Bakland LK. Endodontics. 4th ed. Malvern, PA: Williams & Wilkins; 1994.
12. Doornbusch H, Broersma L, Boering G, et al. Radiographic evaluation of cases referred for surgical endodontics. International Endodontic Journal 2002;35:472–7.
13. Maalouf EM, Gutmann JL. Biological perspectives on the non-surgical endodontic management of periradicular pathosis. International Endodontic Journal 1994;27:154–62.
14. Saunders WP, Saunders EM. Coronal leakage as a cause of failure in root-canal therapy: a review. Endodontics & Dental Traumatology 1994;10:105–8.
15. Rud J, Andreasen JO. A study of failures after endodontic surgery by radiographic, histologic and stereomicroscopic methods. International Journal of Oral Surgery 1972;1: 311–28.
16. Gutmann JL. Clinical, radiographic, and histologic perspectives on success and failure in endodontics. Dental Clinics of North America 1992;36:379–92.
17. Bellizzi R, Loushine R. A clinical atlas of endodontic surgery. Chicago, IL: Quintessence; 1991.
18. Forssell H, Tammisalo T, Forssell K. A follow-up study of apicectomized teeth. Proceedings of the Finnish Dental Society 1988;84:85–93.
19. von Arx T, Fodich I, Bornstein MM. Proximity of premolar roots to maxillary sinus: a radiographic survey using cone-beam computed tomography. Journal of Endodontics 2014;40: 1541–8.
20. Bornstein MM, Wasmer J, Sendi P, et al. Characteristics and dimensions of the Schneiderian membrane and apical bone in maxillary molars referred for apical surgery: a comparative radiographic analysis using limited cone beam computed tomography. Journal of Endodontics 2012;38:51–7.
21. Bornstein MM, Lauber R, Sendi P, et al. Comparison of periapical radiography and limited cone-beam computed tomography in mandibular molars for analysis of anatomical landmarks before apical surgery. Journal of Endodontics 2011;37:151–7.
22. Rubinstein R. Endodontic microsurgery and the surgical operating microscope. Compendium of Continuing Education in Dentistry 1997;18:659–68.
23. Gutmann JL. Parameters of achieving quality anesthesia and hemostasis in surgical endodontics. Anesthesia & Pain Control in Dentistry 1993;2:223–6.
24. Jastak JT, Yagiela JA. Vasoconstrictors and local anesthesia: a review and rationale for use. Journal of the American Dental Association 1983;107:623–30.
25. Malamed SF. Handbook of local anesthesia. 6th ed. St. Louis, MO: Elsevier Mosby; 2012.
26. Gangarosa LP, Halik FJ. A clinical evaluation of local anesthetic solutions containing grades epinephrine concetrations. Archives of Oral Biology 1967;12:611–21.
27. Buckley JA, Ciancio SG, McMullen JA. Efficacy of epinephrine concentration in local anesthesia during periodontal surgery. Journal of Periodontology 1984;55:653–7.
28. Hargreaves KM, Keiser K. New advances in the management of endodontic pain emergencies. Journal of the Californian Dental Association 2004;32:469–73.
29. Troullos ES, Goldstein DS, Hargreaves KM, et al. Plasma epinepherine levels and cardiovascular response to high administered doses of epinepherine in local anesthesia. Anesthesia Progress 1987;34:10–3.
30. Hasse AL, Heng MK, Garret NR. Blood pressure and electrocardiographic response to dental treatment with local anesthesia. Journal of the American Dental Association 1986;113: 639–42.
31. Bennett CR. Monheim's local anesthesia and pain control in dental practice. 7th ed. St. Louis, MO: Mosby; 1984.
32. Roberts DH, Sowray JH. Local analgesia in dentistry. 2nd ed. Bristol, UK: Wright; 1987.
33. Ainamo J, Loe H. Anatomical characteristics of gingiva. A clinical and microscopic study of the free and attached gingiva. Journal of Periodontology 1966;37:5–13.
34. Velvart P. Papilla base incision: a new approach to recession-free healing of the interdental papilla after endodontic surgery. International Endodontic Journal 2002;35:453–60.
35. von Arx T, Alsaeed M, Salvi GE. Five-year changes in periodontal parameters after apical surgery. Journal of Endodontics 2011;37:910–8.
36. von Arx T, Hänni S, Jensen SS. Correlation of bone defect dimensions with healing outcome one year after apical surgery. Journal of Endodontics 2007;33:1044–8.
37. Cambruzzi JV, Marshall FJ. Molar endodontic surgery. Journal of the Canadian Dental Association 1983;49: 61–5.
38. Stashenko P. Role of immune cytokines in the pathogenesis of periapical lesions. Endodontics & Dental Traumatology 1990; 6:89–96.
39. Gutmann JL. Principles of endodontic surgery for the general practitioner. Dental Clinics of North America 1984;28: 895–908.
40. Byers MR, Wheeler EF, Bothwell M. Altered expression of NGF and P75 NGF-receptor by fibroblasts of injured teeth precedes sensory nerve sprouting. Growth Factors 1992;6:41–52.
41. Gutmann JL, Harrison JW. Posterior endodontic surgery: anatomical considerations and clinical techniques. International Endodontic Journal 1985;18:8–34.

42. Peters E, Lau M. Histopathologic examination to confirm diagnosis of periapical lesions: a review. Journal of the Canadian Dental Association 2003;69:598–600.

43. Burkes EJ Jr. Adenoid cystic carcinoma of the mandible masquerading as periapical inflammation. Journal of Endodontics 1975;1:76–8.

44. Copeland RR. Carcinoma of the antrum mimicking periapical pathology of pulpal origin: a case report. Journal of Endodontics 1980;6:655–6.

45. Hutchison IL, Hopper C, Coonar HS. Neoplasia masquerading as periapical infection. British Dental Journal 1990; 168:288–94.

46. Corcoran JF. The importance of periapical biopsy as a diagnostic tool in endodontics. Journal of Michigan Dental Association 1978;60:523–6.

47. Cambruzzi JV, Marshall FJ, Pappin JB. Methylene blue dye: an aid to endodontic surgery. Journal of Endodontics 1985;11:311–4.

48. Luks S. Root end amalgam technic in the practice of endodontics. Journal of the American Dental Association 1956;53:424–8.

49. Rud J, Andreasen JO. Operative procedures in periapical surgery with contemporaneous root filling. International Journal of Oral Surgery 1972;1:297–310.

50. Tidmarsh BG, Arrowsmith MG. Dentinal tubules at the root ends of apicected teeth: a scanning electron microscopic study. International Endodontic Journal 1989;22:184–9.

51. Gilheany PA, Figdor D, Tyas MJ. Apical dentin permeability and microleakage associated with root end resection and retrograde filling. Journal of Endodontics 1994;20:22–6.

52. Nedderman TA, Hartwell GR, Protell FR. A comparison of root surfaces following apical root resection with various burs: scanning electron microscopic evaluation. Journal of Endodontics 1988;14:423–37.

53. Molven O, Halse A, Grung B. Incomplete healing (scar tissue) after periapical surgery–radiographic findings 8 to 12 years after treatment. Journal of Endodontics 1996;22:264–8.

54. von Arx T, Kunz R, Schneider AC, et al. Detection of dentinal cracks after root-end resection: an ex vivo study comparing microscopy and endoscopy with scanning electron microscopy. Journal of Endodontics 2010;36:1563–8.

55. Stropko JJ, Doyon GE, Gutmann JL. Root-end management: resection, cavity preparation, and material placement. Endodontic Topics 2005;11:131–51.

56. Beatty RG. The effect of reverse filling preparation design on apical leakage. Journal of Dental Research 1986;65:259, abstract 805.

57. Vertucci FJ, Beatty RG. Apical leakage associated with retrofilling techniques: a dye study. Journal of Endodontics 1986;12:331–6.

58. Ichesco WR, Ellison RL, Corcoran JF, et al. A spectrophotometric analysis of dentinal leakage in the resected root. Journal of Endodontics 1991;17:503–7.

59. Carrigan PJ, Morse DR, Furst ML, et al. A scanning electron microscopic evaluation of human dentinal tubules according to age and location. Journal of Endodontics 1984;10:359–63.

60. Pashley DH. Smear layer: physiological considerations. Operative Dentistry. Supplement 1984;3:S13–29.

61. Brännström M. Smear layer: pathological and treatment considerations. Operative Dentistry. (Supplement) 1984;3:S35–42.

62. Barry GN, Heyman RA, Elias A. Comparison of apical sealing methods. A preliminary report. Oral Surgery, Oral Medicine, Oral Pathology 1975;39:806–11.

63. Carr GB. Surgical endodontics. In: Cohen S, Burns RC, editors. Pathways of the pulp. 6th ed. St. Louis, MO: Mosby-Year Book; 1994. p. 531–67.

64. Gutmann JL, Saunders WP, Nguyen L, et al. Ultrasonic root-end preparation. Part I. SEM analysis. International Endodontic Journal 1994;27:318–24.

65. Sultan M, Pitt Ford TR. Ultrasonic preparation and obturation of root-end cavities. International Endodontic Journal 1995;28:231–8.

66. Sumi Y, Hattori H, Hayashi K, et al. Ultrasonic root-end preparation: clinical and radiographic evaluation of results. Journal of Oral & Maxillofacial Surgery 1996;54:590–3.

67. Fong CD. A sonic instrument for retrograde preparation. Journal of Endodontics 1993;19:374–5.

68. Lloyd A, Jaunberzins A, Dummer PM, et al. Root-end cavity preparation using the MicroMega Sonic Retro-prep Tip. SEM analysis. International Endodontic Journal 1996;29:295–301.

69. Abedi HR, Van Mierlo BL, Wilder-Smith P, et al. Effects of ultrasonic root-end cavity preparation on the root apex. Oral Surgery, Oral Medicine, Oral Pathology, Oral Radiology, & Endodontics 1995;80:207–13.

70. Saunders WP, Saunders EM, Gutmann JL. Ultrasonic root-end preparation, Part II. Microleakage of EBA root-end fillings. International Endodontic Journal 1994;27:325–9.

71. Gunes B, Ali Aydinbelge H. Effects of ultrasonic root-end cavity preparation with different surgical-tips and at different power-settings on glucose-leakage of root-end filling material. Journal of Conservative Dentistry 2014;17:476–80.

72. Peterson J, Gutmann JL. The outcome of endodontic resurgery: a systematic review. International Endodontic Journal 2001;34:169–75.

73. Peñarrocha-Diago M, Masstre-Ferrin L, Peñarrocha-Oltra D, et al. Influence of hemostatic agents upon the outcome of periapical surgery: dressings with anesthetic and vasoconstrictor or aluminum chloride. Medicina Oral, Patología Oral y Cirugía Bucal 2013;18:e272–8.

74. Jeansonne BG, Boggs WS, Lemon RR. Ferric sulfate hemostasis: effect on osseous wound healing. II. With curettage and irrigation. Journal of Endodontics 1993;19:174–6.

75. Lemon RR, Steele PJ, Jeansonne BG. Ferric sulfate hemostasis: effect on osseous wound healing. Left in situ for maximum exposure. Journal of Endodontics 1993;19:170–3.

76. Witherspoon DE, Gutmann JL. Haemostasis in periradicular surgery. International Endodontic Journal 1996;29:135–49.

77. Frank AL, Glick DH, Patterson SS, et al. Long-term evaluation of surgically placed amalgam fillings. Journal of Endodontics 1992;18:391–8.

78. Dorn SO, Gartner AH. Retrograde filling materials: a retrospective success-failure study of amalgam, EBA, and IRM. Journal of Endodontics 1990;16:391–3.

79. Jesslén P, Zetterqvist L, Heimdahl A. Long-term results of amalgam versus glass ionomer cement as apical sealant after apicectomy. Oral Surgery, Oral Medicine, Oral Pathology, Oral Radiology, & Endodontics 1995;79:101–3.

80. Regan JD, Gutmann JL, Witherspoon DE. Comparison of Diaket and MTA when used as root-end filling materials to support regeneration of the periradicular tissues. International Endodontic Journal 2002;35:840–7.

81. Torabinejad M, Watson TF, Pitt Ford TR. Sealing ability of a mineral trioxide aggregate when used as a root end filling material. Journal of Endodontics 1993;19:591–5.

82. Torabinejad M, Smith PW, Kettering JD, et al. Comparative investigation of marginal adaptation of mineral trioxide aggregate and other commonly used root-end filling materials. Journal of Endodontics 1995;21:295–9.

83. Torabinejad M, Hong CU, Lee SJ, et al. Investigation of mineral trioxide aggregate for root-end filling in dogs. Journal of Endodontics 1995;21:603–8.

84. Torabinejad M, Pitt Ford TR, McKendry DJ, et al. Histologic assessment of mineral trioxide aggregate as a root-end filling in monkeys. Journal of Endodontics 1997;23:225–8.

85. Chong BS, Pitt Ford TR, Hudson MB. A prospective clinical study of Mineral Trioxide Aggregate and IRM when used as root-end filling materials in endodontic surgery. International Endodontic Journal 2003;36:520–6.

86. Saunders WP. A prospective clinical study of periradicular surgery using mineral trioxide aggregate as a root-end filling. Journal of Endodontics 2008;34:660–5.

87. Pitt Ford TR, Andreasen JO, Dorn SO, et al. Effect of IRM root end fillings on healing after replantation. Journal of Endodontics 1994;20:381–5.

88. Crooks WG, Anderson RW, Powell BJ, et al. Longitudinal evaluation of the seal of IRM root end fillings. Journal of Endodontics 1994;20:250–2.

89. Lee SJ, Monsef M, Torabinejad M. Sealing ability of a mineral trioxide aggregate for repair of lateral root perforations. Journal of Endodontics 1993;19:541–4.

90. Pitt Ford TR, Torabinejad M, McKendry D, et al. Use of mineral trioxide aggregate for repair of furcal perforations. Oral Surgery, Oral Medicine, Oral Pathology, Oral Radiology, & Endodontics 1995;79:756–63.

91. Pitt Ford TR, Torabinejad M, Abedi HR, et al. Using mineral trioxide aggregate as a pulp-capping material. Journal of the American Dental Association 1996;127:1491–4.

92. Torabinejad M, Higa RK, McKendry DJ, et al. Dye leakage of four root end filling materials: effects of blood contamination. Journal of Endodontics 1994;20:159–63.

93. Tang HM, Torabinejad M, Kettering JD. Leakage evaluation of root end filling materials using endotoxin. Journal of Endodontics 2002;28:5–7.

94. Apaydin ES, Shabahang S, Torabinejad M. Hard-tissue healing after application of fresh or set MTA as root-end-filling material. Journal of Endodontics 2004;30:21–4.

95. Boyko GA, Melcher AH, Brunette DM. Formation of new periodontal ligament by periodontal ligament cells implanted in vivo after culture in vitro. A preliminary study of transplanted roots in the dog. Journal of Periodontal Research 1981;16:73–88.

96. Boyko GA, Brunette DM, Melcher AH. Cell attachment to demineralized root surfaces in vitro. Journal of Periodontal Research 1980;15:297–303.

97. Register AA. Bone and cementum induction by dentin, demineralized in situ. Journal of Periodontology 1973;44:49–54.

98. Ruse D, Smith DC. Adhesion to bovine dentin – surface characterization. Journal of Dental Research 1991;70:1002–8.

99. Register AA, Burdick FA. Accelerated reattachment with cementogenesis to dentin, demineralized in situ. I. Optimum range. Journal of Periodontology 1975;46:646–55.

100. Codelli GR, Fry HR, Davis JW. Burnished versus nonburnished application of citric acid to human diseased root surfaces: the effect of time and method of application. Quintessence International 1991;22:277–83.

101. Sterrett JD. Optimal citric acid concentration for dentinal demineralization. Quintessence International 1991;22:371–5.

102. Craig KR, Harrison JW. Wound healing following demineralization of resected root ends in periradicular surgery. Journal of Endodontics 1993;19:339–47.

103. Meyers JP, Gutmann JL. Histological healing following surgical endodontics and its implications in case assessment: a case report. International Endodontic Journal 1994;27:339–42.

104. Polson A, Proye GT. Fibrin linkage: a precursor for new attachment. Journal of Periodontology 1983;54:141–7.

105. Ririe CM, Crigger M, Selvig KA. Healing of periodontal connective tissues following surgical wounding and application of citric acid in dogs. Journal of Periodontal Research 1980;15:314–27.

106. Gutmann JL, Pitt Ford TR. Management of the resected root end: a clinical review. International Endodontic Journal 1993;26:273–83.

107. John V, Warner NA, Blanchard SB. Periodontal-endodontic interdisciplinary treatment-a case report. Compendium of Continuing Education in Dentistry 2004;25:601–2, 4–6, 8; quiz 12–3.

108. Kellert M, Chalfin H, Solomon C. Guided tissue regeneration: an adjunct to endodontic surgery. Journal of the American Dental Association 1994;125:1229–33.

109. Pecora G, Kim S, Celletti R, et al. The guided tissue regeneration principle in endodontic surgery: one-year postoperative results of large periapical lesions. International Endodontic Journal 1995;28:41–6.

110. Hirsch JM, Ahlstrom U, Henrikson PA, et al. Periapical surgery. International Journal of Oral Surgery 1979;8:173–85.

111. Skoglund A, Persson G. A follow-up study of apicoectomized teeth with total loss of the buccal bone plate. Oral Surgery, Oral Medicine, Oral Pathology 1985;59:78–81.

112. Velvart P, Peters CI, Peters OA. Soft tissue management: suturing and wound closure. Endodontic Topics 2005;11:179–95.

113. Gutmann JLK. Surgical endodontics: post-surgical care. Endodontic Topics 2005;11:196–205.

114. Halse A, Molven O, Grung B. Follow-up after periapical surgery: the value of the one-year control. Endodontics & Dental Traumatology 1991;7:246–50.

115. Rud J, Andreasen JO, Jensen JF. A multivariate analysis of the influence of various factors upon healing after endodontic surgery. International Journal of Oral Surgery 1972;1:258–71.

116. Reit C. Decision strategies in endodontics: on the design of a recall program. Endodontics & Dental Traumatology 1987;3:233–9.

117. Finn MD, Schow SR, Schneiderman ED. Osseous regeneration in the presence of four common hemostatic agents. Journal of Oral & Maxillofacial Surgery 1992;50:608–12.

118. Pinto VS, Zuolo ML, Mellonig JT. Guided bone regeneration in the treatment of a large periapical lesion: a case report. Practical Periodontics & Aesthetic Dentistry 1995;7:76–81, quiz 2.

119. Benenati FW, Roane JB, Biggs JT, et al. Recall evaluation of iatrogenic root perforations repaired with amalgam and gutta-percha. Journal of Endodontics 1986;12:161–6.

120. Biggs JT, Benenati FW, Sabala CL. Treatment of iatrogenic root perforations with associated osseous lesions. Journal of Endodontics 1988;14:620–4.

121. Trope M, Tronstad L. Long-term calcium hydroxide treatment of a tooth with iatrogenic root perforation and lateral periodontitis. Endodontics & Dental Traumatology 1985;1: 35–8.

122. Walia H, Streiff J, Gerstein H. Use of a hemostatic agent in the repair of procedural errors. Journal of Endodontics 1988;14: 465–8.

123. Fuss Z, Assooline LS, Kaufman AY. Determination of location of root perforations by electronic apex locators. Oral Surgery, Oral Medicine, Oral Pathology, Oral Radiology, & Endodontics 1996;82:324–9.

124. Fuss Z, Trope M. Root perforations: classification and treatment choices based on prognostic factors. Endodontics & Dental Traumatology 1996;12:255–64.

125. Regan JD, Witherspoon DE, Gutmann JL. Prevention, identification and management of tooth perforation. Endodontic Practice 1998;1:24–40.

126. Nicholls E. Treatment of traumatic perforations of the pulp cavity. Oral Surgery 1962;15:603–12.

127. Oswald RJ. Procedural accidents and their repair. Dental Clinics of North America 1979;23:593–616.

128. Sinai IH. Endodontic perforations: their prognosis and treatment. Journal of the American Dental Association 1977;95: 90–5.

129. Young GR. Contemporary management of lateral root perforation diagnosed with the aid of dental computed tomography. Australian Endodontic Journal 2007;33:112–8.

130. American Association of Endodontists. Glossary of endodontic terms. 7th ed. Chicago, IL: American Association of Endodontists; 2003.

131. Weine FS. The case against intentional replantation. Journal of the American Dental Association 1980;100:664–8.

132. Dumsha TC, Gutmann JL. Clinical guidelines for intentional replantation. Compendium of Continuing Education in Dentistry 1985;6:604–8.

133. Scott JN, Zelikow R. Replantation – a clinical philosophy. Journal of the American Dental Association 1980;101: 17–9.

134. Andreasen JO, Rud J, Munksgaard EC. Atlas of replantation and transplantation of teeth. Fribourg. Switzerland: Mediglobe; 1989.

135. Mikkonen M, Kullaa-Mikkonen A, Kotilainen R. Clinical and radiologic re-examination of apicoectomized teeth. Oral Surgery, Oral Medicine, Oral Pathology 1983;55:302–6.

136. Persson G. Periapical surgery of molars. International Journal of Oral Surgery 1982;11:96–100.

137. Aukhil I. Biology of tooth-cell adhesion. Dental Clinics of North America 1991;35:459–67.

138. Bohning BP, Davenport WD, Jeansonne BG. The effect of guided tissue regeneration on the healing of osseous defects in rat calvaria. Journal of Endodontics 1999;25:81–4.

139. Dahlin C, Linde A, Gottlow J, et al. Healing of bone defects by guided tissue regeneration. Plastic & Reconstructive Surgery 1988;81:672–6.

140. Dahlin C, Gottlow J, Linde A, et al. Healing of maxillary and mandibular bone defects using a membrane technique. An experimental study in monkeys. Scandinavian Journal of Plastic & Reconstructive Surgery & Hand Surgery 1990;24: 13–9.

141. Douthitt JC, Gutmann JL, Witherspoon DE. Histologic assessment of healing after the use of a bioresorbable membrane in the management of buccal bone loss concomitant with periradicular surgery. Journal of Endodontics 2001;27:404–10.

142. Blomlöf L, Lindskog S. Cervical root resorption associated with guided tissue regeneration: a case report. Journal of Periodontology 1998;69:392–5.

143. Uchin RA. Use of a bioresorbable guided tissue membrane at an adjunct to bony regeneration in cases requiring endodontic surgical intervention. Journal of Endodontics 1996;22:94–6.

144. Zenobio EG, Shibli JA. Treatment of endodontic perforations using guided tissue regeneration and demineralized freeze-dried bone allograft: two case reports with 2–4 year post-surgical evaluations. Journal of Contemporary Dental Practice 2004;5:131–41.

145. Zorzano LA, Sanchez AL, Chacartegi JE, et al. Guided tissue regeneration procedure applied to the treatment of endodontic-periodontal disease: analysis of a case. Quintessence International 1997;28:87–91.

146. Melcher AH. On the repair potential of periodontal tissues. Journal of Periodontology 1976;47:256–60.

147. Karring T, Nyman S, Lindhe J. Healing following implantation of periodontitis affected roots into bone tissue. Journal of Clinical Periodontology 1980;7:96–105.

148. Karring T, Nyman S, Gottlow J, et al. Development of the biologic concept of guided tissue regeneration – animal and human studies. Periodontology 2000 1993;1:26–35.

149. Nyman S, Gottlow J, Karring T, et al. The regenerative potential of the periodontal ligament. An experimental study in the monkey. Journal of Clinical Periodontology 1982;9:257–65.

150. Gottlow J, Nyman S, Karring T, et al. New attachment formation as the result of controlled tissue regeneration. Journal of Clinical Periodontology 1984;11:494–503.

151. von Arx T, Cochran DL. Rationale for the application of the GTR principle using a barrier membrane in endodontic surgery: a proposal of classification and literature review. International Journal of Periodontics & Restorative Dentistry 2001;21:127–39.

152. Caffesse RG, Mota LF, Quinones CR, et al. Clinical comparison of resorbable and non-resorbable barriers for guided periodontal tissue regeneration. Journal of Clinical Periodontology 1997;24:747–52.

153. Camelo M, Nevins ML, Lynch SE, et al. Periodontal regeneration with an autogenous bone – Bio-Oss composite graft and a Bio-Gide membrane. International Journal of Periodontics & Restorative Dentistry 2001;21:109–19.

154. Rubinstein RA, Kim S. Short-term observation of the results of endodontic surgery with the use of a surgical microscope and Super-EBA as root-end filling material. Journal of Endodontics 1999;25:43–8.

155. Zuolo ML, Ferreira MO, Gutmann JL. Prognosis in periradicular surgery: a clinical prospective study. International Endodontic Journal 2000;33:91–8.

156. Lim LM, Pascon EA, Skribner J, et al. Clinical, radiographic, and histological study of endodontic treatment failures. Oral Surgery, Oral Medicine, Oral Pathology 1991;71:603–11.

157. Nordenram A, Svardstrom G. Results of apicectomy. Swedish Dental Journal 1970;63:593–604.

158. Ray HA, Trope M. Periapical status of endodontically treated teeth in relation to the technical quality of the root filling and the coronal restoration. International Endodontic Journal 1995;28:12–8.

CHAPTER 11

Endodontics in Primary Teeth

F. S. L. Wong

Chapter Contents

Summary

Endodontic treatment of primary teeth can be challenging because of the morphology of the root canal system, difficulties with correct diagnosis and behaviour management issues associated with young patients. The vital, noninfected pulp should be preserved when appropriate. As with any endodontic treatment, the elimination of infection is critical to a successful outcome. The move away from formocresol has led paediatric dentists to advocate for the use of alternative medicaments. Although root canal treatment of the infected primary tooth is often and arguably the best treatment option, it may be challenging or impractical to perform. A referral to a specialist may sometimes be necessary for endodontic management of primary teeth.

Introduction

The basic aims of endodontic treatment of a primary tooth are to help retain the tooth as a space maintainer until the permanent successor erupts, to prevent or treat infection that may cause malformation of its permanent successor and to relieve symptoms, including pain. It is generally accepted that primary teeth, particularly molars, should be retained until they exfoliate naturally to avoid loss of space and crowding of the permanent dentition.

Although the response of primary teeth to infection is similar to that of adult teeth, morphological and physiological differences exist between primary and permanent teeth, resulting in varying techniques for endodontic treatment. In addition, extra care must always be taken when carrying out endodontic treatment, especially on deciduous incisors. Parents must be warned of potential damage to the underlying permanent successor and the risks versus benefits discussed in full. A referral to a specialist paedodontic unit or practice may be necessary for endodontic management of primary teeth.

When deciding on a suitable treatment plan for primary teeth, the clinician must consider whether the tooth should be saved with endodontic treatment, or if extraction is a better option. The following factors should be considered when deciding on treatment.

The following factors are related to the patient:

- Patient cooperation – if a child is uncooperative or unable to cope with treatment in the dental chair, careful thought must be given to the potential benefits versus the risks of carrying out endodontic treatment under general anaesthesia. Although endodontic treatment enjoys a high success rate, the outcome cannot be guaranteed when there are compounding factors. If failure occurs, the child may be subjected to a repeat general anaesthetic just to remove the tooth.
- Medical history – certain medical conditions may determine whether endodontic treatment should be undertaken, e.g. children who are immunosuppressed from receiving chemotherapy and those who are at risk of infective endocarditis; there are concerns about a potential source of infection in the deciduous tooth. Endodontic treatment was previously advocated for children with coagulation disorders to avoid the risk of bleeding associated with an extraction. However, it should only be carried out if their coagulation disorder is mild; haemostatic cover is needed for an extraction but not for endodontic treatment. For those needing haemostatic cover to enable the administration of a local anaesthetic, it may be advisable to extract the tooth rather than risking another episode of needing coagulative factor infusion, e.g. in patients who have severe haemophilia. For any child with a relevant medical history, the medical team should be consulted before deciding on the best treatment option.
- Irregular attenders and poor parental attitude to dentistry – this may lead the clinician to decide against endodontic treatment, resulting from the inability to carry out regular clinical and radiological follow-ups.

The following factors are related to the dentition:

- Extent of dental decay – if the decay is extensive and restoration after endodontic treatment will be difficult, or impossible, then extraction is the treatment of choice.
- Extent of periapical infection – if gross pathological resorption has occurred or the infection is severe, extraction may be the best option.
- Condition of the rest of the dentition – if this is poor and the patient's motivation to change diet and improve oral hygiene is not deemed to be high, extraction is usually recommended.
- Hypodontia – if there is no permanent successor, endodontic treatment may be the best option to keep the space for a future bridge, or an implant.[1] However, the patient should be seen by a multi-disciplinary hypodontia team, which includes an orthodontist, to assess the residual space and timing of extraction, if needed, to allow for space closure.
- Balancing extractions in primary canines and first molars – if the contralateral tooth has been lost, it may be preferable to carry out a 'balancing' extraction rather than perform an endodontic treatment, especially when the arch is crowded.
- Remaining natural lifespan of the tooth – it is generally accepted that primary molar teeth should be retained until they exfoliate naturally to avoid loss of space and crowding of the permanent dentition. However, if physiological root resorption has affected two-thirds or more of the roots, then endodontic treatment is not a sensible option as the tooth is close to being exfoliated and would not cause severe loss of space.

Endodontic Treatment of Primary Teeth

Primary teeth differ morphologically from permanent teeth both in shape and size; pulp space anatomy is covered in Chapter 4. In general, the enamel and dentine are thinner than in a permanent tooth, and the pulp is relatively large. Pulpal changes in response to caries, therefore, occur more rapidly, and bacteria can easily infect the pulp from lesions that appear

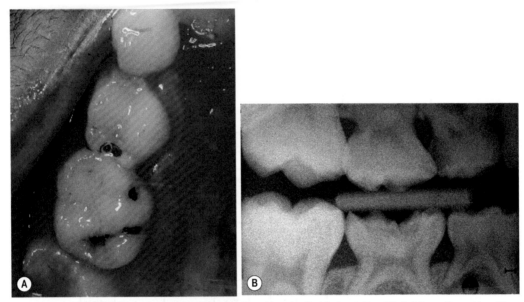

FIGURE 11-1 Clinical appearance of a maxillary primary first molar with caries that looks shallow (A), but the radiographic evidence reveals deep caries extending into the pulp (B).

minimal clinically (Figure 11-1). Multirooted primary molars have fine tapered roots which are flattened mesiodistally to enclose a ribbon-like root canal system, and the canals in single-rooted teeth may become partially calcified with age[2] to produce several intercommunicating canals. Thus, complete instrumentation of the radicular pulp space is difficult. The existence of lateral canals in the furcation of primary molar teeth[3] may contribute to the early spread of infection from the pulp chamber to the interradicular area.[4]

The correct diagnosis of pulpal disease is important as this will determine the type of treatment needed. The diagnosis depends on the combination of a good history, clinical and radiological examination and special tests. However, a clear history of clinical symptoms may be difficult to obtain in young patients because they may be unable to give an accurate pain history; therefore, reliance on parental reporting is usually necessary. Symptoms of irreversible pulpal damage include a history of spontaneous pain, severe pain at night and pain on biting. The clinical examination should begin with assessing the extent of the caries. It has been reported that in the majority of

primary molars with marginal ridge breakdown, there is pulpal inflammation involving the pulp horn adjacent to the carious lesion.[5] The presence of abnormal tooth mobility, intraoral swelling, discharging sinus tracts and tenderness to pressure will indicate the presence of periapical pathosis. In primary teeth, sensitivity testing has been shown to be an unreliable guide to the histological status of the pulp,[6–8] so a combination of the history, clinical and radiological examination is needed to provide an indication of the pulpal status. If the child is cooperative, preoperative radiological examination is invaluable; it provides information regarding root morphology, periapical pathosis, resorption and calcifications, aiding diagnosis and assessment of any local contraindications to endodontic treatment.

Once a diagnosis of the pulpal status is made, the available treatment options may be one of the following:

- indirect pulp capping;
- direct pulp capping;
- pulpotomy;
- pulpectomy;
- extraction.

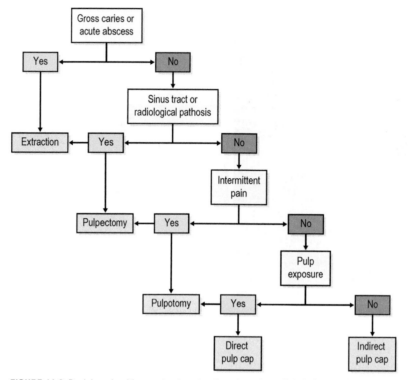

FIGURE 11-2 Decision algorithm on treatment options based on clinical signs and symptoms.

The decision on a treatment option is primarily based on clinical signs and symptoms; a decision algorithm is shown in Figure 11-2. Current concepts of caries management encompass complete, stepwise or partial removal of carious tissue in order to preserve the vitality of the pulp[9] (Figure 11-3). A biological approach of nonremoval, such as sealing the caries in using a preformed metal crown, has been advocated; it is known as the 'Hall technique'.[10–12] Usually, a more conservative treatment approach is advocated unless it is overridden by the severity of the condition or other factors such as the level of cooperation, medical or dental histories.

In all cases, the administration of local anaesthesia and adequate tooth isolation, preferably with a dental dam, are advised. For vital maxillary teeth, infiltration anaesthesia is usually satisfactory, whereas a nerve block or intraligamental injection may be more suitable for mandibular molar teeth. It cannot be overemphasized that a successful treatment outcome is dependent on correct diagnosis, appropriate

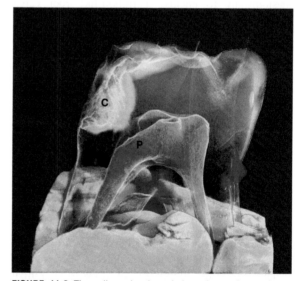

FIGURE 11-3 Three-dimensional rendering of a carious primary molar reconstructed from X-ray tomographic data. Note the pulp (*P*) recedes from the base of the carious lesion (*C*) as a protective response; careful removal of carious tissue will hopefully preserve pulp vitality.

technique and provision of a definitive restoration; ideally, a preformed metal crown, which will provide a good coronal seal, should be provided.[13] If such a restoration is planned, it may be advisable to prepare the tooth and adapt a crown before proceeding with the removal of caries and pulp treatment. This approach has two advantages:

- If the pulp is exposed and a pulp dressing is needed, it does not require the pulp dressing to set fully before the tooth is prepared for the crown. Otherwise, crown preparation may interfere with the dressing or lead to coronal microleakage.
- The removal of caries might alter the tooth so much so that it is more difficult to judge the size of preformed metal crown needed.

After endodontic treatment, all primary teeth should be reviewed and monitored clinically and radiographically until their permanent successors erupt.

INDIRECT PULP CAPPING

Indirect pulp capping is the technique that combines partial caries removal and placement of a therapeutic dressing over residual carious dentine. The aim is to create an environment that is bacteriostatic to allow or promote secondary/reactionary dentine formation within the pulp chamber.[14]

The indications for indirect pulp capping include:

- intermittent and not continuous pain or pain exacerbated by hot and cold stimuli;
- no associated swelling;
- no clinical or radiological evidence of pulpal or periapical disease;
- caries not too extensive to render the tooth unrestorable;
- radiographically >1 mm band of dentine between the base of caries and pulp.

The contraindications include:

- severe pain;
- clinical and/or radiological signs of extensive caries or infection;
- abnormal tooth mobility;
- other patient-related overriding factors.

Technique

After local anaesthesia and appropriate isolation, ideally with a dental dam, access through the overlying enamel is achieved with a bur in a high-speed handpiece. Using a bur in a slow-speed handpiece or a hand excavator, all soft carious dentine can be removed, with particular attention paid to the region along the amelodentinal junction, avoiding any dentine over the pulp if its removal will potentially cause exposure. A layer of hard-setting cement containing calcium hydroxide (e.g. Dycal, Dentsply, Weybridge, Surrey, UK) is then placed on the dentine and sealed with a quick-setting, reinforced zinc oxide-eugenol (e.g. IRM, Dentsply) or glass ionomer cement (e.g. Fuji IX, GC, Tokyo, Japan). A final restoration, preferably a preformed metal crown if the caries lesion involves more than one surface, can then be placed.

A success rate of 92% for indirect pulp capping with calcium hydroxide in primary incisors followed for 42 months has been reported,[15] and a rate of 96% in primary molars after 1 year.[16] Alternatively, an adhesive resin system may be used directly over the dentine, which has shown to have a success rate of 96%[17,18] compared with 83% for calcium hydroxide.[18] The use of glass ionomer, with the additional benefit of fluoride release, placed over the dentine has been reported to have a 93% success rate over 4 years compared with 89% for calcium hydroxide.[19,20]

Some authors have advocated a two-stage procedure in which the tooth is reopened 3 months later and further caries removal is performed.[21] Due to the high success of the one-stage indirect pulp cap, this is no longer considered necessary, and regular review of tooth vitality is preferable to subjecting the patient to subsequent reentry into the tooth.

DIRECT PULP CAPPING

Direct pulp capping describes the technique of covering the site of the pulp exposure with a protective material. It is based on the rationale that bacteria are confined to just below the exposure site. However, if a dentine layer is not clearly visible between the base of the carious lesion and pulp, it is likely that bacteria have entered the pulp space and is unlikely to be confined to just the site of the exposure. Hence, direct pulp capping is generally not advocated for primary teeth because of limited evidence of success in the literature. The only indication for this technique is when pulp tissue has been mechanically exposed as a result of cavity preparation[22] or when the tooth is close to exfoliation.[23]

Technique

The procedure is similar to that for indirect pulp capping. The peripheral caries should be removed first before the caries over the pulp. If there is an exposure and the site is clear of soft caries, it should be irrigated with saline to remove any debris. To control bleeding and keep the pulp moist, a saline-soaked pellet of cotton wool or sponge is compressed over the exposure site to facilitate formation of an intravascular clot,[24,25] as similarly advocated by Cvek for partial pulpotomy of traumatized incisor.[26] If bleeding does not stop after 2 minutes of compression, the pulp is most likely irreversibly damaged. In that case, pulpotomy, instead of direct pulp capping, is more appropriate. If bleeding ceased, the pulp capping material, such as a layer of nonsetting calcium hydroxide (e.g. Ultracal, Ultradent, South Jordan, UT, USA) is gently flowed over the exposure site; this may be followed by a layer of setting calcium hydroxide. The aim of the pulp capping material is to act as a wound dressing and help maintain pulp vitality; calcium hydroxide for example, promotes the formation of a dentine bridge over the exposure site. The cavity can then be sealed with zinc oxide-eugenol followed by a final coronal restoration. Afterward, the tooth should be monitored clinically and radiographically for any signs of subsequent pulp necrosis or extensive resorption, which is indicative of treatment failure.

There is a lack of long-term reports on the outcome of direct pulp capping in primary teeth. Calcium hydroxide as the pulp capping material alone or in conjunction with zinc oxide-eugenol has been widely investigated,[1] but a high incidence of internal resorption has been reported.[27,28] When used to line the pulp after partial pulpotomy in primary molars, a success rate of 83% after 1 year has been reported.[29] The use of dentine bonding systems has also been advocated, with promising results reported.[22,30] Recently, Mineral trioxide aggregate (MTA), a biocompatible material with good sealing properties and higher pH than calcium hydroxide,[31] has been shown to be a better pulp capping material. Favourable results of up to 95% success over 20 months[32] and 80% over 24 months[33] have been reported for direct pulp capping with MTA on primary molars. These reports show that

MTA is emerging as the material of choice for covering pulpal exposures.

PULPOTOMY

Pulpotomy is usually defined as removal of the coronal pulp. However, the suffix '-otomy' means 'cut or open', whereas '-ectomy' means 'removal'. Hence, the procedure would be better termed *(full) coronal pulpectomy*. The rationale is based on the assumption that bacteria that have induced pulpal inflammation and necrosis are confined within the coronal pulp, but the radicular pulp remains healthy. In addition, even if the radicular pulp is not infection free, the pulpotomy medicament, placed over the pulp stumps, has at least bacteriostatic, if not bactericidal, properties to prevent the spread of infection; the primary tooth can be retained until it exfoliates. Based on this rationale, the tooth should be vital. Although nonvital pulpotomy has been proposed in the literature, there is a lack of evidence to support this practice.

The indications for pulpotomy include:
- carious exposure but the tooth restorable;
- radiographically, no obvious band of dentine between the base of the carious lesion and the pulp;
- patient may be experiencing only intermittent pain.

The contraindications for pulpotomy include:
- continuous pain;
- presence of associated swelling or sinus tract;
- extensive caries and the tooth is unrestorable;
- radiological evidence of periapical pathosis and/ or root resorption;
- tooth close to exfoliation.

Technique

The basic technique consists of the following steps:
- Administer local anaesthetic and isolate the tooth, preferably with a dental dam.
- Gain access and remove all periphery caries using a bur in a high-speed handpiece.
- Enter the pulp chamber at the site of the pulp horns (closed to the cusps); avoid the centre of the tooth because of the potential risk of perforating the pulp floor (Figure 11-4A, B).
- Remove the roof of the chamber with an excavator and the bleeding pulp will be visible

(Figure 11-4C, D). If there is no bleeding, the pulp is necrotic so pulpectomy or extraction should be considered.

- Remove the entire contents of the pulp chamber up to the level of the root canal entrance using a slow-speed handpiece or a sharp excavator.
- Thoroughly irrigate the pulp chamber with sterile water, or local anaesthetic solution. It is generally advisable to avoid blowing compressed air into the cavity because of the theoretical risk of surgical emphysema.

- Compress the radicular pulp stumps with a cotton pellet or sponge soaked in saline or sterile water for 30 seconds. For additional disinfection, a 0.2% chlorhexidine gluconate solution may also be used (Figure 11-4E).
- Remove the cotton wool pledge or sponge and place the pulpotomy medicament; in this example, the pulpotomy medicament of 15.5% ferric sulphate is applied using a microbrush to the radicular pulp stumps for about 5 to 10 seconds to achieve haemostasis (Figure 11-4F);

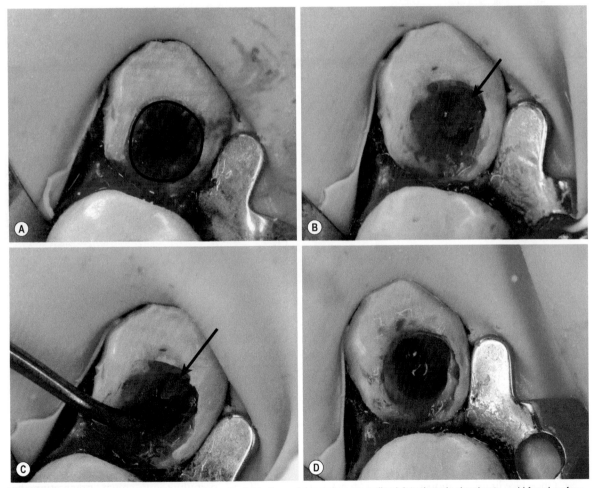

FIGURE 11-4 Pulpotomy procedure. Care should be exercised when gaining access, as outlined, into the pulp chamber to avoid furcal perforation (A); the roof of the pulp is removed with a hand excavator (B, C); coronal pulp tissue is removed from the pulp chamber (D); pressure is applied to the radicular pulp stumps using a saline-soaked cotton wool pellet *Continued*

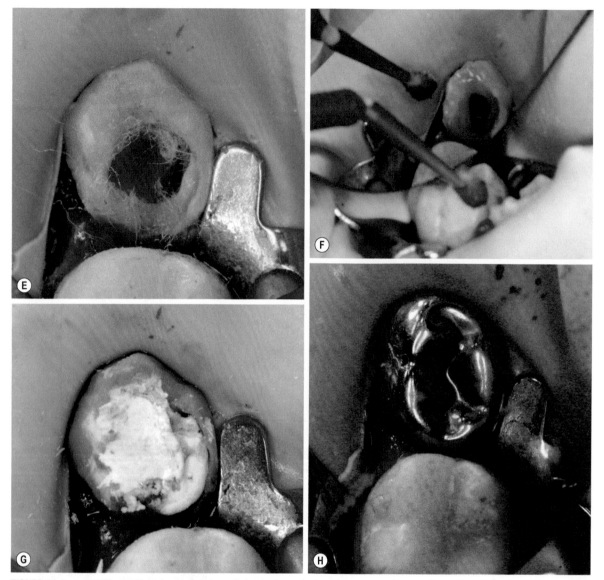

FIGURE 11-4, cont'd (E); 15.5% ferric sulphate is applied onto the radicular pulp stumps using a microbrush (F); the pulp chamber is filled with, for example, zinc oxide-eugenol (G) and the tooth is restored with a preformed metal crown (H).

if bleeding persists, a second application of ferric sulphate may be necessary. However, if the bleeding continues, the radicular pulp is hyperaemic, inflamed and irreversibly damaged so pulpectomy should be considered.

- Once bleeding has stopped, zinc oxide-eugenol cement or alternatives such as MTA is placed into the pulp chamber (Figure 11-4G).

- If the tooth has been prepared for a preformed metal crown before the commencement of the pulpotomy, the crown is then cemented even before the coronal pulp space filling is fully set (Figure 11-4H).
- If no prepulpotomy crown preparation has been carried out, once the coronal pulp space filling is set, the tooth should be prepared and a

preformed metal crown placed. There is evidence that after pulpotomy, placing a crown at the same appointment improves the prognosis of the tooth.

- Monitor the tooth clinically and radiographically until the permanent successor erupts.

Alternative Pulpotomy Techniques

Electrosurgery. A high-frequency unipolar electrosurgery unit (e.g. Whaledent PerFect TCS II, Coltène/Whaledent, Altstätten, Switzerland) may be used to amputate and remove the coronal pulp tissue; it also has the advantages of a coagulation effect to control haemorrhage and avoiding the use of any potentially toxic medicament avoided. However, the heat used to vaporize the tissue may cause root resorption.[34] To minimize heat conduction, the technique can be modified and used only for coagulation of the radicular pulp stumps, after mechanical removal of the coronal pulp tissues.[35] Most reports on the outcome of electrosurgery-assisted pulpotomy are short-term; a 2-year follow-up study indicates that it can have a good clinical (up to 100%) and radiological (95%) success rate.[36] Although there is good potential, more and longer term investigations on electrosurgery-assisted pulpotomy are needed before it is widely adopted.

Lasers. Lasers, including Nd:YAG, Er:YAG, CO_2 and 632/980 nm diode, have also been advocated to assist in the removal of the coronal pulpal tissue; short-term success has been reported.[37,38] However, in some studies, carbonization, necrosis and inflammation of the pulp with little evidence of repair have been shown after laser-assisted pulpotomy.[39–41] A systematic review concluded that there has been only weak evidence that laser application may enhance treatment outcomes of pulpotomy procedures[42]; further studies are needed.

MEDICAMENTS

Medicaments are used in endodontic treatment of primary teeth as wound dressings, tissue fixatives, disinfectants and inflammation suppressants. The choice of medicament to use is very much dependent on the clinical case and, to an extent, an individual operator's preference. However, the general consensus is that the toxic medicament in use in the past should be avoided; some of those listed in the following paragraphs, although included for historical interest, fall into this category.

Formocresol

Buckley[43] formulated a solution containing equal parts of formalin and tricresol to treat the putrescent pulp. It was later developed as a commercial solution containing 19% formaldehyde, and 35% cresol in a glycerine/water vehicle (Buckley's formocresol, Cosby Laboratories, Burbank, CA, USA) for treatment of the exposed pulp of primary teeth. The aim of this treatment technique is to fix the coronal portion of the radicular pulp and to maintain vitality of the remaining apical portion. The technique involves dampening a piece of sterile cotton wool pledget with this solution and placing it in contact with the radicular pulp stump for 4 minutes. Formocresol acts through its aldehyde group and binds to the amino acids of protein and bacteria to prevent autolysis and hydrolysis, thereby rendering tissue inert (i.e., fixing the tissue).[44,45]

Although for many years it was regarded as the gold standard medicament for pulpotomy of primary teeth, there is increasing concern about the toxicity, both local and systemic, of formocresol. Experimental animal studies have shown that absorption of formocresol from multiple pulpotomy sites can be sufficient to induce early tissue injury in the kidneys and liver.[46–49] This has led to the use of a 20% (1 : 5) diluted solution of formocresol to reduce its absorption.[50,51] Although it could be argued that the minute quantity of formocresol used as a medicament should mean the risk is less, or even negligible, the classification of formaldehyde as a carcinogen by the International Agency for Research on Cancer (IARC) in 2004 has led to questions about the continuing use of formocresol, especially in children. It has also prompted the search for alternative medicaments with similar or better success rates. Case control and cohort studies of workers exposed to formaldehyde daily have shown an association between formaldehyde exposure and nasopharyngeal cancer and leukaemia. The use of alternative medicaments has been debated within the literature amid growing unease. Reevaluation of the research regarding safety of formaldehyde may have concluded that there was inconsequential risk of carcinogenesis associated with the use of formaldehyde in endodontics in primary teeth.[52,53] However, the majority of paediatric dentists have moved away from formocresol in preference of alternative medicaments.[54–56]

Glutaraldehyde

Glutaraldehyde has been advocated as an alternative to formocresol because of its lower toxicity; it molecular size is larger than formaldehyde, and as a result diffusion through the tissues is reduced.[57,58] When 2% unbuffered glutaraldehyde was used, over 96% clinical success was reported after 42 months.[59] Other concentrations of glutaraldehyde have also been proposed following similarly clinically successful outcome.[60] A 90% clinical success rate was reported after 1 year, where 2% buffered glutaraldehyde was applied for 5 minutes in pulpotomies, but at follow-up after 2 years there was a failure rate of 18% as a result of internal resorption[61]; the authors concluded that the relatively high failure rate reported in this study does not justify recommending a 2% buffered glutaraldehyde solution as a substitute to formocresol. Although glutaraldehyde was proposed as a replacement for formocresol, questions remain about its safety since on a weight-for-weight basis there is little difference in toxicity between formocresol and glutaraldehyde.[62,63] Hence, at present this medicament is not widely used.

Ferric Sulphate

Ferric sulphate is an astringent and haemostatic agent that agglutinates blood protein to form a metal-protein barrier. It has been recorded that the use of ferric sulphate was invented in the late 1840s by Leon Monsel, a French military pharmacist, to help arrest bleeding of soldiers in battle. It is commonly used in dentistry for control of bleeding during surgery, or for gingival retraction. When applied directly to pulp tissue, a ferric ion-protein complex is formed which blocks the cut vessels mechanically. Although not a fixative, having only bacteriostatic properties, ferric sulphate is used to control haemorrhage by gentle intermittent application of a 15.5% solution for up to 15 seconds. The short application time is a clear advantage when treating children.

It has been proposed that the failure of pulpotomy is caused by the formation of an extravascular blood clot.[25] When the host defense system attempts to dissolve this fibrin clot, the inflammatory process also causes internal resorption. The rationale for using ferric sulphate is that its astringent property promotes the formation of an intravascular blood clot, avoiding or minimizing the activation of the inflammatory cells.[64]

Since ferric sulphate lacks bactericidal properties, an overlying protective material is required to provide a hermetic seal to prevent any ingress of bacteria. Even with this theoretical drawback, the success rate of ferric sulphate, with zinc oxide-eugenol as the lining/base material, is comparable to that of formocresol,[65,66] achieving a clinical success rate of 97% after 3 years.[67]

Calcium Hydroxide

Calcium hydroxide has a high pH and is widely used for indirect and direct pulp capping because it can induce dentine bridge formation. The application of pure calcium hydroxide to the cut pulp stumps after haemorrhage control was previously favoured for pulpotomy of primary teeth.[68] However, the work of Magnusson[69,70] cast doubt over the use of this material in primary teeth.

It has also been reported that if bleeding is well controlled, the success rate of calcium hydroxide pulpotomy can be comparable to that of formocresol.[71] However, most studies concluded that, comparatively, it performs poorly as a pulpotomy medicament.[67,72–75]

Mineral Trioxide Aggregate

MTA is chemically related to Portland cement, consisting of a mixture of dicalcium silicate, tricalcium silicate, tricalcium aluminate, gypsum and tetracalcium aluminoferrite, with an addition of bismuth oxide to increase its radiopacity.[76] It was originally formulated as a root-end filling material for apical surgery[77] and its properties include[78–80]:

- biocompatibility;
- hydrophilic;
- high pH, 12.5;
- bactericidal;
- low solubility;
- adequate compressive strength;
- resistance to marginal leakage;
- potential to promote healing and induce hard tissue barrier formation;
- resistance to marginal leakage.

The original MTA is grey in colour but it is now available in white. The MTA powder is mixed with sterile water to form a paste and then placed over the pulp stumps once haemostasis has been achieved. The setting time has been report to vary from 45 to 175 minutes. Due to its long setting time, the initial compressive strength is low. To improve its handling properties and increase setting time, new formulations have come on the market, with some manufacturers claiming that their version can set adequately after 15 minutes. Glass ionomer, or composite resin, can be placed directly over partially set MTA with no adverse reactions.[81,82] It is therefore advisable to restore the tooth immediately with a preformed metal crown or a composite resin restoration. Although it has been reported that MTA can cause tooth discolouration, this is not a problem if a preformed metal crown is placed after pulpotomy.

The clinical success rate of MTA is reported to be high, reaching 100% over 24 months of observation.[83,84] No internal resorption was found, but 41% were reported to have pulp canal obliteration.[85] Recent reviews all concluded that MTA is the best pulpotomy medicament for primary teeth.[72,78,86] The major drawback of MTA seems to be its relative higher cost compared with other pulpotomy medicaments.

Calcium Silicates

Calcium silicates have similar properties to that of MTA, but their setting time is shorter (12 minutes) and their compressive strength is higher by comparison.[87] Biodentine (Septodont, St. Maur-des-Fossés, France), first marketed in 2009, is claimed by its manufacturer to be a bioactive material suitable for use as a dentine substitute. The powder is composed of tricalcium silicate, dicalcium silicate, calcium carbonate and oxide filler, iron oxide shade and zirconium oxide as the radiopacifier. The liquid consists of calcium chloride as an accelerator and a hydrosoluble polymer that serves as a water reducing agent. Current reports on Biodentine are limited to animal studies[88,89] and case reports. However, its potential to replace MTA has been recognized by some reviewers.[90,91] Longer-term studies are needed to ascertain the efficacy of this material.

Corticosteroids

Corticosteroid may be used to suppress inflammation for the short-term purpose of desensitizing the pulp, for example, when the pulp is so inflamed and hyperaemic that adequate local anaesthesia is not achievable. A corticosteroid-antibiotic preparation (e.g. Ledermix, Haupt Pharma GmbH, Wolfratshausen, Germany, or Odontopaste, Australian Dental Manufacturing, Brisbane, Australia) may be useful for treating the inflamed, but not infected pulp, when it is too painful to allow pulp tissue removal. It is placed directly over the exposed pulp followed by a temporary dressing. The tooth is then revisited a week or so later, and pulp removal is then carried out. Corticosteroid compounds should only be used in carefully selected cases and never as a substitute for proper pulp treatment.

Bone Morphogenic Proteins

Bone morphogenic proteins (BMPs) are a family of growth factors discovered after the observation that demineralized bone matrix can stimulate new bone when implanted in an ectopic site such as muscle.[92] With the development of molecular biology, these factors were isolated and their physiological roles investigated. A number of BMPs are capable of inducing reparative dentine, and recombinant human BMPs have been used experimentally.[93] Although these materials have clear advantages in regenerative endodontics,[94] further development is needed for BMPs to be used as a medicament in pulpotomy.

Antibiotics

The concept of 'Lesion Sterilization and Tissue Repair' (LSTR) was developed in which a combination of antibiotics is used to disinfect the infected root canal system without the need for instrumentation. A similar concept of a mixture of antibiotics is also used, albeit for pulp space revascularization when managing necrotic or infected immature permanent teeth after trauma (see Chapter 12).

Studies on primary teeth with infected root canals and periapical lesions, in which a mixture of antibiotics (metronidazole, ciprofloxacin and minocycline) was placed at the orifices of root canals or in the pulp chamber, reported promising results.[95,96] However, available research is still limited, and this technique is not currently recommended as there is a concern about the overuse and abuse of antibiotics.

PULPECTOMY

Nonvital primary teeth may be retained successfully with pulpectomy, but it may be technically difficult to carry out due to the fine, ribbon-like canals and the high incidence of accessory canals. Greater care should also be exercised to avoid instrumentation through the apex lest the underlying, developing permanent successor is damaged. Pulpal necrosis, alveolar swelling, interradicular or periapical radiolucency are not contraindications in this treatment modality. However, contraindications include the presence of a large facial swelling, the tooth is unrestorable, or the patient has a high caries risk, or is medically compromised. Root canal treatment provides the most satisfactory method of retaining the restorable primary tooth where infection extends to the radicular pulp; extraction remains the only other option. The whole procedure may be completed in one visit when there is no infection, or over multiple visits if infection is present (Figure 11-5).

Technique

- Administer local anaesthetic and isolate the tooth, preferably with a dental dam.
- Gain access and remove all periphery caries using a bur in a high-speed handpiece.
- Enter the pulp chamber at the site of the pulp horns (closed to the cusps); avoid the centre of the tooth because of the potential risk of perforating the pulp floor.

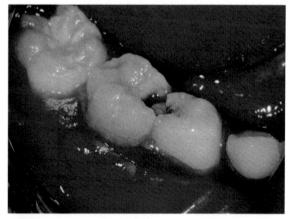

FIGURE 11-5 A buccal draining abscess related to two carious deciduous molars.

- Remove the roof of the pulp with an excavator.
- Remove all the tissues in the pulp chamber and identify the root canal orifices.
- Instrument the root canals with small files (ISO sizes 15 and 20) to within 2 mm of the radiographic apex.
- Irrigate the root canals with 1% sodium hypochlorite solution. Alternatively, 0.2% chlorhexidine gluconate may be used but it has no tissue-solvent properties.
- Dry the canals with sterile paper points.
- If treatment is carried out over more than one visit, the canals may be dressed with nonsetting calcium hydroxide and a temporary filling.
- The canals are obturated (see list of obturating materials), and the pulp chamber is filled with zinc oxide-eugenol or glass ionomer cement.
- The tooth is then restored with a preformed metal crown.
- The tooth is monitored until it exfoliates and the permanent successor erupts.

Obturating Materials.   There is no agreed consensus as to the preferred root canal filling material, but it should have the following properties:

- nonirritant to the periapical tissues and the underlying, developing permanent tooth;
- resorption at a rate similar to that of the deciduous tooth;
- antiseptic properties.

Resorbable materials based on pure zinc oxide-eugenol, calcium hydroxide and iodoform paste have been used successfully.[97-101] A study comparing the long-term outcomes of ferric sulphate pulpotomy and root canal treatment of vital, caries-exposed deciduous molars reported that root canal-treated molars demonstrated significantly greater survival than ferric sulphate pulpotomy-treated molars 3 years postoperatively.[102] Vitapex (Neo Dental, Federal Way, WA, USA) a premixed calcium hydroxide and iodoform paste, or Kri paste, another iodoform-based material, have been shown to have better clinical results than zinc oxide-eugenol.[98,103] Concerns have also been expressed that zinc oxide-eugenol cement is not completely resorbable. One study showed that pure calcium hydroxide paste had the least clinical success rate compared with zinc oxide-eugenol or Vitapex.[100] It is reported that overfilling the canal leads a higher failure rate compared with underfilling.[103]

Learning Outcomes

After completing this chapter the reader should be able to recognize and discuss the:

- endodontic challenges of treating the primary dentition and the patient management issues associated with the young patient;
- importance and difficulties of correct diagnosis and its influence on treatment planning;
- factors to consider when deciding whether endodontic treatment is appropriate;
- various endodontic treatment procedures for primary teeth;
- medicaments used in endodontic treatment of primary teeth;
- importance of eliminating infection in order to secure a successful endodontic treatment outcome.

REFERENCES

1. Rodd HD, Waterhouse PJ, Fuks AB, et al. Pulp therapy for primary molars. International Journal of Paediatric Dentistry 2006;16(Suppl. 1):S15–23.
2. Hibbard ED, Ireland RL. Morphology of the root canals of the primary molar teeth. Journal of Dentistry for Children 1957;24:250–7.
3. Winter GB. Abscess formation in connection with deciduous molar teeth. Archives of Oral Biology 1962;7:373–9.
4. Wrbas KT, Kielbassa AM, Hellwig E. Microscopic studies of accessory canals in primary molar furcations. Journal of Dentistry for Children 1997;64:118–22.
5. Duggal MS, Nooh A, High A. Response of the primary pulp to inflammation: a review of the Leeds studies and challenges for the future. European Journal of Paediatric Dentistry 2002;3:111–4.
6. McDonald RE. Diagnostic aids and vital pulp therapy for deciduous teeth. Journal of the American Dental Association 1956;53:14–22.
7. Mumford JM. Pain perception threshold on stimulating human teeth and the histological condition of the pulp. British Dental Journal 1967;123:427–33.
8. Asfour MA, Millar BJ, Smith PB. An assessment of the reliability of pulp testing deciduous teeth. International Journal of Paediatric Dentistry 1996;6:163–6.
9. Ricketts D, Lamont T, Innes NP, et al. Operative caries management in adults and children. Cochrane Database Syst Rev 2013;(3):CD003808.
10. Innes N, Evans D, Hall N. The Hall technique for managing carious primary molars. Dental Update 2009;36:472–4, 477–8.
11. Innes N, Evans D, Stirrups D. The Hall technique. British Dental Journal 2008;205:167–8.
12. Innes N, Evans D, Stirrups D. The Hall Technique; a randomized controlled clinical trial of a novel method of managing carious primary molars in general dental practice: acceptability of the technique and outcomes at 23 months. BMC Oral Health 2007;7:18.
13. Holan G, Fuks AB, Ketlz N. Success rate of formocresol pulpotomy in primary molars restored with stainless steel crown vs amalgam. Pediatric Dentistry 2002;24:212–6.
14. Shovelton DS. The maintenance of pulp vitality. British Dental Journal 1972;133:95–101.
15. Coll JA, Josell S, Nassof S, et al. An evaluation of pulpal therapy in primary incisors. Pediatric Dentistry 1988;10:178–84.
16. Al-Zayer MA, Straffon LH, Feigal RJ, et al. Indirect pulp treatment of primary posterior teeth: a retrospective study. Pediatric Dentistry 2003;25:29–36.
17. Gruythuysen RJ, van Strijp AJ, Wu MK. Long-term survival of indirect pulp treatment performed in primary and permanent teeth with clinically diagnosed deep carious lesions. Journal of Endodontics 2010;36:1490–3.
18. Falster CA, Araujo FB, Straffon LH, et al. Indirect pulp treatment: in vivo outcomes of an adhesive resin system vs calcium hydroxide for protection of the dentin-pulp complex. Pediatric Dentistry 2002;24:241–8.
19. Marchi JJ, de Araujo FB, Fröner AM, et al. Indirect pulp capping in the primary dentition: a 4-year follow-up study. Journal of Clinical Pediatric Dentistry 2006;31:68–71.
20. Massara ML, Alves JB, Brandao PR. Atraumatic restorative treatment: clinical, ultrastructural and chemical analysis. Caries Research 2002;36:430–6.
21. Vij R, Coll JA, Shelton P, et al. Caries control and other variables associated with success of primary molar vital pulp therapy. Pediatric Dentistry 2004;26:214–20.
22. Ranly DM, Garcia-Godoy F. Current and potential pulp therapies for primary and young permanent teeth. Journal of Dentistry 2000;28:153–61.
23. Fuks AB. Current concepts in vital primary pulp therapy. European Journal of Paediatric Dentistry 2002;3:115–20.
24. Schroder U, Granath LE. On internal dentine resorption in deciduous molars treated by pulpotomy and capped with calcium hydroxide. Odontologisk Revy 1971;22:179–88.
25. Schroder U. Effect of an extra-pulpal blood clot on healing following experimental pulpotomy and capping with calcium hydroxide. Odontologisk Revy 1973;24:257–68.
26. Cvek M. A clinical report on partial pulpotomy and capping with calcium hydroxide in permanent incisors with complicated crown fracture. Journal of Endodontics 1978;4:232–7.
27. Starkey PE. Methods of preserving primary teeth which have exposed pulps. ASDC Journal of Dentistry for Children 1963;30:219–24.
28. Kopel HM. Considerations for the direct pulp capping procedure in primary teeth: a review of the literature. Journal of Dentistry for Children 1992;59:141–9.
29. Schroder U, Szpringer-Nodzak M, Janicha J, et al. A one-year follow-up of partial pulpotomy and calcium hydroxide capping in primary molars. Endodontics and Dental Traumatology 1987;3:304–6.
30. Kopel HM. The pulp capping procedure in primary teeth 'revisited'. Journal of Dentistry for Children 1997;64:327–33.

31. Torabinejad M, Chivian N. Clinical applications of mineral trioxide aggregate. Journal of Endodontics 1999;25:197–205.

32. Fallahinejad Ghajari M, Asgharian Jeddi T, Iri S, et al. Treatment outcomes of primary molars direct pulp capping after 20 months: a randomized controlled trial. Iranian Endodontic Journal 2013;8:149–52.

33. Hilton TJ, Ferracane JL, Mancl L. Comparison of CaOH with MTA for direct pulp capping: a PBRN randomized clinical trial. Journal of Dental Research 2013;92(7 Suppl.):16S–22S.

34. Shulman ER, McIver FT, Burkes EJ Jr. Comparison of electrosurgery and formocresol as pulpotomy techniques in monkey primary teeth. Pediatric Dentistry 1987;9:189–94.

35. Ruemping DR, Morton TH Jr, Anderson MW. Electrosurgical pulpotomy in primates—a comparison with formocresol pulpotomy. Pediatric Dentistry 1983;5:14–8.

36. Khorakian F, Mazhari F, Asgary S, et al. Two-year outcomes of electrosurgery and calcium-enriched mixture pulpotomy in primary teeth: a randomised clinical trial. European Archives of Paediatric Dentistry 2014;15:223–8.

37. Yadav P, Indushekar K, Saraf B, et al. Comparative evaluation of ferric sulfate, electrosurgical and diode laser on human primary molars pulpotomy: an 'in-vivo' study. Laser Therapy 2014;23:41–7.

38. Durmus B, Tanboga I. In vivo evaluation of the treatment outcome of pulpotomy in primary molars using diode laser, formocresol, and ferric sulphate. Photomedicine and Laser Surgery 2014;32:289–95.

39. Jukic S, Anić I, Koba K, et al. The effect of pulpotomy using CO2 and Nd:YAG lasers on dental pulp tissue. International Endodontic Journal 1997;30:175–80.

40. Shoji S, Nakamura M, Horiuchi H. Histopathological changes in dental pulps irradiated by CO2 laser: a preliminary report on laser pulpotomy. Journal of Endodontics 1985;11:379–84.

41. Elliott RD, Roberts MW, Burkes J, et al. Evaluation of the carbon dioxide laser on vital human primary pulp tissue. Pediatric Dentistry 1999;21:327–31.

42. De Coster P, Rajasekharan S, Martens L. Laser-assisted pulpotomy in primary teeth: a systematic review. International Journal of Paediatric Dentistry 2013;23:389–99.

43. Buckley JP. A rational treatment for putrescent pulps. Dental Review 1904;18:1193–7.

44. Loos PJ, Straffon LH, Han SS. Biological effects of formocresol. Journal of Dentistry for Children 1973;40:193–7.

45. Loos PJ, Han SS. An enzyme histochemical study of the effect of various concentrations of formocresol on connective tissues. Oral Surgery, Oral Medicine and Oral Pathology 1971; 31:571–85.

46. Myers DR, Pashley DH, Whitford GM, et al. Tissue changes induced by the absorption of formocresol from pulpotomy sites in dogs. Pediatric Dentistry 1983;5:6–8.

47. Myers DR, Pashley DH, Whitford GM, et al. The acute toxicity of high doses of systemically administered formocresol in dogs. Pediatric Dentistry 1981;3:37–41.

48. Pashley EL, Myers DR, Pashley DH, et al. Systemic distribution of 14C-formaldehyde from formocresol-treated pulpotomy sites. Journal of Dental Research 1980;59:602–8.

49. Myers DR, Shoaf HK, Dirksen TR, et al. Distribution of 14C-formaldehyde after pulpotomy with formocresol. Journal of the American Dental Association 1978;96:805–13.

50. Morawa AP, Straffon LH, Han SS, et al. Clinical evaluation of pulpotomies using dilute formocresol. Journal of Dentistry for Children 1975;42:360–3.

51. Fuks AB, Bimstein E. Clinical evaluation of diluted formocresol pulpotomies in primary teeth of school children. Pediatric Dentistry 1981;3:321–4.

52. Milnes AR. Is formocresol obsolete? A fresh look at the evidence concerning safety issues. Journal of Endodontics 2008;34(7 Suppl.):S40–6.

53. Milnes AR. Persuasive evidence that formocresol use in pediatric dentistry is safe. Journal of the Canadian Dental Association 2006;72:247–8.

54. Ni Chaollai A, Monteiro J, Duggal MS. The teaching of management of the pulp in primary molars in Europe: a preliminary investigation in Ireland and the UK. European Archives of Paediatric Dentistry 2009;10:98–103.

55. Srinivasan V, Patchett CL, Waterhouse PJ. Is there life after Buckley's formocresol? Part I — a narrative review of alternative interventions and materials. International Journal of Paediatric Dentistry 2006;16:117–27.

56. Patchett CL, Srinivasan V, Waterhouse PJ. Is there life after Buckley's formocresol? Part II - development of a protocol for the management of extensive caries in the primary molar. International Journal of Paediatric Dentistry 2006;16: 199–206.

57. Davis MJ, Myers R, Switkes MD. Glutaraldehyde: an alternative to formocresol for vital pulp therapy. Journal of Dentistry for Children 1982;49:176–80.

58. 's-Gravenmade EJ. Some biochemical considerations of fixation in endodontics. Journal of Endodontics 1975;1: 233–7.

59. Garcia-Godoy F. A 42-month clinical evaluation of glutaraldehyde pulpotomies in primary teeth. Journal of Pedodontics 1986;10:148–55.

60. Tsai TP, Su HL, Tseng LH. Glutaraldehyde preparations and pulpotomy in primary molars. Oral Surgery, Oral Medicine and Oral Pathology 1993;76:346–50.

61. Fuks AB, Bimstein E, Guelmann M, et al. Assessment of a 2 percent buffered glutaraldehyde solution in pulpotomized primary teeth of schoolchildren. Journal of Dentistry for Children 1990;57:371–5.

62. Sun HW, Feigal RJ, Messer HH. Cytotoxicity of glutaraldehyde and formaldehyde in relation to time of exposure and concentration. Pediatric Dentistry 1990;12:303–7.

63. Feigal RJ, Messer HH. A critical look at glutaraldehyde. Pediatric Dentistry 1990;12:69–71.

64. Fuks AB, Eidelman E, Cleaton-Jones P, et al. Pulp response to ferric sulfate, diluted formocresol and IRM in pulpotomized primary baboon teeth. Journal of Dentistry for Children 1997;64:254–9.

65. Fuks AB, Holan G, Davis JM, et al. Ferric sulfate versus dilute formocresol in pulpotomized primary molars: long-term follow up. Pediatric Dentistry 1997;19:327–30.

66. Fei AL, Udin RD, Johnson R. A clinical study of ferric sulfate as a pulpotomy agent in primary teeth. Pediatric Dentistry 1991;13:327–32.

67. Huth KC, Hajek-Al-Khatar N, Wolf P, et al. Long-term effectiveness of four pulpotomy techniques: 3-year randomised controlled trial. Clinical Oral Investigations 2012;16: 1243–50.

68. Berk H. Effect of calcium-hydroxide methyl cellulose paste on the dental pulp. Journal of Dentistry for Children 1950; 17:65–8.

69. Magnusson B. Therapeutic pulpotomy in primary molars—clinical and histological follow-up. I. Calcium hydroxide paste as wound dressing. Odontologisk Revy 1970;21:415–31.

70. Magnusson B. Therapeutic pulpotomy in primary molars—clinical and histological follow-up. II. Zinc oxide-eugenol as wound dressing. Odontologisk Revy 1971;22:45–54.

71. Waterhouse PJ, Nunn JH, Whitworth JM. An investigation of the relative efficacy of Buckley's formocresol and calcium hydroxide in primary molar vital pulp therapy. British Dental Journal 2000;188:32–6.

72. Lin PY, Chen HS, Wang YH, et al. Primary molar pulpotomy: a systematic review and network meta-analysis. Journal of Dentistry 2014;42:1060–77.

73. Huth KC, Paschos E, Hajek-Al-Khatar N, et al. Effectiveness of 4 pulpotomy techniques—randomized controlled trial. Journal of Dental Research 2005;84:1144–8.

74. Sonmez D, Sari S, Cetinbas T. A comparison of four pulpotomy techniques in primary molars: a long-term follow-up. Journal of Endodontics 2008;34:950–5.

75. Moretti AB, Sakai VT, Oliveira TM, et al. The effectiveness of mineral trioxide aggregate, calcium hydroxide and formocresol for pulpotomies in primary teeth. International Endodontic Journal 2008;41:547–55.

76. Camilleri J, Montesin FE, Brady K, et al. The constitution of mineral trioxide aggregate. Dent Mater 2005;21:297–303.

77. Torabinejad M, Hong CU, McDonald F, et al. Physical and chemical properties of a new root-end filling material. Journal of Endodontics 1995;21:349–53.

78. Rao A, Shenoy R. Mineral trioxide aggregate—a review. Pediatric Dentistry 2009;34:1–7.

79. Parirokh M, Torabinejad M. Mineral trioxide aggregate: a comprehensive literature review. Part I: chemical, physical, and antibacterial properties. Journal of Endodontics 2010;36:16–27.

80. Torabinejad M, Parirokh M. Mineral trioxide aggregate: a comprehensive literature review. Part II: leakage and biocompatibility investigations. Journal of Endodontics 2010;36:190–202.

81. Tunc ES, Sönmez IS, Bayrak S, et al. The evaluation of bond strength of a composite and a compomer to white mineral trioxide aggregate with two different bonding systems. Journal of Endodontics 2008;34:603–5.

82. Ballal S, Venkateshbabu N, Nandini S, et al. An in vitro study to assess the setting and surface crazing of conventional glass ionomer cement when layered over partially set mineral trioxide aggregate. Journal of Endodontics 2008;34:478–80.

83. Jayam C, Mitra M, Mishra J, et al. Evaluation and comparison of white mineral trioxide aggregate and formocresol medicaments in primary tooth pulpotomy: clinical and radiographic study. Journal of the Indian Society of Pedodontics and Preventive Dentistry 2014;32:13–8.

84. Farsi N, Alamoudi N, Balto K, et al. Success of mineral trioxide aggregate in pulpotomized primary molars. Journal of Clinical Pediatric Dentistry 2005;29:307–11.

85. Eidelman E, Holan G, Fuks AB. Mineral trioxide aggregate vs. formocresol in pulpotomized primary molars: a preliminary report. Pediatric Dentistry 2001;23:15–8.

86. Asgary S, Shirvani A, Fazlyab M. MTA and ferric sulfate in pulpotomy outcomes of primary molars: a systematic review and meta-analysis. Journal of Clinical Pediatric Dentistry 2014;39:1–8.

87. Grech L, Mallia B, Camilleri J. Investigation of the physical properties of tricalcium silicate cement-based root-end filling materials. Dental Materials 2013;29:e20–8.

88. Shayegan A, Jurysta C, Atash R, et al. Biodentine used as a pulp-capping agent in primary pig teeth. Pediatric Dentistry 2012;34:e202–8.

89. Zanini M, Sautier JM, Berdal A, et al. Biodentine induces immortalized murine pulp cell differentiation into odontoblast-like cells and stimulates biomineralization. Journal of Endodontics 2012;38:1220–6.

90. Rajasekharan S, Martens LC, Cauwels RG, et al. Biodentine material characteristics and clinical applications: a review of the literature. European Archives of Paediatric Dentistry 2014;15:147–58.

91. Malkondu Ö, Karapinar Kazandağ M, Kazazoğlu E. Review on biodentine, a contemporary dentine replacement and repair material. BioMed Research International 2014;2014:160951. doi:10.1155/2014/160951.

92. Urist MR. Bone: formation by autoinduction. Science 1965;150:893–9.

93. Nakashima M. Induction of dentin formation on canine amputated pulp by recombinant human bone morphogenetic proteins (BMP)-2 and -4. Journal of Dental Research 1994;73:1515–22.

94. Nakashima M, Akamine A. The application of tissue engineering to regeneration of pulp and dentin in endodontics. Journal of Endodontics 2005;31:711–8.

95. Takushige T, Cruz EV, Asgor Moral A, et al. Endodontic treatment of primary teeth using a combination of antibacterial drugs. International Endodontic Journal 2004;37:132–8.

96. Burrus D, Barbeau L, Hodgson B. Treatment of abscessed primary molars utilizing lesion sterilization and tissue repair: literature review and report of three cases. Pediatric Dentistry 2014;l36:240–4.

97. Barcelos R, Santos MP, Primo LG, et al. ZOE paste pulpectomies outcome in primary teeth: a systematic review. Journal of Clinical Pediatric Dentistry 2011;35:241–8.

98. Mortazavi M, Mesbahi M. Comparison of zinc oxide and eugenol, and Vitapex for root canal treatment of necrotic primary teeth. International Journal of Paediatric Dentistry 2004;14:417–24.

99. Cerqueira DF, Mello-Moura AC, Santos EM, et al. Cytotoxicity, histopathological, microbiological and clinical aspects of an endodontic iodoform-based paste used in pediatric dentistry: a review. Journal of Clinical Pediatric Dentistry 2008;32:105–10.

100. Ozalp N, Saroglu I, Sonmez H. Evaluation of various root canal filling materials in primary molar pulpotomies: an in vivo study. American Journal of Dentistry 2005;18:347–50.

101. Barja-Fidalgo F, Moutinho-Ribeiro M, Oliveira MA, et al. A systematic review of root canal filling materials for deciduous teeth: is there an alternative for zinc oxide-eugenol? ISRN Dentistry 2011;2011:367318.

102. Casas MJ, Kenny DJ, Johnston DH, et al. Long-term outcomes of primary molar ferric sulfate pulpotomy and root canal therapy. Pediatric Dentistry 2004;26:44–8.

103. Holan G, Fuks AB. A comparison of pulpectomies using ZOE and KRI paste in primary molars: a retrospective study. Pediatric Dentistry 1993;15:403–7.

CHAPTER 12

Endodontic Aspects of Traumatic Injuries

A. Sigurdsson and C. Bourguignon

Chapter Contents

Summary

For all dental traumatic injuries, correct diagnosis, timely and appropriate treatment and follow-up are essential to achieve a favourable outcome. The management of traumatized teeth requires team effort, involving general dentists, paediatric dentists, oral surgeons and other frontline emergency service personnel. Endodontic specialists often participate in the effort to preserve the pulp and retain the tooth at a later stage. An informed and coordinated effort from all team members ensures that the patient receives the most appropriate and effective care. The emphasis on postinjury treatment may differ depending on the patient's age and the stage of development of the dentition. For young patients with permanent teeth, the focus has to be on the preservation of pulpal vitality, periodontal ligament healing and saving the tooth at all possible costs. This is essential because unless pulpal vitality is preserved, there is no further root development, and the immature tooth cannot attain structural strength. For younger children with primary teeth, the emphasis has to be on limiting further damage to the underlying permanent tooth bud, resulting in tooth malformation, impaction or eruption disturbances. In addition, clinicians should always bear in mind the possibility of nonaccidental injury in cases of trauma.

Introduction

This chapter focuses on emergency and endodontic aspects of traumatic injuries of teeth and does not attempt to cover dental traumatology comprehensively. For that, the reader is advised to consult a textbook on dental traumatology and current guidelines of the International Association for Dental Traumatology (IADT).[1-3]

In dental trauma, taking a complete history, a full account and performing a thorough examination are essential to ensure correct diagnosis, appropriate treatment and achieve the best possible outcome. The pulp status of all involved teeth must be assessed and their vitality maintained wherever possible. It should be borne in mind that vital teeth may be unresponsive to sensibility testing immediately after traumatic injury.[4] Maintaining dental pulp vitality is covered in Chapter 5.

History, Examination and Immediate Management

A dental injury should always be considered and dealt with as an emergency. However, before focusing on the dental injuries, management of the patient's medical condition, for example, any severe bleeding, or respiratory problems, takes priority. Often the dentist is the first healthcare professional to see the patient after a head injury. Any dental trauma is, by definition, a head injury. Therefore, assessment of possible brain concussion and/or haemorrhage has to be carried out before any dental treatment. According to a meta-analysis, the prevalence of intracranial haemorrhage after a mild head injury is 8%, and the onset of symptoms can be delayed for minutes to hours.[5] The most common signs of serious cerebral concussion, or haemorrhage are loss of consciousness, posttraumatic amnesia, nausea and/or vomiting, fluid discharge from the ear/nose, situational confusion, blurred vision, or uneven pupils and speech difficulties, including slurred speech.[6] If there are any signs of brain injury, immediate referral to a hospital, or other appropriate medical facilities, takes priority, and the dental trauma is then a secondary issue.

The dental injury must be evaluated thoroughly by careful clinical and radiographic investigation. It is recommended to follow a checklist to ensure that all necessary information regarding the patient and injury is collected (Table 12-1). A diagnosis can then be made and appropriate treatment provided. Inconsistencies between the history and injuries sustained, particularly if accompanied by late presentation, should

TABLE 12-1 **Fact Finding**
1. Patient's name, age, gender, address, contact numbers and, for young patients, their weight.
2. Any central nervous system symptoms after the injury?
3. General health, including medical history or any medications.
4. ***WHEN*** did the injury occur?
5. ***WHERE*** did the injury occur?
6. ***HOW*** did the injury occur?
7. Any treatment elsewhere?
8. History of previous dental injuries.
9. Is there any disturbance/s in the bite?
10. Do the teeth react to thermal changes, sweet or sour sensitivity?
11. Are the teeth sore to touch or during eating?
12. Is there spontaneous pain from the teeth?

alert the clinician to the possibility of nonaccidental injury.[7] Healthcare providers, including dentists, are in a unique position in the detection, intervention and prevention of violence and physical abuse, which is reported to be a significant public health problem, especially for females, young children and the elderly.[7] Injuries to the head, neck and/or mouth are clearly visible to the dental team during clinical examination. A recent review of the anatomical distribution of nonaccidental injuries in cases of violence and abuse against the elderly showed that 23% of the injuries were located in maxillofacial, dental and neck areas.[8] Everyone involved with the management of dental trauma should, therefore, be familiar with diagnostic and assessment tools for identifying victims of such injuries of all ages.[9]

A detailed account of when, where and how the injury occurred must be investigated and recorded before any treatment decisions; the patient, parents, or other accompanying person should be questioned. The circumstances of the accident may have legal implications, and photographic documentation should ideally be obtained as long as appropriate emergency treatment is not unnecessarily delayed. The time interval between injury and presentation for care can influence the treatment choices and may for instance, be critical to the successful replantation of an avulsed tooth. Where the injury happened may suggest possible

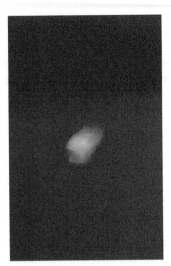

FIGURE 12-1 Radiograph of a tooth fragment embedded in the lacerated lip. The radiographic film was placed in the vestibule behind the lip, and the radiation dosage was adjusted accordingly. The fragment was subsequently removed from the lip after administration of a local anaesthetic and reattached to the fractured tooth by bonding with composite resin.

contamination of open wounds and the need for tetanus prophylaxis. The way the injury occurred may provide indication of its type and extent. Any signs of previous injury or treatment should be investigated and recorded. The medical history must be reviewed or updated. General and systemic illnesses and indications/contraindications to endodontics are covered in Chapter 2.

Clinical examination should include assessment and palpation of the soft tissues and facial skeleton. Disturbances to the occlusion, including deviation in mouth opening or closing movements, and/or inability to open normally as before may indicate jaw fracture or condylar displacement. Any extraoral soft tissue injury should be noted, and the possible presence of embedded foreign bodies considered; radiological examination may be necessary to facilitate its location (Figure 12-1). Suturing of soft tissues should be delayed until the injured teeth have been treated, especially in cases of luxation and avulsion, unless there is severe bleeding from the wound.

Infractions, fractures, pulpal exposures, mobility, or displacement are noted along with any colour changes. Lost pieces of fractured teeth should be accounted for

in case they are embedded in soft tissue, or have been swallowed, or inhaled. Adjacent, apparently unaffected teeth should always be included in the investigations as some injuries may go unnoticed.

Mobility and percussion testing should be carried out as they may indicate damage to the supporting tissues. Responses to pulp sensibility testing should be recorded; the results provide a baseline for later comparison. Injured pulps have the potential to recover but may remain unresponsive to sensibility testing for up to 3 months after trauma.[10] Therefore, the lack of response to sensibility testing after the injury should not be taken as an indication for immediate root canal treatment. In addition, some studies show that in severely luxated teeth, intracanal blood flow can be detected quite some time before their pulps responding to electric pulp testing.[11,12]

With regard to radiographical examination of an injured tooth, the IADT guidelines suggest taking:

- periapical radiograph with a 90-degree horizontal angle with a central beam through the tooth in question, using a paralleling device;
- occlusal view;
- periapical radiograph with lateral angulations from the mesial or distal aspect of the tooth in question.

If a root fracture is suspected, radiographs with different horizontal angulations should be taken. For primary teeth, an occlusal film alone is usually sufficient.

Cone beam computed tomography (CBCT) can provide enhanced visualization of many dental injuries, particularly root fractures and lateral luxations, and aid monitoring of healing and complications. Since CBCT may not be easily accessible, its use is not considered routine. Particularly for younger patients, because of the increased radiation dosage, discretion in the use of radiographs is recommended.[1,13–15]

Once a thorough clinical and radiographical examination has been completed, a diagnosis can be made and recorded for each injured tooth; the importance of this cannot be overstated. The outcome of treatment is dependent on correct diagnosis. This is to prevent inappropriate emergency treatment, which may be easily initiated at this stage[16] and should be avoided at all costs.

Classification of Traumatic Injuries

Trauma may cause the following damage to teeth:

- infraction of enamel, craze lines, or cracks in the clinical crown but with no tooth tissue loss;
- uncomplicated crown fracture;
- complicated crown fracture;
- crown–root fracture;
- root fracture;
- luxation injuries (concussion, subluxation, extrusion, lateral luxation, intrusion and avulsion).

Each tooth can potentially sustain multiple types of injury in the same accident. If several teeth are involved, each tooth can suffer a different type of injury.

Effects of Trauma on Dental Tissues and Treatment Objectives

The highest incidence of dental trauma occurs in anterior teeth and in children while their teeth are still immature.[17] Immature teeth have larger pulp spaces, more open apices and shorter but wider and more opened dentinal tubules. Infection may readily spread to the pulp, even if only the clinical crown is fractured, thereby arresting further tooth development. An immature tooth with a necrotic pulp is also prone to fracture, especially at the cervical region.[18] Consequently, one of the main objectives in the management of dental trauma is to maintain or reestablish pulp space vitality. Favourable periodontal healing and avoiding tooth loss at all costs, especially in children and teenagers, are also important goals.

Emergency Management of Permanent Teeth

FRACTURES

Enamel Infractions and Fractures

Infractions, also called enamel cracks and fractures, rarely require operative treatment, but the pulpal status should be monitored. Bacteria rarely enter the pulp through enamel infractions. Fractures of enamel may be either smoothed over or repaired with composite resin. The likelihood of pulp canal obliteration, or pulp necrosis occurring is low.[19] The chance of pulp damage is increased if there is an associated luxation of the tooth.[20]

Uncomplicated Crown Fracture: Enamel and Enamel–Dentine Fracture without Pulp Exposure

When only the enamel edge of the crown breaks off without any dentine exposure, treatment is performed solely for aesthetic and comfort reasons.[21] There is no need to rush to treat either. If the fractured fragment is found, it may be possible to rebond it back in place. If it is lost, composite resin, or just contouring the sharp edges may be the treatment of choice. When the fracture involves dentine as well, it is important to realize that because teeth of children or teenagers are likely to have larger pulps and wider dentinal tubules, exposed dentine can therefore result in damage to the pulp. Bacterial plaque can easily grow on the exposed dentine surface and can cause pulpal inflammation, which may lead to pulp necrosis. Etching and bonding composite resin onto the exposed dentine restores appearance and does not hinder subsequent monitoring of pulp vitality. There is no need to cap the exposed dentine as long as the remaining dentine thickness covering the pulp is 0.5 mm or more.[22,23] However, if it is estimated that the dentine thickness is less than 0.5 mm (usually the pulp horn may be discernible through the intact dentine), it has been shown that placing a calcium hydroxide base/liner on the deepest part of the dentine protects the underlying odontoblasts much better than etching and bonding directly on the thin dentine.[24]

The fractured fragment may be successfully reattached with composite resin after etching the enamel of both fragments and bonding it to the tooth. The key to reliable reattachment of the fractured fragment is the close approximation of the two portions so that there is a minimal layer of composite (flowable or nano filled) between the fragments. If it is necessary to place a calcium hydroxide base/liner on the dentine exposure, a dimple needs to be made in the fractured fragment to match the base/liner thickness. Once the fragment has been reattached, it has been recommended to cut a shallow chamfer at the junction where the two pieces meet. Then, the junction of contact is re-etched, bonded and additional composite flowed into the cut chamfer. This will increase the strength of the reattachment and help hide the fracture

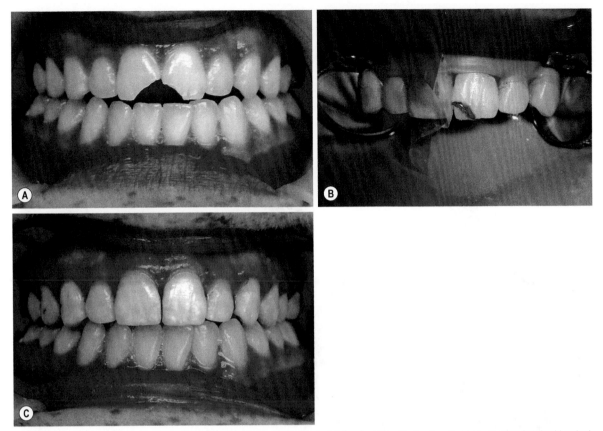

FIGURE 12-2 (A) Crown fractures of maxillary central incisors. (B) Under dental dam isolation, the fracture line was chamfered and acid etched, and both tooth fragments were bonded back using nano-filled composite resin. (C) Clinical view immediately after rebonding of the fragments.

line (Figure 12-2).[25,26] The bonding strength is also increased by rehydrating in advance the fractured fragment in water for 30 minutes if it was kept dry before arriving at the dental practice.[27]

The occurrence of pulp canal obliteration, or pulp necrosis is low after fractures involving dentine, provided the dentinal tubules are effectively covered.[19] The chance of pulp damage is increased if there is an associated luxation of the tooth.[20,28]

Complicated Crown Fracture: Enamel and Dentine Fracture with Pulp Exposure

Immature Teeth. In immature teeth, the treatment is directed at maintaining pulp vitality to allow continued tooth maturation, thus reducing the risk of subsequent root fracture or complex endodontic

treatment.[28] The pulp can be treated conservatively as it has a good blood supply and rarely becomes necrotic.[29,30] Partial pulpotomy is the treatment of choice.[29,31–33] The advantages of partial pulpotomy over direct pulp capping are that inflamed pulp tissue and adjacent infected dentine are removed.

Local anaesthesia, without vasoconstriction if at all possible, is necessary to carry out the pulpotomy. The tooth must be isolated with a dental dam to exclude salivary or aerosol contaminants. The pulp is removed with a diamond bur in a high-speed turbine handpiece using copious water spray. This causes less damage than a bur at slow speed, or an excavator (Figure 12-3).[30,34,35] Pulp removal is usually confined to the superficial 2 mm since infection and/or inflammation does not normally extend beyond this level.[31]

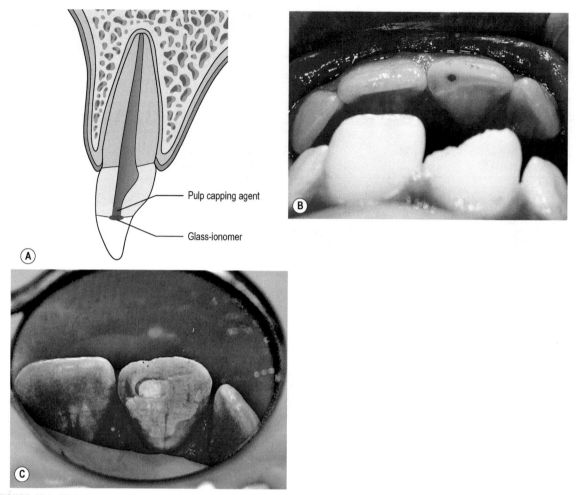

FIGURE 12-3 (A) In partial pulpotomy, it is advisable to cut an approximately 2-mm deep cavity into the pulp chamber with a high-speed diamond bur with copious irrigation. The cavity is then filled with a pulp capping material, such as a thick paste of calcium hydroxide, which is then domed over with glass ionomer cement. The tooth and fragment may then be acid etched; the fragment is reattached with composite resin or alternatively, the fracture built up with composite resin. (B) Clinical example of a complicated crown fracture with the mesial pulp horn exposed. (C) Same tooth after partial removal of the exposed, inflamed pulp, creation of the 2-mm deep cavity and placement of a calcium hydroxide layer.

Haemorrhage is arrested by placing a cotton pellet or preferably sponge soaked in saline on the pulp stump with light pressure for a few minutes. The wound is then covered with a thick calcium hydroxide (mixed with saline or anaesthetic solution) paste. For some years now, Mineral trioxide aggregate (MTA) has been recommended for pulp capping in anterior teeth.[33,36,37] However, it has been realized that both grey and white MTA can cause discolouration or grey staining

of teeth; therefore, MTA is no longer recommended for anterior teeth if discolouration is a concern.[38,39] After the placement of the calcium hydroxide cap, a domed-shaped layer of resin-modified glass ionomer cement is placed over the cap, before restoring with composite resin ensure that it is in place. At the same time, etching and bonding is carried out to the rest of the exposed dentine and enamel. A hard tissue barrier will form beneath the dressing and be visible on a radiograph in some weeks to months later in most cases.[32,35] This treatment has a high success rate; the pulp may be expected to remain vital and healthy.[29,31] Root canal treatment is not needed subsequent to pulpotomy unless pulp necrosis and infection develops.[34]

Mature Teeth. If a crown fracture occurs and exposes the pulp of a mature tooth, conservative treatment by partial pulpotomy is the first treatment option. However, when the entire clinical crown has been lost, pulpal extirpation, root canal filling and construction of a post-retained crown is usually indicated.

Crown–Root Fractures

Uncomplicated Crown–Root Fractures. In these types of extensive fractures, the coronal fragment is usually retained by the periodontal ligament. These teeth have a poor prognosis, especially if the fracture line is a long way subgingival on the palatal aspect. It is necessary to remove the fragment so that the extent of the fracture can be assessed and sealed. Leaving the piece in place, with some stabilization, is usually not a long-term solution because bacteria will colonize the fracture line, creating periodontal and pulpal complications. When the fracture does not extend too far subgingivally, it is possible to restore the tooth without crown lengthening. Otherwise, periodontal surgery, orthodontic extrusion or extraction and repositioning of the tooth in a more incisal location need to be considered in order to expose the fracture margin and allow restoration of the tooth. In an immature permanent tooth with an exposed pulp, where the fracture does not extend far subgingivally, partial pulpotomy should be carried out (as described earlier). When root loss is more extensive, the tooth will be difficult to restore, and the prognosis is poor.

If it is possible to cover the exposed root surface, the treatment of the crown fracture should follow the same guidelines as previously mentioned. Where the prognosis is poor, extraction of the remaining root is necessary if it is infected; otherwise, elective decoronation, or root submersion may be used to preserve the alveolar ridge in case of a growing child or teenager.[40,41]

Root Fractures

Root fractures are relatively uncommon. The coronal fragment may be mobile, extruded, or laterally luxated. The apical fragment, almost without exception, remains vital. There is a good possibility that the coronal fragment will recover its vitality if it is repositioned within a few hours after the injury. Thus, it does not require endodontic treatment as part of emergency or later treatment (Figure 12-4).[42]

If there is no mobility, or displacement of the coronal fragment, no splint is required.[43,44] If the tooth is displaced, or mobile, immediate treatment consists of repositioning the coronal fragment and splinting for 4 weeks. When the crown of a fractured maxillary incisor is severely palatally displaced, the apical portion of the coronal fragment is likely to be wedged in the facial cortical plate. To reposition, it has to be pulled slightly down and then rotated into correct alignment. Just forcing it facially will not allow the two root halves to approximate; correctly repositioned, this treatment has a high success rate.[45]

Pulp necrosis, if it occurs, is invariably confined to the coronal fragment.[42,46,47] No response to thermal and electrical stimuli is common. There will be a radiolucency in the bone around the tooth at the fracture line if the coronal pulp becomes necrotic, or a radiolucency (or internal root resorption) at the fracture line within the root of the coronal fragment only, unless there is definite evidence to implicate involvement of the apical fragment. If the apical fragment is nonvital, surgical removal is usually indicated.

LUXATION INJURIES

A luxation injury is characterized by damage to the supporting tissues of the tooth. The tooth may be displaced. There may be severance of the vessels and nerves at the apex. Prognosis for pulp recovery is reduced if there is a concomitant crown fracture as this is a potential route for entry of microbes.[17,48–50]

Concussion

This is an injury to the supporting tissues without loosening, or displacement of the tooth. The tooth is sensitive to percussion. Lasting pulp damage is rare, especially in an immature tooth, but the pulp may be

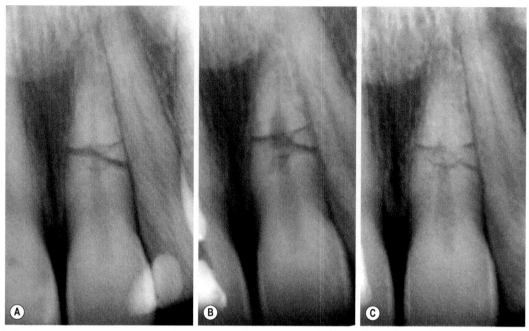

FIGURE 12-4 Root fracture of a maxillary central incisor. (A) Radiograph taken immediately after repositioning of the luxated coronal fragment and splinting. (B) Six-month recall radiograph showing extensive internal root resorption at the fracture line. However, there is no bone loss lateral to the fracture line and the pulp responded positively to sensibility testing. Hence, a 'wait and see' approach was adopted. (C) Five-year recall radiograph, fracture healing is obvious, and the root fractured tooth still responds normally to sensibility testing. Therefore, no endodontic treatment was needed.

unresponsive to sensibility testing for some months posttrauma.[51]

Subluxation

With subluxation, the tooth is loosened in its socket but not displaced. Pulp survival rate has been reported to be 90% for immature teeth and 75% for mature teeth.[51] It can take weeks or months to obtain normal responses to sensibility testing. The clinician has to look out for possible signs of pulpal necrosis and infection.[1]

Extrusive Luxation

If the extrusion is severe, the pulpal vessels and nerves are usually severed. In an immature tooth, quickly repositioned after injury, revascularization followed by the obliteration of the pulp space is the likely outcome. In a mature tooth, pulp necrosis is more common.[51]

Lateral Luxation

Lateral luxations can occur with or without apical dislocation. Mandibular anterior teeth can be severely laterally luxated, with minimal movement of the apex from its original place (Figure 12-5). Lateral luxation with apical dislocation is common for maxillary anterior teeth; the tooth crown is displaced palatally, and the apex breaks through the cortical plate facially and is locked in the bone. To confirm that the apex is locked, when the tooth is percussed with a mirror handle, it will emit a high pitched or metallic tone. To reposition the tooth, the locked apex has to be freed first; this is accomplished by gently pulling the tooth down with fingers, or with extraction forceps. Once freed from the apical lock, the tooth will easily return to its original position (Figure 12-6). Alternatively, this may be facilitated by pushing down on the apex, through the buccal cortical plate, to make it move incisally and then gently into the correct position.

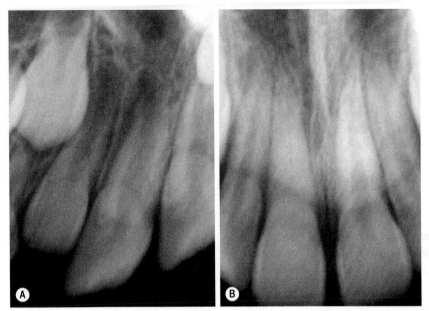

FIGURE 12-5 (A) Severe lateral luxation of the immature maxillary right central incisor. The tooth was repositioned and followed up according to the International Association for Dental Traumatology's recommendations. (B) Three-year recall radiograph showing continued tooth development but severe calcification of the pulp chamber (root canal obliteration). The tooth does not respond to cold testing but responds to electric pulp testing.

FIGURE 12-6 In lateral luxation with apical dislocation, the apex is likely to be displaced through the buccal cortical bone plate. (A) Applying force solely in a buccal direction will not allow proper repositioning of the tooth back into its socket. (B) The apex has to be freed first by pulling or pushing the tooth downward coronally and second by rotating the tooth into its correct position.

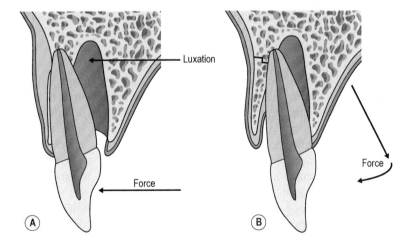

Pulp space healing, most often by revascularization, may be expected in 70% of immature teeth for this type of injury.[51]

Intrusive Luxation

This is one of the most severe luxation injuries. The tooth is forced into its socket, crushing the supporting structures, the blood vessels and nerve fibres that supply the pulp. The tooth, wedged in the supporting bone, displays a lack of mobility and a ringing tone on percussion. Radiographs will show an absence of periodontal ligament space. Immature teeth might re-erupt spontaneously.[52–54] If there is no evidence of eruption after 3 weeks, rapid orthodontic repositioning should be undertaken. In cases of severe intrusion (>6 mm) of a mature permanent tooth, immediate surgical repositioning should be considered as there is little hope for spontaneous re-eruption.[55,56] Accessing the clinical crown for endodontic treatment is essential in these teeth as there is no hope for pulpal survival. In immature teeth, approximately 60% become nonvital and do not recover after this injury.[51] Intruded teeth are prone to resorption, so the patient should be followed up carefully as the rate of complications is high (see 'Posttrauma Complications').

AVULSION

Emergency Management of Avulsion Injuries on Site (Outside the Dental Surgery)

Immediate Replantation. The length of time the tooth spent outside its socket ('extraalveolar time') is the most critical factor influencing the survival of an avulsed and replanted tooth, particularly if the root surface was allowed to dehydrate because the tooth was left in open air.[57,58] Therefore, the aim of treatment is always to replant the tooth back into its socket as quickly as possible. Education of the public on what to do in case of dental trauma is vitally important. Posters like the one from IADT are available and can be widely distributed as part of public education (Figure 12-7).

The public should be advised that if the root surface is heavily contaminated by debris, it should not be removed by scrapping or wiping but rather by just rinsing the tooth for a few seconds under running water. Gentle management of the root surface is important in order to preserve all the remaining viable periodontal ligament and cementum cells. If there is still residual debris or if no water is available, the tooth should be replanted as it is. Replantation should be carried out by holding the tooth by its crown and placing it back into its socket gently. The patient can then bite gently on a piece of cloth, handkerchief, or on anything convenient so as to keep the tooth in place. If some resistance is met during repositioning, there may be an alveolar bone fracture. The tooth should not be forcibly repositioned but rather soaked in transport medium, milk, or saliva, and the patient (and the tooth) brought to the dental practice as soon as possible.

Storing the Avulsed Tooth in Transport Medium before Replantation. If it is not feasible to replant the tooth immediately at the site of the accident, care must be taken to store it in proper conditions to increase the chances of survival of the periodontal ligament cells still attached to the root surface. Specially formulated transport media in containers designed for tooth transportation include the Save-A-Tooth (Phoenix-Lazerus, Inc., Pottstown, PA, USA) kit and the DentoSafe (Dentosafe BmbH, Iserlohn, Germany) tooth rescue box. Alternatively, milk or physiological saline is the second best transport media.[2] If none of these transport media are available, the avulsed tooth should be placed in the vestibule of the mouth in contact with saliva as it is better than keeping the tooth dry or in water.[59,60] Water should not be used as a transport medium because it is hypotonic and of incompatible osmolarity to the surviving cells on the root surface.[60] Massive and rapid cell lysis starts within minutes of the tooth being placed in tap water.

By far the best alternative to the specialized transport media is milk. It is usually and readily available; it maintains a high percentage of viable cell count for at least 3 hours, and it has an osmolarity and a pH close to ideal for cell survival. Additionally, pasteurized milk is relatively free of bacteria.[61] Refrigeration of the milk with the avulsed tooth is unnecessary.[59]

Emergency Management of Avulsion Injuries at the Dental Surgery

Patient Examination. If the tooth was replanted before the patient arrived at the dental practice, it will be loose and in most cases, will have the tendency to drift out of the tooth socket. If the tooth was not replanted before the patient's arrival at the dental practice, then its storage condition needs to be immediately assessed on arrival. If it was not stored in proper conditions, it should be placed immediately in the best available specialized storage medium, milk or saline while a thorough examination of all the patient's injuries is performed.

Socket Manipulation. Replanting the tooth into a coagulum that has formed in the empty socket has not been shown to be detrimental to healing; however, the clot may impede proper tooth repositioning.[62] It is therefore, advisable to gently rinse the socket with sterile saline before attempting replantation. Once the

Save your tooth

Most of your permanent teeth may be saved if you know what to do after a blow to the mouth

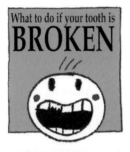

What to do if your tooth is BROKEN

  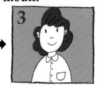

1	2	3
Find the piece of tooth	The piece can be glued on	For this to be possible, seek attention immediately from a dentist

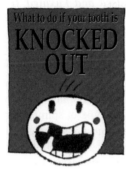

What to do if your tooth is KNOCKED OUT

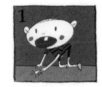 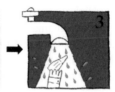

1	2	3
Find the tooth	Hold it by the crown	(Plug the sink) Rinse in cold tap water

4
FOLLOW ONE OF THESE ALTERNATIVES:

   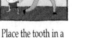

a	b	c
Put the tooth back in its place	Place the tooth in a cup of milk or saline	When milk is not available, place the tooth in the mouth between the cheeks and gums

 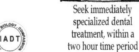

5
Seek immediately specialized dental treatment, within a two hour time period

Dental Trauma Education
and Prevention Campaign,
Children's Dental
Traumatology Service
Faculty of Dentistry
University of Valparaiso
Chile
Tel. 56 - 32 - 508 690 - 1
Fax 56 - 32 - 508 696
e-mail: cliinffo@uv.cl

UNIVERSIDAD DE VALPARAISO CHILE

IADT
International Association
of Dental Traumatology

Colgate

FIGURE 12-7 English version of an educational 'Save Your Tooth' poster from the International Association for Dental Traumatology (IADT); available free for public use in 14 different languages.

socket is cleared, the wall of the socket needs to be assessed. If collapsed, a blunt instrument like a mirror handle should be gently inserted into the socket and pressure applied to the collapsed walls to reposition and reopen the alveolus.

Root Manipulation. Depending on the duration of the extraalveolar drying time and on the stage of root development, there are four main treatment pathways for an avulsed tooth.[2] If the tooth was kept dry for less than 1 hour or up 3 to 4 hours in an appropriate storage medium, then it should be replanted as soon as possible. However, if the tooth was kept dry for longer than 1 hour, then there is almost no chance of periodontal ligament survival; additional steps need to be taken to slow down the root resorption process, which is likely to occur after replantation. Periodontal ligament cell death when exposed to air reaches critical levels after approximately 30 minutes and then increases exponentially after 45 to 60 minutes, up to a point where only a few viable cells remain on the root surface after 60 to 90 minutes in a dry environment.[63–65]

Extraalveolar Dry Time Less Than 1 Hour or Tooth Stored in Appropriate Storage Medium

Closed Apex. The tooth should be replanted as soon as possible after the debris has been gently washed off with a stream of sterile saline.

Open Apex. Teeth with an apical foramen larger than 1.1 mm have the potential for pulpal revascularization after replantation.[66–68] The rate of revascularization has been reported to be between 18% and 40%.[68,69] The extraalveolar time, as well as bacterial contamination are additional factors which will influence the rate of revascularization.[70] If bacterial contamination is reduced by soaking the tooth in doxycycline, there is a very significant increase in complete revascularization.[70] Therefore, it is now recommended to soak a tooth with an open apex in a solution of doxycycline (1 mg in approximately 10 mL of physiological saline) for 5 minutes before replantation. Recent animal studies suggest that covering the root with minocycline (available as Arestin Microspheres, Oral Pharma, Inc., Warminster, PA, USA or Dentomycin, Henry Schein UK Holdings Ltd., Kent, UK) will further aid revascularization compared with a doxycycline soak.[71]

Extraalveolar Time More Than 1 Hour

Closed Apex. In these situations, there is a minimum amount of vital cells left on the root surface. Current recommendations include scraping off the layer of dead cells and the remnants of the periodontal ligament and then soaking the tooth in 2% sodium fluoride for 20 minutes.[2] This will not prevent root resorption, only possibly slowing it down.

Open Apex. Replantation of teeth with an open apex and extended extraalveolar dry time has the worst prognosis. It might be beneficial to perform root canal treatment before replanting such a tooth as a result of difficulty in hermetically obturating the apical portion of the root canal via a traditional, orthograde access.

Splinting of Avulsed and Luxated Teeth. One of the keys to success in treatment of most luxation and avulsion injuries is the use of an appropriate splint and a suitable duration of splinting (Table 12-2). It has been shown that a rigid splint placed after tooth avulsion was significantly associated with ankylosis.[72] Through the years, various splints have been recommended; however, the type of splint is not as critical as long as it allows some physiological movement of the injured tooth/teeth.[43,73] The splint has to be placed such that the patient can easily maintain good oral hygiene, especially around the injured tooth/teeth.

TABLE 12-2 **Recommended Splinting Time for Different Types of Dental Trauma**[1,2]	
Type of Injury	**Splinting Time**
Subluxation	2 weeks (if splint was needed)
Extrusive luxation	2 weeks
Lateral luxation	2 weeks
Intrusion	4 weeks
Root fracture (middle or apical 1/3)	4 weeks
Root fracture (cervical 1/3)	Up to 4 months
Alveolar fracture	4 weeks
Avulsion (<60 min extraoral drying time)	2 weeks
Avulsion (>60 min extraoral drying time)	4 weeks

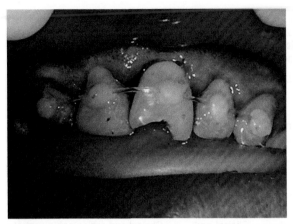

FIGURE 12-8 After repositioning of traumatized teeth, it is advisable to ask the patient to bite into rolled and softened wax so that the displaced teeth remain stable and in an optimum position while the splint is applied. In this case, the maxillary right central incisor was avulsed and the left central incisor was severely laterally luxated; a 30-lb fishing line and composite were used for splinting.

Any soft wire or monofilament line (e.g. fishing line 20–30 lbs/9–14 kg, 0.4–0.5 mm diameter) can be attached with composite on the facial surface of the tooth, and it is recommended to extend, if at all possible, the splint to two adjacent teeth on either side. While the splint is being applied, it is advisable to have the patient bite into softened pink wax that has been double or triple rolled to ensure that the tooth/teeth are in optimal position (Figure 12-8). Once the splint has been placed, a radiograph should be taken to confirm proper repositioning, and the occlusion may need to be adjusted as well. Splinting times for each type of injury are shown in Table 12-2.

Endodontic Treatment Considerations at the Emergency Visit. Root canal treatment of luxated teeth should not be initiated at the emergency visit. It is not recommended either to initiate root canal treatment of avulsed teeth at the time of injury except maybe in cases of open apices with extended drying time (>60 min). This is because every effort should be made to minimize the duration of the extraoral time. Additionally, it has been shown that placing calcium hydroxide too early into the root canal system might be detrimental to the healing processes of the periodontal ligament.[74]

Systemic Treatment

Antibiotics. The prescription of systemic penicillin, if the patient is not allergic to it, after the replantation of an avulsed tooth has been recommended for the last 20 years.[75] IADT now recommends the prescribing of doxycycline at the appropriate dosage for age and weight, twice a day for 1 week after replantation for anyone older than 12 years of age. For younger patients, the appropriate dosage of phenoxymethyl-penicillin (Penicillin V) is still recommended,[2] if the patient is not allergic to it. Special precautions should be taken not to prescribe tetracycline-based antibiotics to women who are pregnant or nursing because of the risks of birth defects, teeth discolouration and delayed bone growth. Systemic antibiotics are not particularly recommended by IADT for luxations or other traumatic injuries.

Analgesics. In most cases of dental trauma, non-prescription strength, over-the-counter, nonsteroidal antiinflammatory drugs such as ibuprofen are sufficient.

Instructions to the Patient. The need for good oral hygiene should be emphasized to the patient. However, pain from the splint and fear of causing additional harm may make the patient reluctant or even unable to brush and floss the affected area efficiently. Thus, mouth rinsing with chlorhexidine is recommended twice a day for at least 1 week or for as long as the splint is in place. Tetanus prophylaxis should be checked and administered, or a booster recommended if necessary.

Prognosis Assessment at the Emergency Visit. The patient and/or parents must be warned about the likely prognosis of the injured teeth and the need for follow-up appointments (see Tables 12-3 and 12-4, later in this chapter). The patient should be aware that even if the crown of the tooth appears normal and in its correct alignment, the root is the important structure in determining tooth survival. The discussion should be candid and honest, based on the knowledge of the accident's circumstances, extraoral time and all other factors; the patient should be informed of the likelihood of tooth survival, and care must be taken not to be overly optimistic.

Review at 7 to 10 Days Post Replantation of the Avulsed Tooth. All avulsed and luxated teeth need to

TABLE 12-3	Recommended Follow-Up Regimen after Tooth Fractures				
Posttrauma Period	Uncomplicated Crown Fracture	Complicated Crown Fracture	Uncomplicated Crown–Root Fracture	Complicated Crown–Root Fracture	Root Fracture
4 weeks					Splint removal* Clinical and radiographic control
6–8 weeks	Clinical and radiographic control	Clinical and radiographic control	Clinical and radiographic control	Clinical and radiographic control	Clinical and radiographic control
4 months					Splint removal** Clinical and radiographic control
6 months					Clinical and radiographic control
1 year	Clinical and radiographic control	Clinical and radiographic control	Clinical and radiographic control	Clinical and radiographic control	Clinical and radiographic control
Yearly for 5 years					Clinical and radiographic control

*Splint removal in case of apical third and midroot fractures.
**Splint for root fracture near the cervical area recommended for up to 4 months.

be reevaluated 7 to 10 days after trauma. The splint is only removed at the end of this follow-up visit. In most instances, endodontic treatment should be initiated if the tooth has a closed apex.

The pulp of open apex teeth has the potential to revascularize. Therefore, these teeth should not be endodontically treated at this point, unless there are already signs of infection, or if the extraoral time was more than 1 hour.

Posttrauma Complications

ROOT CANAL OBLITERATION

Root canal obliteration is quite a common occurrence after most types of dental injuries and is considered a favourable mode of healing.[76,77] Endodontic treatment is not recommended electively when root canal obliteration is noticed on a radiograph and should only be performed if pain, or a radiolucency develops (see Figure 12-5). However, root canal obliteration can cause colour changes in the clinical crown.

PULPAL NECROSIS

There are two main consequences of pulpal necrosis: (1) cessation of root development and (2) bacterial

contamination of the pulpal space. The bacterial contamination will become the driving force behind root resorption and destruction of the surrounding bone if not prevented, or addressed, in a timely fashion.

EXTERNAL ROOT RESORPTION

Under normal circumstances, permanent teeth do not resorb; this appears to result from the antiresorptive properties of the precementum on the external surface of the root and of the predentine on the internal surface of the root.[78] If these layers are scraped off or severely damaged during the dental injury, the underlying dentine becomes exposed and at risk of being resorbed[79] as one of the consequences of damage to the periodontium.

Surface Root Resorption

Surface root resorption probably occurs after all luxation injuries.[80,81] It is the most benign form of all resorptions, and it is self-limiting. As it is difficult to visualize the resorption radiographically, where it appears as localized rough areas on the root surface, it is frequently undiagnosed.

If the pulp is vital there is no need for endodontic treatment. If the pulp is necrotic or if its vitality is

TABLE 12-4 Recommended Follow-Up Regimen after Luxation and Avulsion

Time	Concussion	Subluxation	Extrusion	Lateral Luxation	Intrusion	Avulsion	Alveolar Fracture
7–10 days						Initiate root canal treatment for teeth with closed apex	
2 weeks		Splint removal (if applied for subluxation) Clinical and radiographic control	Splint removal Clinical and radiographic control	Splint removal Clinical and radiographic control	Splint removal Clinical and radiographic control	Splint removal* Clinical and radiographic control	
4 weeks	Clinical and radiographic control	Clinical and radiographic control	Clinical and radiographic control	Clinical and radiographic control	Clinical and radiographic control	Splint removal** Clinical and radiographic control	Splint removal Clinical and radiographic control
6–8 weeks	Clinical and radiographic control	Clinical and radiographic control	Clinical and radiographic control	Clinical and radiographic control	Clinical and radiographic control	Clinical and radiographic control	Clinical and radiographic control
6 months	Clinical and radiographic control	Clinical and radiographic control	Clinical and radiographic control	Clinical and radiographic control	Clinical and radiographic control	Clinical and radiographic control	Clinical and radiographic control
1 year	Clinical and radiographic control	Clinical and radiographic control	Clinical and radiographic control	Clinical and radiographic control	Clinical and radiographic control	Clinical and radiographic control	Clinical and radiographic control
Yearly for 5 years			Clinical and radiographic control	Clinical and radiographic control	Clinical and radiographic control	Clinical and radiographic control	Clinical and radiographic control

*For teeth that had <60 minutes extraoral dry time.
**For teeth that had >60 minutes extraoral dry time.

questionable, then those root surface irregularities are likely to be related to the onset of inflammatory root resorption and immediate endodontic treatment is required.

Replacement Root Resorption

Replacement root resorption or ankylosis occurs when there has been very significant damage to the periodontal ligament, cementum and precementum after injuries, such as avulsions and severe types of luxations. Osteoclasts, followed by osteoblasts, come into direct contact with dentine, and it is gradually replaced with normal bone.

Radiographically, the root starts to fade away, and no clear periodontal ligament space is seen. In advanced stages the root disappears (Figure 12-9). Replacement root resorption can be seen as early as 2 weeks after trauma, but in most cases it may be noticed within 2 years. Replacement root resorption has also been reported to occur up to 10 years

posttrauma.[64,82] The high-pitched metallic percussion sound elicited is often the earliest diagnostic sign of ankylosis before any resorptive changes are detected radiographically.[83,84]

Currently, there is no treatment for replacement root resorption.[85] Involved teeth pose a problem for growing children because fusion of the root to the bone render them immobile and does not allow them to advance with the neighbouring teeth as the alveolus grows; thus, they become infrapositioned. Decoronation and intentional replantation have been suggested as temporary measures to maintain the alveolar ridge, but these measures do not save the tooth itself (Figure 12-10).[86]

In the decoronation technique the crown of the tooth is removed, and the gingiva is covered over the remaining root, allowing it to be gradually replaced by bone.[40,41,87] This procedure will allow alveolar bone to continue its vertical growth and preserve some of the alveolar thickness, facilitating the placement of an

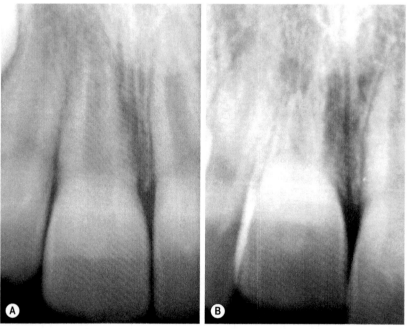

FIGURE 12-9 Example of replacement root resorption (ankylosis) where the periodontal ligament and root structure is replaced with bone so that over time all the root structure is lost. (A) Four-month recall radiograph of the maxillary right central incisor after avulsion and replantation. Some signs of ankylosis can be seen radiographically, and the tooth exhibits a high-pitched metallic sound to percussion. (B) 18-month recall radiograph showing progression of ankylosis. The tooth and the bone are fused without any detectable periodontal ligament space in between. In addition, the tooth is becoming infrapositioned.

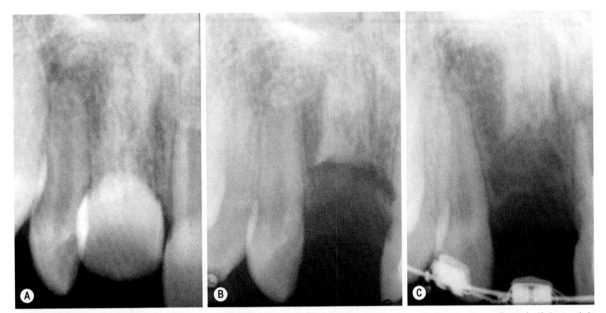

FIGURE 12-10 Decoronation of an ankylosed and infrapositioned maxillary right central incisor. (A) Preoperative radiograph. If the tooth is not extracted or treated, in a growing child, it will lead to a serious defect of the alveolar ridge. (B) Postoperative radiograph immediately after the tooth was decoronated slightly below the crestal bone level in an attempt to allow alveolar growth and to maintain the alveolar ridge; the root is left *in situ*. (C) Review radiograph 2 years later. Over time the ankylosed root will continue to resorb; however, the bone volume is better maintained than if extraction was performed. The decoronation procedure allowed continuation of vertical alveolar bone growth, and bone formation incisal to the root remnant is evident; orthodontic treatment is in progress.

implant after the growth spurt and, ideally, as late as possible in life.

Inflammatory Root Resorption

Inflammatory root resorption occurs when there is serious damage to the precementum, cementum and to the periodontal ligament (Figure 12-11). This will allow osteo/odontoclastic direct contact with the dentine surface.[80] This clastic activity is further enhanced and maintained as a result of pulp necrosis and infection in the root canal space.[88] When the protective cementum layer is lost, bacteria and bacterial elements such as endotoxins have a clear pathway, through the dentinal tubules, to reach the root surface, thereby stimulating a rapid inflammatory response. In children aged 6 to 10 years, this type of root resorption is usually aggressive because the dentinal tubules of incisor teeth are larger, and the distance from the pulp canal to the root surface is shorter.[57,89]

Radiographically, inflammatory root resorption can be seen as early as 2 weeks after the injury,

especially in young teeth.[57,90] It may appear, initially, as if the periodontal ligament space is wider and irregular on both the alveolar bone and on the root side. Subsequently, distinctive radiolucent lesions will form on the root surface and in the adjacent bone.

The clinician should be alert for these signs as it may be possible to treat, or reduce inflammatory root resorption if it is diagnosed early. The key to successful treatment is to completely disinfect the root canal space. Calcium hydroxide intracanal medication has been shown to be beneficial in the treatment of inflammatory root resorption.[2,91,92] Once the root canal space is disinfected, the periodontal ligament width may return to normal and follow the new contours of the root surface (see Figure 12-11).

Cervical Root Resorption

In essence, cervical root resorption is a subclassification of inflammatory root resorption, appearing immediately below the epithelial attachment of the

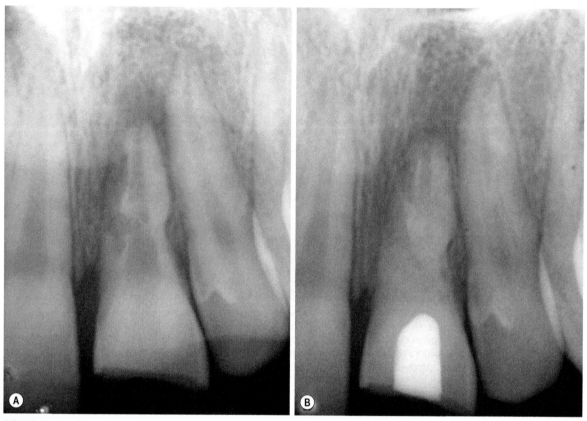

FIGURE 12-11 Inflammatory root resorption. (A) Diagnostic radiograph 4 months after trauma. Damage to certain areas of the periodontal ligament has resulted in resorption lesions appearing as radiolucent areas both on the root and in the adjacent bone. This type of resorption is related to infection within the root canal system. Treatment consists of endodontic treatment with long-term calcium hydroxide dressing in the root canal space. (B) Review radiograph 5 months after commencement of endodontic treatment. The lost root structure will not reappear; however, the radiolucent areas have disappeared, and a normal periodontal ligament width is becoming reestablished.

tooth (Figure 12-12). It seems to be a delayed reaction to some kind of a trauma close to the cemento-enamel junction, or close to wherever the epithelial attachment terminates.[93] The exact pathogenesis is unknown, but histologically it resembles inflammatory root resorption. The aetiology does not seem related to the status of the pulpal space, as cervical root resorption occurs equally in vital and in nonvital teeth.

Radiographic evaluation reveals a radiolucent area in the cervical area of the tooth adjacent to the crestal bone. The lesion usually develops confined within dentine, without perforating the protective layers of precementum and predentine. CBCT is a valuable method of assessing the extension of the resorption and determining the best treatment approach.

Treatment of cervical root resorption can be complex. If the pulp is necrotic and infected, endodontic treatment should be performed. However, if the pulp is vital, endodontic treatment will not arrest the progression of the lesion.[78,94] Periodontal surgery may be attempted; the entire lesion then needs to be exposed, all resorptive tissue removed and the defect restored with, for example, composite resin (e.g. Geristore, Den-Mat, Santa Maria, CA, USA). In these situations there is, obviously, a risk that the tooth may end up with an untreatable periodontal pocket. Sometimes, extraction of the tooth may be the only treatment option.

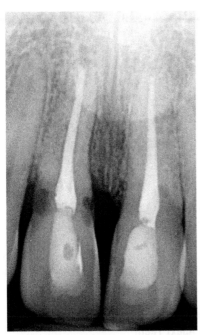

FIGURE 12-12 Cervical root resorption is usually a late complication of dental trauma. The maxillary central incisors were severely luxated, endodontic treatment was started and calcium hydroxide was placed in the root canals 10 days posttrauma and left for 6 weeks. At review 4 years posttrauma, cervical root resorption in the maxillary right central incisor is evident just below the level of the epithelial attachment.

INTERNAL ROOT RESORPTION

Internal resorption is a rare complication of dental trauma. The pulp chamber and/or the canal become gradually enlarged by giant cells action at the dentinal surface. A zone of necrotic pulp tissue is usually found coronal to the resorbing tissue.[95] Due to the resorptive tissue being supplied by blood vessels coming through the apex, endodontic treatment will arrest the progression of the resorption, and should, therefore, be instituted as soon as possible after diagnosis. Endodontic treatment can become quite complicated because of the resorption defect.

Some external root resorptions can easily be misdiagnosed as internal. Taking supplementary mesial and distal eccentric radiographs is helpful to making a differential diagnosis. In external resorptions the resorptive area will appear less radiolucent than the root canal, which remains distinguishable; CBCT investigation can also be useful.[95]

Posttrauma Follow-Ups

FREQUENCY OF CALLS

All traumatized teeth should be carefully reevaluated periodically after the injury, irrespective of its apparent severity. Tables 12-3 and 12-4 show the IADT's recommendations for a recall schedule after each type of injury.[1,2]

ENDODONTIC EVALUATION AND MANAGEMENT OF INJURED TEETH

Pulp Status Evaluation and Diagnosis

It is important to remember that a tooth can sustain multiple injuries at the same time and this may affect the outcome. For example, a luxation injury can occur in combination with an uncomplicated crown fracture.[48,49,96,97]

After emergency treatment, it is essential to monitor the tooth closely to ensure that the pulp has survived (see Tables 12-3 and 12-4). If published guidelines are followed, more favourable outcomes can be expected compared with cases treated without complying with the guidelines.[98] At every review appointment, radiographs need to be taken. Also, there is a need to look out for clinical signs and symptoms associated with pulp necrosis. The pulp may remain unresponsive to sensibility testing for several months; however, if no other signs are evident it is advisable not to intervene but, rather, schedule further recalls, especially if the patient's tooth is immature. Additional signs to look for are colour changes of the crown, alteration to the width of the periodontal ligament, appearance of a periapical lesion and other signs of infection such as the presence of a fistula, tissue swelling and/or pain.[46,76,99–101] If in doubt about the status of the pulp, a timely referral to a specialist is strongly recommended because root resorption associated with necrotic and infected pulp space can result in rapid and irreversible loss of root structure in a matter of weeks.

Keeping the Pulp Alive and Favouring Spontaneous Pulp Space Revascularization

As mentioned previously in this chapter, one of the main goals of posttraumatic management is the maintenance of pulp space vitality. For instance, if proper emergency treatment is provided to a crown-fractured immature tooth, the pulp has a high chance of remaining vital because of the larger vascular supply and larger apical opening; pulpal survival, or spontaneous pulp space revascularization is a possibility subsequent to severe luxation injuries,[68,102] and this is a desirable mode of healing. However, while waiting for revascularization, the tooth has to be monitored closely, against the risk of pulp necrosis, infection and root resorption, which can severely compromise the tooth.

Endodontic Treatment of Necrotic Teeth

Signs and symptoms of pulp necrosis and infection include: pain, swelling or discomfort, fistula, excessive mobility, sensitivity to palpation and percussion, periapical radiolucency, colour changes, persistent unresponsiveness to sensibility testing, or failure of root development. Once the pulp has been diagnosed with certainty as being necrotic, endodontic treatment should be instituted as soon as possible. The endodontic approach will be dictated by the stage of root development, type of injury and time elapsed since the traumatic episode. Treatment often involves an apexification procedure (see later).

Endodontic Treatment of Necrotic Mature (Closed Apex) Teeth

In decreasing order, the most severe injury to the periodontal ligament and pulp are intrusion and avulsion, lateral luxation, extrusion, subluxation and concussion. When there is little or no chance of pulp survival in a mature tooth, endodontic treatment should be initiated between 7 to 10 days posttrauma in order to prevent the necrotic pulp from becoming infected.[1,2] Endodontic treatment should not be started at the emergency visit for two reasons. First, additional manipulation of the tooth soon after the injury could further traumatize the periodontal ligament.[2,74] Second, the application of calcium hydroxide too early can have a detrimental effect on periodontal ligament healing.[74]

Since a luxated or avulsed tooth may still exhibit some mobility 7 to 10 days after trauma, it is advisable to commence endodontic treatment while the tooth is still splinted. The splint can be removed at the end of the appointment, if so indicated.[1,2]

For all endodontic treatment, dental dam isolation should be used. It is not advisable to clamp the traumatized tooth but, rather, dental dam retention will have to rely on clamping adjacent teeth, using Wedjets (Hygienic, Coltène/Whaledent, Cuyahoga Falls, OH, USA) stabilizing cords, or dental floss.

Currently, the most widely accepted intracanal medicament is calcium hydroxide paste, either premixed, or mixed with chlorhexidine, or sterile water.[91,103–105] It has been shown that if calcium hydroxide is placed into the root canal system of a traumatized tooth before becoming infected (within about 2 weeks posttrauma) and kept in place for 2 weeks, the treatment outcome is favourable.[106] If endodontic treatment is started later and an established infection exists before the placement of calcium hydroxide, it is recommended that the calcium hydroxide remains in place for several months before the final root canal obturation; this is in order to reduce the risk of inflammatory root resorption.[107]

Endodontic Treatment of Necrotic Immature (Opened Apex) Teeth

As the pulp is needed for root development in an immature tooth, it is good clinical practice to monitor its status and consider the pulp as vital until there is clear evidence demonstrating the contrary (at least two signs and symptoms indicating pulp necrosis and infection). Only when the confirmed diagnosis is necrotic a pulp should endodontic treatment be initiated.[1,2] Several approaches exist: classical apexification, MTA apexification, or the 'revascularization' procedures.

Classical Apexification. The classical apexification procedure of a tooth with an open apex involves cleaning and repeated placement of a calcium hydroxide dressing into the root canal to stimulate the formation of a hard tissue barrier at the apical portion of the root. After this biological calcified barrier has been formed, it is possible to obturate the canal system without the risk of overextending the root filing material.[108,109]

It is a prerequisite to disinfect the canal space to create a suitable environment for stimulating apical barrier formation. Disinfection is achieved by thorough, but gentle irrigation with sodium hypochlorite solution and by placing, spinning into the root canal space, a relatively thin mixture (less than toothpaste consistency) of calcium hydroxide (powder mixed with chlorhexidine solution). It is not recommended to include barium sulphate, as a radiopacifier, in the mixture because it prevents the assessment of the thoroughness of calcium hydroxide placement. After about 3 weeks, the patient is recalled, and the thin calcium hydroxide mixture removed by gentle irrigation. At this appointment, a thicker, almost dry mixture of calcium hydroxide and sterile saline is packed, using pluggers, or inverted gutta-percha cones, to the full length of the root. A radiograph is taken to confirm that a dense filling of calcium hydroxide, all the way to the apex, is in place. A temporary restoration with reinforced zinc oxide-eugenol cement, such as intermediate restorative material (IRM; Dentsply, Milford, DE, USA), should then be placed in the access cavity.

The patient should be recalled every 3 months and the density of the mixture evaluated radiographically. Currently, it is not recommended to replace the mixture if it appears to be intact at these recall appointments.[2] The time required to achieve the apical barrier formation varies between 6 and 24 months with an average of 1 year and 7 months.[110] Once the presence of the barrier has been confirmed both radiographically and clinically, the final root canal obturation can be carried out (Figure 12-13).

MTA Apexification. In the last 20 years the use MTA as an artificial apical plug has gained popularity in order to allow root canal obturation sooner than with the classical apexification approach.[111] However, it is important to note that MTA has minimal bactericidal effect on several bacterial species.[112,113] Given that bacteria are the single most important contributory factor to maintaining inflammatory root resorption, it is strongly advised to follow a two- to three-step apexification approach when the canal space is likely to be infected. The protocol involves, at the first visit, disinfecting and medicating the root canal for 7 to 14 days with a thin calcium hydroxide paste. At the second visit, an apical barrier is created by compacting MTA into the apical area. CollaCote (Integra, Plainsboro, NJ, USA), or calcium sulphate sponges can be placed apically beforehand to act as a matrix and to help prevent extrusion of MTA. A wet cotton pellet is then placed in contact with the MTA for at least a few hours or days to promote setting. At the third visit, the rest of the canal is obturated (Figure 12-14).

It is a delicate process to place MTA correctly at the apex. An operating microscope is needed, as magnification and good lighting are essential. MTA seems to have a good biocompatibility; however, both the grey

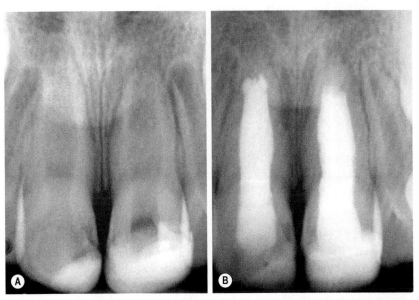

FIGURE 12-13 Classical apexification of nonvital immature maxillary central incisors. (A) Preoperative radiograph showing the very immature central incisors. (B) In this 2-year follow-up radiograph after apexification treatment with calcium hydroxide and canal obturation, the apical calcified barriers are clearly visible.

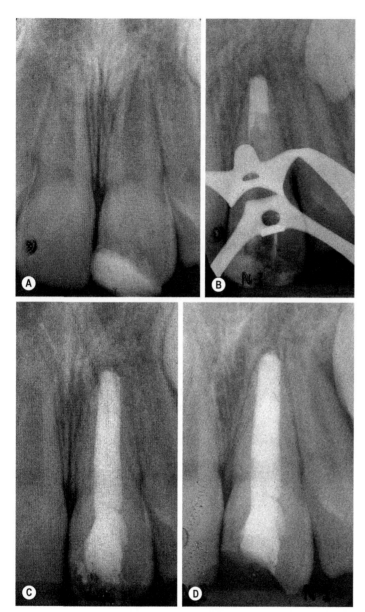

FIGURE 12-14 MTA apexification. (A) The maxillary left central incisor has become nonvital after a traumatic injury; the root canal is wider than that of the right central incisor, signifying that the tooth has been nonvital for some time. (B) The root canal has been disinfected and the apical 4 mm filled with MTA. (C) The canal was then back-filled with gutta-percha, and the neck of the tooth was filled with etched and bonded composite resin. (D) One year later, healing has taken place.

and white versions have the inconvenience of causing unaesthetic discolouration of teeth, even when used as an apexification material.

Pulp Space Revascularization of Necrotic, Infected Teeth. Until recently it was thought that there was no possibility of promoting regrowth of vital tissue into infected root canal spaces in teeth with open apices.[69,114,115] It has now been realized that, under

certain conditions, it is possible not only to heal periapical lesions associated with necrotic and immature teeth but more interestingly to also stimulate tissue growth inside the canal space of these teeth (Figure 12-15).[116,117] This is accomplished by reducing the bacterial load, first by thorough irrigation and then by intracanal placement of either a dual or triple mix of antibiotics (metronidazole, ciprofloxacin and,

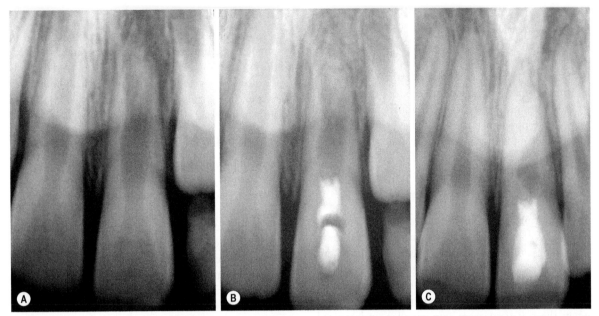

FIGURE 12-15 Pulp space revascularization treatment of an infected immature maxillary left central incisor. (A) Preoperative radiograph with a history of trauma 5 months earlier. Endodontic treatment was started, and a triple antibiotic paste was placed in the canal and left for 3 weeks. At the next session, a blood clot was induced in the root canal space, a capping material was placed over the blood clot and the access cavity was sealed with reinforced zinc-oxide eugenol cement. (B) Four-month recall radiograph; the patient was symptom-free, and there were radiographic signs of periapical healing. (C) Four-year recall radiograph; the patient remained symptom-free and, interestingly, there were signs of both apical growth and lateral thickening within the root canal space.

possibly, minocycline) or, alternatively, a calcium hydroxide dressing for a few weeks.[118–121] The key to success is to be able to disinfect the canal space and then to create a scaffolding for the in-growing tissue.[122] Presently, the scaffolding is created by allowing a blood clot to form at the second appointment, after the disinfecting paste has been washed out. Once a clot has started to organize itself, a double seal is placed in the access cavity, close to the level of the cervical area. The use of a bioceramic material is recommended to cap the blood clot, and then a conventional restoration is placed on top.[118] The success rate of this procedure, where the root end continues to grow and/or mature, has been reported to be between 27% and 55%, and the survival rate of such teeth much higher.[120,123,124] If the tooth does not respond to treatment, then the traditional apexification procedure is still an option. It is important to remember that the response of the tooth to this revascularization procedure can take months if not years to occur.[123]

Endodontic Treatment in the Prevention and Treatment of Inflammatory Root Resorption. Calcium hydroxide, as an intracanal medication, has proven to be effective in halting the progression of external inflammatory root resorption, especially if detected early (see Figure 12-11).[125,126]

Calcium hydroxide paste should be used in a thick, almost dry consistency. It should be checked and renewed every 3 months if it is washed out. Treatment should be continued until all signs of inflammatory root resorption have ceased and until a normal periodontal ligament width has been reestablished. This can take anywhere from 6 to 24 months. The access cavity of the tooth should be temporized with an appropriate restorative material such as IRM (Dentsply), as it is of upmost importance to reduce coronal microleakage and keep bacteria away of the root canal space.

Postendodontic Access Restoration of Traumatized Teeth. Nonvital immature teeth have thin roots with weak dentine walls and are especially at risk of root fracture at the neck of the tooth.[109,127] The cervical area of the tooth may be reinforced using etched and bonded composite resin, allowing space if indicated, for a post.[126,128] If little coronal tooth structure remains, a fibre post may be bonded into the root canal. Metallic posts should be avoided. Compared with metal posts, fibre posts have the advantage of some flexibility; if it fails, it is more likely to become de-cemented rather than cause a root fracture.[129]

Management of Injured Primary Teeth

When a primary tooth is injured, avoiding damage to the successional tooth is the main concern. Damage to the successional tooth may occur either mechanically at the time of injury, during treatment, or as a result of postinjury infection.[130] Young children may be uncooperative, particularly after a traumatic injury when the soft tissues are sore, swollen and bruised. Thus, immediate treatment should be kept to what is strictly necessary.

The following recommendations for primary teeth are based on the latest IADT guidelines.[3]

CROWN FRACTURES

Enamel fractures should be smoothed, whereas fractures into dentine should be covered with glass ionomer if at all possible, and in the case of large missing fragments, a composite build-up may be performed. If the pulp has been exposed and there is sufficient cooperation and tooth structure left, a partial pulpotomy using calcium hydroxide as a pulp capping agent is suitable followed by restoration; this does not need to be at the emergency visit.[3,31,131] Lack of maturity and coping ability of the child might necessitate extraction of the tooth. The technique of pulp capping is covered in the section on permanent teeth. Root canal treatment of primary teeth is covered in Chapter 11. An infected primary tooth should not be left untreated as the infection may cause damage to the underlying permanent successor.

In case of primary tooth crown–root fracture, the broken-off fragment should be removed if it only involves a small part of the root and it is possible to restore the tooth; otherwise, extraction is recommended.[3]

INTRAALVEOLAR ROOT FRACTURES

These fractures are less common in primary than in permanent teeth. Active intervention is rarely required. If the coronal fragment is very loose or if pulp necrosis and infection develops, extraction is usually indicated; however, the apical fragment is normally left *in situ* to resorb naturally.

LUXATED PRIMARY TEETH

In general, a conservative approach to management is adopted with primary teeth. Laterally luxated primary teeth will frequently reposition naturally in time by occlusal and muscular forces. If a laterally luxated tooth interferes with the occlusion, the injury is mild and there is no risk to the permanent successor, it may be carefully repositioned.[3] If the root apex is directed palatally toward the developing permanent tooth, the primary tooth should then be extracted. If a tooth is very mobile and in danger of being inhaled, or if occlusal interference is too great, it should be extracted. Intruded teeth will usually re-erupt albeit sometimes over several months. If the pulp becomes nonvital and infected, root canal treatment may be considered.

AVULSED PRIMARY TEETH

Replantation of avulsed primary teeth is not normally carried out because of the potential risk of direct physical damage to the underlying developing permanent tooth, or damage from later infection of the pulp; however, in rare and selected cases it might be successfully done.[132]

TOOTH DISCOLOURATION IN PRIMARY TEETH

Pulp damage is a frequent complication of injuries, and as a result, primary teeth may discolour. Immediate discolouration indicates bleeding in the pulp and the possibility of repair. Unless associated infection exists, root canal treatment is not indicated.[133] Later darkening of the tooth signifies pulp necrosis, and if there is associated infection, root canal treatment or extraction is indicated. Later, yellow discolouration indicates pulp canal obliteration and no intervention is required.

Learning Outcomes

After reading this chapter, the reader should be able to recognize and discuss the:

- correct diagnosis and treatment planning process in cases of trauma;
- classification of traumatic injuries;
- effects of trauma on the dental tissues;
- treatment objectives and the importance of maintaining pulpal vitality wherever possible;
- emergency management of traumatic injuries;
- likely posttrauma complications and follow-up regime;
- need for referral to a specialist in complex cases.

REFERENCES

1. DiAngelis AJ, Andreasen JO, Ebeleseder KA, et al. International Association of Dental Traumatology guidelines for the management of traumatic dental injuries: 1. Fractures and luxations of permanent teeth. Dental Traumatology 2012;28: 2–12.
2. Andersson L, Andreasen JO, Day P, et al. International Association of Dental Traumatology guidelines for the management of traumatic dental injuries: 2. Avulsion of permanent teeth. Dental Traumatology 2012;28:88–96.
3. Malmgren B, Andreasen JO, Flores MT, et al. International Association of Dental Traumatology guidelines for the management of traumatic dental injuries: 3. Injuries in the primary dentition. Dental Traumatology 2012;28:174–82.
4. Skieller V. The prognosis for young teeth loosened after mechanical injuries. Acta Odontologica Scandinavica 1960;18: 171–3.
5. Hofman PA, Nelemans P, Kemerink GJ, et al. Value of radiological diagnosis of skull fracture in the management of mild head injury: meta-analysis. Journal of Neurology, Neurosurgery, and Psychiatry 2000;68:416–22.
6. McCrory P, Meeuwisse WH, Aubry M, et al. Consensus statement on concussion in sport: the 4th International Conference on Concussion in Sport, Zurich, November 2012. Journal of Athletic Training 2013;48:554–75.
7. Thompson LA, Tavares M, Ferguson-Young D, et al. Violence and abuse: core competencies for identification and access to care. Dental Clinics of North America 2013;57: 281–99.
8. Murphy K, Waa S, Jaffer H, et al. A literature review of findings in physical elder abuse. Canadian Association of Radiologists Journal 2013;64:10–4.
9. Everett RJ, Kingsley K, Demopoulos CA, et al. Awareness and beliefs regarding intimate partner violence among first-year dental students. Journal of Dental Education 2013;77: 316–22.
10. Gopikrishna V, Tinagupta K, Kandaswamy D. Comparison of electrical, thermal, and pulse oximetry methods for assessing pulp vitality in recently traumatized teeth. Journal of Endodontics 2007;33:531–5.
11. Gazelius B, Olgart L, Edwall B. Restored vitality in luxated teeth assessed by laser Doppler flowmeter. Endodontics and Dental Traumatology 1988;4:265–8.
12. Lee JY, Yanpiset K, Sigurdsson A, et al. Laser Doppler flowmetry for monitoring traumatized teeth. Dental Traumatology 2001;17:231–5.
13. Venskutonis T, Plotino G, Juodzbalys G, et al. The importance of cone-beam computed tomography in the management of endodontic problems: a review of the literature. Journal of Endodontics 2014;40:1895–901.
14. May JJ, Cohenca N, Peters OA. Contemporary management of horizontal root fractures to the permanent dentition: diagnosis—radiologic assessment to include cone-beam computed tomography. Journal of Endodontics 2013;39:S20–5.
15. Pauwels R, Cockmartin L, Ivanauskaite D, et al. Estimating cancer risk from dental cone-beam CT exposures based on skin dosimetry. Physics in Medicine and Biology 2014; 59:3877–91.
16. Andreasen FM, Andreasen JO. Diagnosis of luxation injuries: the importance of standardized clinical, radiographic and photographic techniques in clinical investigations. Endodontics and Dental Traumatology 1985;1:160–9.
17. Lauridsen E, Hermann NV, Gerds TA, et al. Pattern of traumatic dental injuries in the permanent dentition among children, adolescents, and adults. Dental Traumatology 2012; 28:358–63.
18. Cvek M. Prognosis of luxated non-vital maxillary incisors treated with calcium hydroxide and filled with gutta-percha. A retrospective clinical study. Endodontics and Dental Traumatology 1992;8:45–55.
19. Stalhane I, Hedegard B. Traumatized permanent teeth in children aged 7-15 years. Svensk Tandlakare Tidskrift 1975;68: 157–69.
20. Ravn JJ. Follow-up study of permanent incisors with enamel-dentin fractures after acute trauma. Scandinavian Journal of Dental Research 1981;89:355–65.
21. Ravn JJ. Follow-up study of permanent incisors with enamel fractures as a result of an acute trauma. Scandinavian Journal of Dental Research 1981;89:213–7.
22. About I, Murray PE, Franquin JC, et al. The effect of cavity restoration variables on odontoblast cell numbers and dental repair. Journal of Dentistry 2001;29:109–17.
23. Murray PE, About I, Lumley PJ, et al. Odontoblast morphology and dental repair. Journal of Dentistry 2003;31:75–82.
24. Hebling J, Giro EM, Costa CA. Human pulp response after an adhesive system application in deep cavities. Journal of Dentistry 1999;27:557–64.
25. De Santis R, Prisco D, Nazhat SN, et al. Mechanical strength of tooth fragment reattachment. Journal of Biomedical Materials Research 2001;55:629–36.
26. Stellini E, Stomaci D, Zuccon A, et al. Tooth fragment reattachment through the use of a nano-filled composite resin. European Journal of Paediatric Dentistry 2010;11:77–81.
27. Capp CI, Roda MI, Tamaki R, et al. Reattachment of rehydrated dental fragment using two techniques. Dental Traumatology 2009;25:95–9.
28. Robertson A, Andreasen FM, Andreasen JO, et al. Long-term prognosis of crown-fractured permanent incisors. The effect of stage of root development and associated luxation injury. International Journal of Paediatric Dentistry 2000;10:191–9.
29. Cvek M. A clinical report on partial pulpotomy and capping with calcium hydroxide in permanent incisors with complicated crown fracture. Journal of Endodontics 1978;4:232–7.
30. Heide S, Mjor IA. Pulp reactions to experimental exposures in young permanent monkey teeth. International Endodontic Journal 1983;16:11–9.
31. Heide S, Kerekes K. Delayed direct pulp capping in permanent incisors of monkeys. International Endodontic Journal 1987;20:65–74.
32. Fuks AB, Cosack A, Klein H, et al. Partial pulpotomy as a treatment alternative for exposed pulps in crown-fractured

permanent incisors. Endodontics and Dental Traumatology 1987;3:100–2.

33. Nair PN, Cuncan HF, Pitt-Ford TR, et al. Histological, ultrastructural and quantitative investigations on the response of healthy human pulps to experimental capping with mineral trioxide aggregate: a randomized controlled trial. International Endodontic Journal 2008;41:128–50.

34. Cvek M, Lundberg M. Histological appearance of pulps after exposure by a crown fracture, partial pulpotomy, and clinical diagnosis of healing. Journal of Endodontics 1983;9: 8–11.

35. Granath LE, Hagman G. Experimental pulpotomy in human bicuspids with reference to cutting technique. Acta Odontologica Scandinavica 1971;29:155–63.

36. Ford TR, Torabinejad M, Abedi HR, et al. Using mineral trioxide aggregate as a pulp-capping material. Journal of the American Dental Association (1939) 1996;127:1491–4.

37. Farsi N, Alamoudi N, Balto K, et al. Clinical assessment of mineral trioxide aggregate (MTA) as direct pulp capping in young permanent teeth. The Journal of Clinical Pediatric Dentistry 2006;31:72–6.

38. Belobrov I, Parashos P. Treatment of tooth discoloration after the use of white mineral trioxide aggregate. Journal of Endodontics 2011;37:1017–20.

39. Felman D, Parashos P. Coronal tooth discoloration and white mineral trioxide aggregate. Journal of Endodontics 2013; 39:484–7.

40. Sigurdsson A. Decoronation as an approach to treat ankylosis in growing children. Pediatric Dentistry 2009;31:123–8.

41. Malmgren B. Ridge preservation/decoronation. Journal of Endodontics 2013;39:S67–72.

42. Zachrisson BU, Jacobsen I. Long-term prognosis of 66 permanent anterior teeth with root fracture. Scandinavian Journal of Dental Research 1975;83:345–54.

43. Andreasen JO, Andreasen FM, Mejare I, et al. Healing of 400 intra-alveolar root fractures. 2. Effect of treatment factors such as treatment delay, repositioning, splinting type and period and antibiotics. Dental Traumatology 2004;20:203–11.

44. Cvek M, Tsilingaridis G, Andreasen JO. Survival of 534 incisors after intra-alveolar root fracture in patients aged 7-17 years. Dental Traumatology 2008;24:379–87.

45. Jacobsen I, Kerekes K. Diagnosis and treatment of pulp necrosis in permanent anterior teeth with root fracture. Scandinavian Journal of Dental Research 1980;88:370–6.

46. Andreasen FM. Pulpal healing after luxation injuries and root fracture in the permanent dentition. Endodontics and Dental Traumatology 1989;5:111–31.

47. Andreasen JO, Ahrensburg SS, Tsilingaridis G. Root fractures: the influence of type of healing and location of fracture on tooth survival rates - an analysis of 492 cases. Dental Traumatology 2012;28:404–9.

48. Lauridsen E, Hermann NV, Gerds TA, et al. Combination injuries 2. The risk of pulp necrosis in permanent teeth with subluxation injuries and concomitant crown fractures. Dental Traumatology 2012;28:371–8.

49. Lauridsen E, Hermann NV, Gerds TA, et al. Combination injuries 3. The risk of pulp necrosis in permanent teeth with extrusion or lateral luxation and concomitant crown fractures without pulp exposure. Dental Traumatology 2012;28: 379–85.

50. Viduskalne I, Care R. Analysis of the crown fractures and factors affecting pulp survival due to dental trauma. Stomatologija 2010;12:109–15.

51. Andreasen FM, Pedersen BV. Prognosis of luxated permanent teeth—the development of pulp necrosis. Endodontics and Dental Traumatology 1985;1:207–20.

52. Andreasen JO, Bakland LK, Andreasen FM. Traumatic intrusion of permanent teeth. Part 2. A clinical study of the effect of preinjury and injury factors, such as sex, age, stage of root development, tooth location, and extent of injury including number of intruded teeth on 140 intruded permanent teeth. Dental Traumatology 2006;22:90–8.

53. Andreasen JO, Bakland LK, Andreasen FM. Traumatic intrusion of permanent teeth. Part 3. A clinical study of the effect of treatment variables such as treatment delay, method of repositioning, type of splint, length of splinting and antibiotics on 140 teeth. Dental Traumatology 2006;22: 99–111.

54. Andreasen JO, Bakland LK, Matras RC, et al. Traumatic intrusion of permanent teeth. Part 1. An epidemiological study of 216 intruded permanent teeth. Dental Traumatology 2006; 22:83–9.

55. Tsilingaridis G, Malmgren B, Andreasen JO, et al. Intrusive luxation of 60 permanent incisors: a retrospective study of treatment and outcome. Dental Traumatology 2012;28: 416–22.

56. Alkhalifa JD, Alazemi AA. Intrusive luxation of permanent teeth: a systematic review of factors important for treatment decision-making. Dental Traumatology 2014;30:169–75.

57. Andreasen JO, Hjorting-Hansen E. Replantation of teeth. I. Radiographic and clinical study of 110 human teeth replanted after accidental loss. Acta Odontologica Scandinavica 1966; 24:263–86.

58. Andreasen JO, Hjorting-Hansen E. Replantation of teeth. II. Histological study of 22 replanted anterior teeth in humans. Acta Odontologica Scandinavica 1996;24:287–306.

59. Hiltz J, Trope M. Vitality of human lip fibroblasts in milk, Hanks balanced salt solution and Viaspan storage media. Endodontics and Dental Traumatology 1991;7:69–72.

60. Blomlof L, Otterskog P, Hammarstrom L. Effect of storage in media with different ion strengths and osmolalities on human periodontal ligament cells. Scandinavian Journal of Dental Research 1981;89:180–7.

61. Blomlof L. Milk and saliva as possible storage media for traumatically exarticulated teeth prior to replantation. Swedish Dental Journal (Supplement) 1981;8:1–26.

62. Andreasen JO. The effect of removal of the coagulum in the alveolus before replantation upon periodontal and pulpal healing of mature permanent incisors in monkeys. International Journal of Oral Surgery 1980;9:458–61.

63. Andreasen JO. Analysis of pathogenesis and topography of replacement root resorption (ankylosis) after replantation of mature permanent incisors in monkeys. Swedish Dental Journal 1980;4:231–40.

64. Andreasen JO. A time-related study of periodontal healing and root resorption activity after replantation of mature permanent incisors in monkeys. Swedish Dental Journal 1980;4: 101–10.

65. Andreasen JO. Effect of extra-alveolar period and storage media upon periodontal and pulpal healing after replantation of mature permanent incisors in monkeys. International Journal of Oral Surgery 1981;10:43–53.

66. Kling M, Cvek M, Mejare I. Rate and predictability of pulp revascularization in therapeutically reimplanted permanent incisors. Endodontics and Dental Traumatology 1986;2: 83–9.

67. Skoglund A, Tronstad L. Pulpal changes in replanted and autotransplanted immature teeth of dogs. Journal of Endodontics 1981;7:309–16.

68. Cvek M, Cleaton-Jones P, Austin J, et al. Pulp revascularization in reimplanted immature monkey incisors—predictability and the effect of antibiotic systemic prophylaxis. Endodontics and Dental Traumatology 1990;6:157–69.

69. Ohman A. Healing and sensitivity to pain in young replanted human teeth. an experimental, clinical and histological study. Odontologisk Tidskrift 1965;73:166–227.

70. Cvek M, Cleaton-Jones P, Austin J, et al. Effect of topical application of doxycycline on pulp revascularization and periodontal healing in reimplanted monkey incisors. Endodontics and Dental Traumatology 1990;6:170–6.

71. Ritter AL, Ritter AV, Murrah V, et al. Pulp revascularization of replanted immature dog teeth after treatment with minocycline and doxycycline assessed by laser Doppler flowmetry, radiography, and histology. Dental Traumatology 2004;20:75–84.

72. Andreasen JO. Periodontal healing after replantation of traumatically avulsed human teeth. Acta Odontologica Scandinavica 1975;33:325–35.

73. Kahler B, Heithersay GS. An evidence-based appraisal of splinting luxated, avulsed and root-fractured teeth. Dental Traumatology 2008;24:2–10.

74. Lengheden A, Blomlof L, Lindskog S. Effect of immediate calcium hydroxide treatment and permanent root-filling on periodontal healing in contaminated replanted teeth. Scandinavian Journal of Dental Research 1991;99:139–46.

75. Hammarstrom L, Blomlof L, Feiglin B, et al. Replantation of teeth and antibiotic treatment. Endodontics and Dental Traumatology 1986;2:51–7.

76. Andreasen FM, Zhijie Y, Thomsen BL, et al. Occurrence of pulp canal obliteration after luxation injuries in the permanent dentition. Endodontics and Dental Traumatology 1987;3:103–15.

77. Jacobsen I. Sangnes G. Traumatized primary anterior teeth. Prognosis related to calcific reactions in the pulp cavity. Acta Odontologica Scandinavica 1978;36:199–204.

78. Trope M. Root resorption of dental and traumatic origin: classification based on etiology. Practical Periodontics and Aesthetic Dentistry 1998;10:515–22.

79. Mandel U, Viidik A. Effect of splinting on the mechanical and histological properties of the healing periodontal ligament in the vervet monkey (*Cercopithecus aethiops*). Archives of Oral Biology 1989;34:209–17.

80. Andreasen JO, Reinholdt J, Riis I, et al. Periodontal and pulpal healing of monkey incisors preserved in tissue culture before replantation. International Journal of Oral Surgery 1978;7:104–12.

81. Hammarstrom L, Lindskog S. General morphological aspects of resorption of teeth and alveolar bone. International Endodontic Journal 1985;18:93–108.

82. Andreasen JO, Borum MK, Jacobsen HL, et al. Replantation of 400 avulsed permanent incisors. 4. Factors related to periodontal ligament healing. Endodontics and Dental Traumatology 1995;11:76–89.

83. Andersson L, Blomlof L, Lindskog S, et al. Tooth ankylosis. Clinical, radiographic and histological assessments. International Journal of Oral Surgery 1984;13:423–31.

84. Campbell KM, Casas MJ, Kenny DJ, et al. Diagnosis of ankylosis in permanent incisors by expert ratings, Periotest and digital sound wave analysis. Dental Traumatology 2005;21:206–12.

85. De Souza RF, Travess H, Newton T, et al. Interventions for treating traumatised ankylosed permanent front teeth. Cochrane Database of Systematic Reviews 2015;(12):CD007820.

86. Malmgren B, Cvek M, Lundberg M, et al. Surgical treatment of ankylosed and infrapositioned reimplanted incisors in adolescents. Scandinavian Journal of Dental Research 1984;92:391–9.

87. Malmgren B. Decoronation: how, why, and when? Journal of the California Dental Association 2000;28:846–54.

88. Andreasen JO, Kristerson L. Evaluation of different types of autotransplanted connective tissues as potential periodontal ligament substitutes. An experimental replantation study in monkeys. International Journal of Oral Surgery 1981;10:189–201.

89. Andreasen JO. Relationship between surface and inflammatory resorption and changes in the pulp after replantation of permanent incisors in monkeys. Journal of Endodontics 1981;7:294–301.

90. Andreasen JO. Analysis of topography of surface and inflammatory root resorption after replantation of mature permanent incisors in monkeys. Swedish Dental Journal 1980;4:135–44.

91. Cvek M. Treatment of non-vital permanent incisors with calcium hydroxide. II. Effect on external root resorption in luxated teeth compared with effect of root filling with gutta-pucha. A follow-up. Odontologisk Revy 1973;24:343–54.

92. Forghani M, Mashhoor H, Rouhani A, et al. Comparison of pH changes induced by calcium enriched mixture and those of calcium hydroxide in simulated root resorption defects. Journal of Endodontics 2014;40:2070–3.

93. Trope M. Cervical root resorption. Journal of the American Dental Association (1939) 1997;128:56S–59S.

94. Heithersay GS. Invasive cervical resorption following trauma. Australian Endodontic Journal 1999;25:79–85.

95. Patel S, Ricucci D, Durak C, et al. Internal root resorption: a review. Journal of Endodontics 2010;36:1107–21.

96. Wang C, Qin M, Guan Y. Analysis of pulp prognosis in 603 permanent teeth with uncomplicated crown fracture with or without luxation. Dental Traumatology 2014.

97. Lauridsen E, Hermann NV, Gerds TA, et al. Combination injuries 1. The risk of pulp necrosis in permanent teeth with concussion injuries and concomitant crown fractures. Dental Traumatology 2012;28:364–70.

98. Bucher K, Neumann C, Thiering E, et al. Complications and survival rates of teeth after dental trauma over a 5-year period. Clinical Oral Investigations 2013;17:1311–8.

99. Andreasen FM. Transient root resorption after dental trauma: the clinician's dilemma. Journal of Esthetic and Restorative Dentistry 2003;15:80–92.

100. Hermann NV, Lauridsen E, Ahrensburg SS, et al. Periodontal healing complications following concussion and subluxation injuries in the permanent dentition: a longitudinal cohort study. Dental Traumatology 2012;28:386–93.

101. Hermann NV, Lauridsen E, Ahrensburg SS, et al. Periodontal healing complications following extrusive and lateral luxation in the permanent dentition: a longitudinal cohort study. Dental Traumatology 2012;28:394–402.

102. Andreasen JO. Etiology and pathogenesis of traumatic dental injuries. A clinical study of 1,298 cases. Scandinavian Journal of Dental Research 1970;78:329–42.

103. Bystrom A, Claesson R, Sundqvist G. The antibacterial effect of camphorated paramonochlorophenol, camphorated phenol and calcium hydroxide in the treatment of infected root canals. Endodontics and Dental Traumatology 1985;1: 170–5.

104. Haapasalo HK, Siren EK, Waltimo TM, et al. Inactivation of local root canal medicaments by dentine: an in vitro study. International Endodontic Journal 2000;33:126–31.

105. Sjogren U, Figdor D, Spangberg L, et al. The antimicrobial effect of calcium hydroxide as a short-term intracanal dressing. International Endodontic Journal 1991;24:119–25.

106. Trope M, Yesilsoy C, Koren L. Effect of different endodontic treatment protocols on periodontal repair and root resorption of replanted dog teeth. Journal of Endodontics 1992;18: 492–6.

107. Trope M, Moshonov J, Nissan R, et al. Short vs. long-term calcium hydroxide treatment of established inflammatory root resorption in replanted dog teeth. Endodontics and Dental Traumatology 1995;11:124–8.

108. Steiner JC, Cathey GM. Inducing root end closure of nonvital permanent teeth. Journal of Dentistry for Children 1968;35: 47–54.

109. Kerekes K, Heide S, Jacobsen I. Follow-up examination of endodontic treatment in traumatized juvenile incisors. Journal of Endodontics 1980;6:744–8.

110. Kleier DJ, Barr ES. A study of endodontically apexified teeth. Endodontics and Dental Traumatology 1991;7:112–17.

111. Steinig TH, Regan JD, Gutmann JL. The use and predictable placement of Mineral Trioxide Aggregate in one-visit apexification cases. Australian Endodontic Journal 2003;29:34–42.

112. Estrela C, Bammann LL, Estrela CR, et al. Antimicrobial and chemical study of MTA, Portland cement, calcium hydroxide paste, Sealapex and Dycal. Brazilian Dental Journal 2000;11: 3–9.

113. Torabinejad M, Hong CU, Pitt-Ford TR, et al. Antibacterial effects of some root end filling materials. Journal of Endodontics 1995;21:403–6.

114. Myers WC, Fountain SB. Dental pulp regeneration aided by blood and blood substitutes after experimentally induced periapical infection. Oral Surgery, Oral Medicine, and Oral Pathology 1974;37:441–50.

115. Ostby BN. The role of the blood clot in endodontic therapy. An experimental histologic study. Acta Odontologica Scandinavica 1961;19:324–53.

116. Iwaya SI, Ikawa M, Kubota M. Revascularization of an immature permanent tooth with apical periodontitis and sinus tract. Dental Traumatology 2001;17:185–7.

117. Banchs F, Trope M. Revascularization of immature permanent teeth with apical periodontitis: new treatment protocol? Journal of Endodontics 2004;30:196–200.

118. Trope M. Treatment of the immature tooth with a non-vital pulp and apical periodontitis. Dental Clinics of North America 2010;54:313–24.

119. Sato I, Ando-Kurihara N, Kota K, et al. Sterilization of infected root-canal dentine by topical application of a mixture of ciprofloxacin, metronidazole and minocycline in situ. International Endodontic Journal 1996;29:118–24.

120. Nagata JY, Gomes BP, Rocha Lima TF, et al. Traumatized immature teeth treated with 2 protocols of pulp revascularization. Journal of Endodontics 2014;40:606–12.

121. Hoshino E, Kurihara-Ando N, Sato I, et al. In-vitro antibacterial susceptibility of bacteria taken from infected root dentine to a mixture of ciprofloxacin, metronidazole and minocycline. International Endodontic Journal 1996;29:125–30.

122. Thibodeau B, Teixeira F, Yamauchi M, et al. Pulp revascularization of immature dog teeth with apical periodontitis. Journal of Endodontics 2007;33:680–9.

123. Jeeruphan T, Jantarat J, Yanpiset K, et al. Mahidol study 1: comparison of radiographic and survival outcomes of immature teeth treated with either regenerative endodontic or apexification methods: a retrospective study. Journal of Endodontics 2012;38:1330–6.

124. Khademi AA, Dianat O, Mahjour F, et al. Outcomes of revascularization treatment in immature dog's teeth. Dental Traumatology 2014;30:374–9.

125. Cvek M, Sundstrom B. Treatment of non-vital permanent incisors with calcium hydroxide. V. Histologic appearance of roentgenographically demonstrable apical closure of immature roots. Odontologisk Revy 1974;25:379–91.

126. Trope M, Maltz DO, Tronstad L. Resistance to fracture of restored endodontically treated teeth. Endodontics and Dental Traumatology 1985;1:108–11.

127. Cvek M, Mejare I, Andreasen JO. Healing and prognosis of teeth with intra-alveolar fractures involving the cervical part of the root. Dental Traumatology 2002;18:57–65.

128. Rabie G, Trope M, Garcia C, et al. Strengthening and restoration of immature teeth with an acid-etch resin technique. Endodontics and Dental Traumatology 1985;1:246–56.

129. Mannocci F, Machmouridou E, Watson TF, et al. Microtensile bond strength of resin-post interfaces created with interpenetrating polymer network posts or cross-linked posts. Medicina Oral, Patologia Oral y Cirugia Bucal 2008;13:E745–52.

130. Andreasen JO, Ravn JJ. The effect of traumatic injuries to primary teeth on their permanent successors. II. A clinical and radiographic follow-up study of 213 teeth. Scandinavian Journal of Dental Research 1971;79:284–94.

131. Holan G, Eidelman E, Fuks AB. Long-term evaluation of pulpotomy in primary molars using mineral trioxide aggregate or formocresol. Pediatric Dentistry 2005;27:129–36.

132. Holan G. Long-term effect of different treatment modalities for traumatized primary incisors presenting dark coronal discoloration with no other signs of injury. Dental Traumatology 2006;22:14–7.

133. Holan G. Replantation of avulsed primary incisors: a critical review of a controversial treatment. Dental Traumatology 2013;29:178–84.

CHAPTER 13

Marginal Periodontitis and the Dental Pulp

I. Rotstein

Chapter Contents

Summary

Endodontic–periodontal diseases often present challenges to the clinician in their diagnosis, treatment and prognosis assessment. Aetiological factors, such as microorganisms, as well as contributing factors, such as trauma, root resorption, perforation and dental malformation, play a role in the development and progression of such diseases. Treatment and prognosis of endodontic–periodontal diseases vary and are dependent on the aetiology, pathogenesis and correct recognition of each specific condition. Therefore, understanding the interrelationship between endodontic and periodontal diseases will enhance the clinician's ability to establish correct diagnosis, assess the prognosis of the teeth involved and select a treatment plan based on biological and clinical evidence.

Introduction

The dental pulp and periodontium are intimately related and connected via exposed dentinal tubules, lateral, or accessory canals, and the apical foramen.[1–14] These communications can influence the propagation of pathogens from one tissue to the other.[15–18] Exposed dentinal tubules in areas devoid of cementum may serve as viable communication pathways between the dental pulp and periodontal ligament. Exposure of dentinal tubules may occur as a result of developmental defects, disease and after periodontal, or surgical, procedures. Radicular dentinal tubules extend from the pulp to the cemento-dentinal junction (CDJ). They run a relatively straight course and range in size from 1 to 3 μm in diameter.[13] The diameter of the tubules decreases with age, or as a response to chronic low-grade stimuli, causing apposition of highly mineralized peritubular dentine. The number of dentinal tubules varies from approximately 8000 mm^2 at the CDJ to 57 000 mm^2 at the pulpal end. In the cervical area of the root, the number of dentinal tubules is approximately 15 000 mm^2.[13]

When the cementum and enamel do not meet at the cemento-enamel junction (CEJ), these tubules remain exposed, thereby creating potential pathways of communication between the pulp and periodontal ligament. Patients experiencing cervical dentine hypersensitivity are an example of such a phenomenon. Fluid and irritants may flow through patent dentinal tubules. In the absence of an intact enamel or cementum layer, the pulp can become exposed to irritants and microbes originating from the oral environment and progressing via the gingival sulcus, or periodontal pocket. Experimental studies demonstrated that soluble material from bacterial plaque applied to exposed dentine could cause pulpal inflammation, indicating that dentinal tubules may provide direct access between the periodontium and pulp.[19]

Scanning electron microscopic studies have demonstrated that dentine exposure at the CEJ occurred in approximately 18% of teeth in general and in 25% of anterior teeth in particular.[20] In addition, the same tooth may have different CEJ characteristics presenting dentine exposure on one surface, whereas the other surfaces may be covered with cementum.[21] The exposed CEJ area is susceptible to the progression of endodontic pathogens, as well as to the effect of scaling and root planing on cementum integrity, trauma and bleaching-induced pathosis.[22-25] Scaling and root planning were based on the previous concept that the cementum is infected, and, hence, must be removed to promote periodontal health; the aim of root surface debridement, which is currently practised, is to disrupt the microbial biofilm and remove factors that promote plaque retention. Apart from the exposed CEJ, other areas of dentinal communication may be through developmental grooves located both palato-gingivally and apically.[25] Often not covered by cementum, the base of these grooves is, therefore, exposed to contamination.

Lateral and accessory canals can be present anywhere along the length of the root. Their presence, incidence and location have been well documented in animal and human teeth using a variety of methods, including dye perfusion, injection of impression materials, microradiography, light microscopy and scanning electron microscopy.[2,4,6,8,10,14,26] It is estimated that 30% to 40% of all teeth have other smaller canal systems, and the majority of them are found in the apical third of the root. It was reported that 17% of teeth presented multiple canal systems in the apical third of the root, about 9% had them in the middle third and less than 2% had them in the coronal third.[4] However, it seems that the incidence of periodontal disease associated with these types of canals is relatively low. A study of 1000 human teeth with extensive periodontal disease found only 2% of such canals associated with the involved periodontal pockets.[8]

Other canal systems in the furcation of molars may also be a direct pathway of communication between the pulp and periodontium.[6,10] The incidence of accessory canals may vary from 23% to 76%.[2,4,27] These accessory canals contain connective tissue and blood vessels that connect the circulatory system of the pulp to that of the periodontium. However, not all these canals extend the full length from the pulp chamber to the floor of the furcation.[27]

Pulpal inflammation may cause inflammatory reaction in the interradicular periodontal tissues.[28] The presence of these patent smaller canals is a potential pathway for the spread of microorganisms and their toxic byproducts from the pulp to the periodontal ligament and vice-versa, resulting in inflammation of the involved tissues.

The apical foramen is the main route of communication between the pulp and periodontium. Microbial and inflammatory byproducts may exit readily through the apical foramen to cause periapical pathosis. The apex is also a potential portal of entry of inflammatory byproducts from deep periodontal pockets into the pulp. Pulp inflammation, or pulp necrosis, extends into the periapical tissues, causing a local inflammatory response often associated with bone and root resorption. Endodontic treatment aims to eliminate the intraradicular aetiological factors, thereby leading to healing of the affected periapical tissues.[17,18,29,30]

Effect of Inflamed Pulp on the Periodontium

When the pulp becomes inflamed, it elicits an inflammatory response in the periodontal ligament at the apical foramen and/or adjacent to smaller openings of the root canal system.[31] Inflammatory byproducts of pulpal origin may permeate through the apex, smaller canals in the apical third of the root canal system, or exposed dentinal tubules and trigger an inflammatory vascular response in the periodontium.[32–39] Among those are living pathogens such as certain bacteria strains, including spirochetes, fungi and viruses,[32,33,35,39–44] as well as nonliving pathogens.[43,45–48] Many of these are pathogens similarly encountered in periodontal inflammatory disease. In certain cases, pulpal disease will stimulate epithelial growth, affecting the integrity of the periapical tissues.[49,50]

In an experimental study, defects of different sizes were created on root surfaces of extracted lateral incisors with open and mature apices. The canals were either infected, or filled with calcium hydroxide, and the teeth replanted. It was observed that intrapulpal infection promoted marginal epithelial downgrowth on the denuded dentine surface after 20 weeks.[51] The effects of endodontic pathogens on marginal periodontal wound healing on dentinal surfaces surrounded by healthy periodontal ligament have also been assessed.[52] It was found that in infected teeth the defect was covered by 20% more epithelium. It appears that the pathogens in a necrotic canal can stimulate epithelial downgrowth along denuded dentine surfaces with marginal communication.

The effect of endodontic infection on periodontal probing depth and the presence of furcation involvement in mandibular molars have also been investigated.[53] Patients presenting with periapical lesions on both roots of molars had a significantly greater probing depth compared with teeth without periapical lesions. It was suggested that root canal inflammation in molars involved with marginal periodontitis might potentiate periodontitis progression by pathogens spreading through accessory canals and dentinal tubules, causing more attachment loss in the furcation.

Periodontal pathogens in pulp and periodontal diseases affecting the same tooth were studied by means of 16S RNA gene-directed polymerase chain reaction (PCR).[54] Specific PCR methods were used to detect *Aggregatibacter actinomycetemcomitans*, *Tannerella forsythia*, *Eikenella corrodens*, *Fusobacterium nucleatum*, *Porphyromonas gingivalis*, *Prevotella intermedia* and *Treponema denticola*. These pathogens were found in all endodontic samples. In chronic apical periodontitis and chronic marginal periodontitis, similar pathogens were also found. Therefore, it appears that periodontal pathogens often accompany endodontic infections and support the concept that endodontic–periodontal interrelationships are a critical pathway for both diseases. In addition, foreign bodies and materials may pass into the periapical tissues. Extrinsic foreign bodies, including foreign lipids, cellulose granulomas and iatrogenic materials, can cause a direct inflammatory response.[17]

Effect of Marginal Periodontitis on the Pulp

The effect of periodontal inflammation on the pulp is controversial and conflicting studies abound.[3,5,12,19,28,55–60] One study suggested that marginal periodontitis has no effect on the pulp at least, until it involves the apex.[3] On the other hand, several studies suggested that the effect of periodontal disease on the pulp is degenerative in nature. The effects include an increase in calcifications, fibrosis and collagen resorption, as well as a direct inflammatory action.[9,11] It appears that the pulp is usually not severely affected by periodontal disease until recession has opened an accessory canal to the oral environment. At that stage, pathogens leaking from the oral cavity through the accessory canal into the pulp may cause a chronic inflammatory reaction followed by pulpal necrosis. However, as long as the accessory canals are protected by sound cementum, necrosis does not usually occur. Additionally, if the microvasculature of the apical foramen remains intact, the pulp will retain its vitality.[9] However, once the apical vasculature is compromised, the pulp will lose its vitality; this is shown in cases of teeth with primary periodontal lesions with secondary endodontic involvement (see later). The effect of periodontal treatment on the pulp is similar during root surface debridement, or periodontal surgery, if accessory canals are opened to the oral environment. In such cases, pathogenic invasion and secondary inflammation and necrosis of the pulp can occur.

Classification

There are many ways of classifying the so-called endodontic–periodontal (endo–perio) lesions.[19,28,29,61–63] For differential diagnostic and treatment purposes, they are best classified as endodontic, periodontal or combined diseases.[17,18] They include:

- primary endodontic lesion;
- primary periodontal lesion;
- combined lesions.

The combined lesions include:

- primary endodontic lesion with secondary periodontal involvement;
- primary periodontal lesion with secondary endodontic involvement;
- true combined lesions.

This classification is based on the theoretical pathways explaining how these lesions are formed.[63] By understanding the pathogenesis, the clinician can then suggest an appropriate course of treatment and better assess the prognosis.

PRIMARY ENDODONTIC LESION

An acute exacerbation of a chronic periapical lesion on a tooth with a necrotic pulp may drain coronally through the periodontal ligament into the gingival sulcus (Figure 13-1A). This condition may mimic a periodontal abscess. However, it is only periodontal in that it passes through the periodontal ligament space (Figures 13-2 through 13-5). In reality, it is a sinus tract resulting from pulpal disease. Therefore, it is essential that a gutta-percha cone be inserted into the sinus tract and that one or more radiographs are taken to track the origin of the lesion. When the sinus tract is probed, it is usually narrow and lacks width. A similar situation occurs where drainage from the apex of a molar tooth extends coronally into the furcation area (Figure 13-6). Direct extension of inflammation from the pulp may also occur in the furcation area of a nonvital tooth when accessory canals are present (Figure 13-7). Primary endodontic lesions usually heal after root canal treatment. The sinus tract extending into the gingival sulcus or furcation usually disappears within a few weeks, once the necrotic pulp has been treated. It is important to recognize that an attempt to provide periodontal treatment for this condition will result in failure if the necrotic pulp has not been diagnosed and treated.

PRIMARY PERIODONTAL LESION

These lesions (see Figure 13-1C) are caused by marginal periodontitis, which progresses apically along the root surface until the apical region is reached. In such conditions, pulp sensitivity testing will be within normal limits (Figures 13-8 and 13-9). In addition, a wide pocket can be probed, possibly becoming

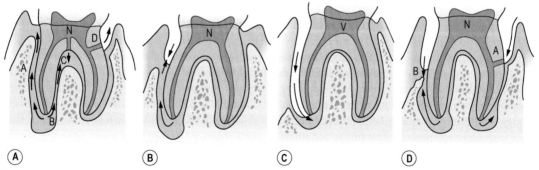

FIGURE 13-1 Classification of endodontic–periodontal lesions. (A) Primary endodontic lesions: pathway extending from the apex to gingival sulcus via the periodontium (*A*); apex to furcation (*B*); lateral canal to furcation (*C*) and lateral canal to pocket (*D*). (B) Primary endodontic lesion with secondary periodontal involvement. (C) Primary periodontal lesion extending to the apex. (D) Primary periodontal lesion with secondary endodontic involvement via a lateral canal (*A*). Combined lesion resulting from coalescence of separate lesions (*B*). N = Necrotic pulp; V = vital pulp.

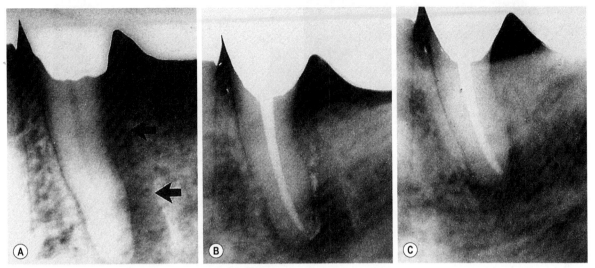

FIGURE 13-2 Primary endodontic lesion. Mandibular premolar with a radiolucency along the distal surface of the root. (A) Pretreatment, the lesion (*arrowed*) drained through the gingival sulcus. (B) Immediately after the treatment, the root canal sealer can be observed in the lesion. (C) Six months later, there is evidence of healing and bone filling.

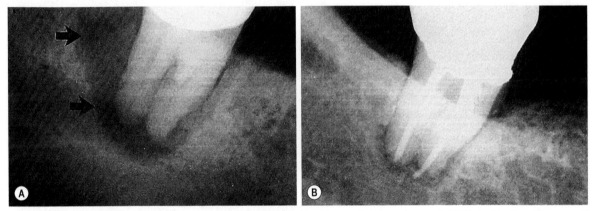

FIGURE 13-3 (A) Mandibular molar with a narrow probable distal pocket and large radiolucency (*arrowed*). (B) Marked healing at 1-year recall confirming that the original 'pocket' was of endodontic origin.

progressively shallower as the probe is moved laterally. There is also evidence of the presence of plaque and frequently calculus. The prognosis in this condition depends wholly on the stage of the marginal periodontitis and the efficacy of periodontal treatment. The clinician must also be aware of the radiographic appearance of marginal periodontitis associated with developmental radicular anomalies (see later).

COMBINED LESIONS

Primary Endodontic Lesion with Secondary Periodontal Involvement

If a suppurating primary endodontic lesion remains untreated after a period of time, it may become secondarily involved with marginal periodontal breakdown (see Figure 13-1B). Biofilm forms at the gingival

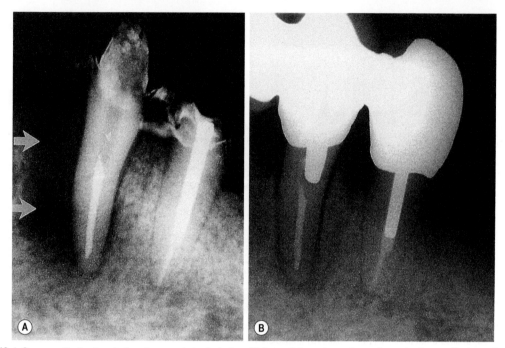

FIGURE 13-4 Success after treatment of a primary endodontic lesion. (A) Immediate postoperative radiograph of a mandibular canine showing mesial radiolucency (*arrowed*). (B) Radiograph at 15 months posttreatment showing healing.

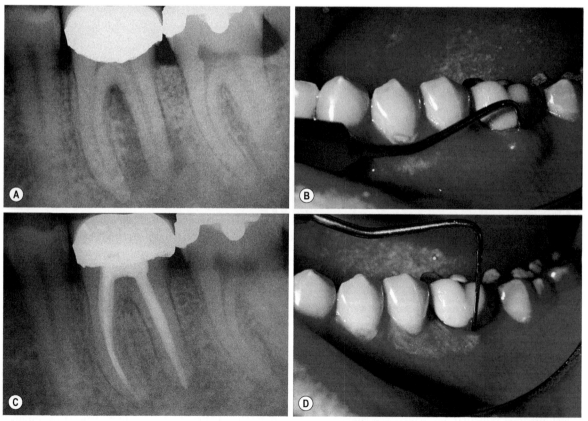

FIGURE 13-5 Mandibular molar with apical lesion extending into root furcation. (A) Preoperative radiograph showing furcal and distal radiolucency. (B) Clinical photograph of gingival swelling and a periodontal probe in the furcation. (C) A 1-year recall radiograph showing marked reduction of furcal and distal radiolucencies. (D) Clinical photograph showing minimal pocket depth on the buccal. Healing occurred after root canal treatment alone.

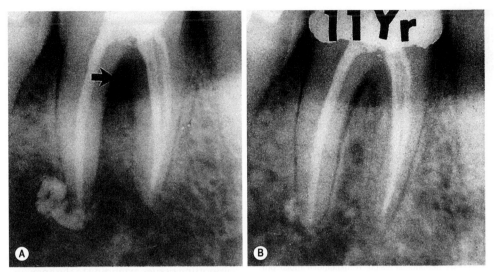

FIGURE 13-6 Mandibular molar where apical involvement extends into the furcation (*arrowed*). (A) Immediately after root canal treatment, excess sealer is present at the apex of the distal root. (B) Radiograph 11 years later showing apical and furcation healing.

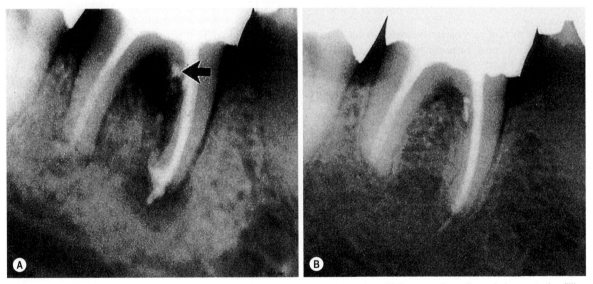

FIGURE 13-7 Primary endodontic lesion with a lateral canal demonstrated in the furcation. (A) Postoperative radiograph demonstrating filling material passing through openings into the furcation (*arrowed*). (B) After 18 months, complete healing of the lesions at the apex and adjacent to the lateral canal is evident.

margin of the sinus tract and leads to marginal peri-odontitis. When plaque or calculus is encountered on probing, the treatment and prognosis of the tooth are altered; the tooth now requires both endodontic and periodontal treatments. If the endodontic treatment is adequate, prognosis depends on the severity of the

marginal periodontal damage and the efficacy of peri-odontal treatment. With endodontic treatment alone, only part of the lesion will heal to the level of the secondary periodontal lesion.

Primary endodontic lesions with secondary perio-dontal involvement may also occur as a result of root

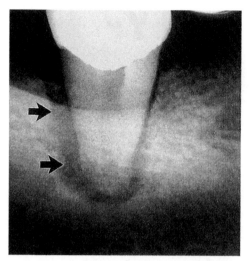

FIGURE 13-8 Primary periodontal lesion. A mandibular molar presented with a probable distal pocket (*arrowed*). Pulp testing was positive, indicating a lesion of periodontal origin.

perforation during root canal treatment or because of misalignment of pins, or posts during coronal restoration (Figure 13-10). Symptoms may be acute, with periodontal abscess formation associated with pain, swelling, pus exudation, pocket formation and tooth mobility. A more chronic response may sometimes occur without pain and involves the sudden appearance of a pocket with bleeding on probing, or exudation of pus. When the root perforation is situated close to the alveolar crest, it may be feasible to raise a flap, repair the defect with an appropriate filling material, and subsequently reposition the flap apically to expose the repaired perforation site. In deeper perforations or in the roof of the furcation, immediate internal repair of the perforation and infection control is essential for better prognosis. Many materials have been in use for this purpose; Mineral trioxide aggregate (MTA), for example, is most widely used with good results.[64–66]

Root fractures may also present as primary endodontic lesions with secondary periodontal involvement. These typically occur with a root-treated tooth (Figure 13-11), often with a post supported crown *in situ*. The signs may range from a local deepening of a periodontal pocket to more acute periodontal abscess formation. In addition, root fractures have become an

increasing problem with molar teeth that have been treated by root resection. In a study of 100 patients, a total of 38 teeth failed during the 10-year period of observation, and 47% of the failures were a result of root fractures, with the vast majority being in mandibular molar teeth.[67,68]

Primary Periodontal Lesion with Secondary Endodontic Involvement

The apical progression of a periodontal pocket can continue until the apex is reached. As a result, the pulp may become necrotic because of irritants permeating via a lateral canal or the apical foramen (see Figure 13-1D). In a single-rooted tooth, the prognosis is usually poor, unlike the primary endodontic lesion. In molar teeth, not all roots may suffer the same loss of supporting tissues extending to the apex, in which case the possibility of root resection should be considered.

The treatment of marginal periodontitis can also lead to secondary endodontic involvement. Lateral or accessory canals and dentinal tubules can be opened to the oral environment by root surface debridement, or surgical flap procedures (Figures 13-12 and 13-13). For example, a blood vessel within a lateral canal may be severed by a curette during treatment. Additionally, pulp changes resulting from marginal periodontitis were observed when the main apical foramen was involved.[9] Provided the blood supply through the apex is intact, the pulp has a strong capacity for survival (see Figure 13-10).

There is a correlation between cultivable microorganisms from the root canals of human caries-free teeth with advanced periodontitis and those from associated periodontal pockets.[8,69,70] The microorganisms from the periodontal pocket are a possible source for root canal infection. Support for this concept has come from research in which cultured samples obtained from the pulp tissue and radicular dentine of periodontally involved human teeth showed bacterial growth in 87% of the cases.[55,71] It is likely that the reservoir of bacteria in the dentine and pulp can contribute to the failure of periodontal treatment. A possibility also exists that these teeth may develop pulpal necrosis.

Sometimes, there is lack of correlation between marginal periodontitis and pulp involvement.[58] The histological status of the pulps of periodontally

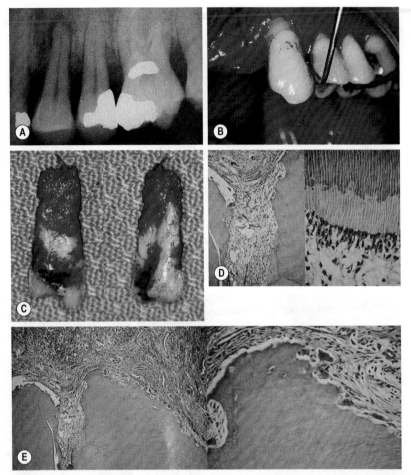

FIGURE 13-9 Primary periodontal lesion. (A) Preoperative radiograph of maxillary first premolar with a periapical lesion but no obvious endodontic aetiology. (B) Clinical photograph with periodontal probe in place. The pulp will respond normally to pulp sensitivity testing. (C) Two views of the extracted tooth. Note mesial anatomical groove along the root. (D) Micrographs showing vital pulp in the tooth. (E) Micrographs showing inflammatory resorption and periodontitis.

involved teeth was similar to control teeth with a normal periodontium.[67] Despite conflicting opinions from various research studies[19,60] from a clinical standpoint, it seems that plaque-associated marginal periodontitis rarely causes significant pathological changes in the pulp, and this remains true until the periodontal pocket reaches a portal of entry to the pulp either via dentinal tubules, lateral/accessory canals, or the apical foramen.

True Combined Lesions

These lesions (see Figure 13-1D) occur where an endodontic lesion, progressing coronally, becomes continuous with a plaque-infected periodontal pocket progressing apically.[18,63] The degree of attachment loss in this type of lesion is, invariably, large and the prognosis guarded. The prognosis is particularly poor in single rooted teeth, but the situation may be salvaged in molars by sectioning the tooth, if all the roots are not as severely involved. Healing of apical periodontitis may be anticipated after successful endodontic treatment. The periodontal component of this lesion may, or may not, respond to periodontal treatment, depending on the severity of involvement (Figure 13-14). The radiographical appearance of true combined endodontic-periodontal lesions may be similar

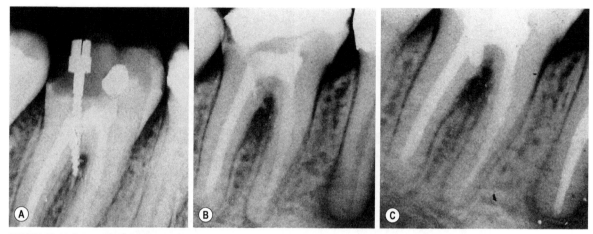

FIGURE 13-10 Primary endodontic lesion with secondary periodontal involvement. (A) A screw post has perforated the furcation area of a mandibular second molar. (B) After 6 months, furcation bone loss is evident. (C) The perforation was treated from within the tooth and the pocket debrided. Some new bone has formed in the furcation. Clinically, no pocket can be probed.

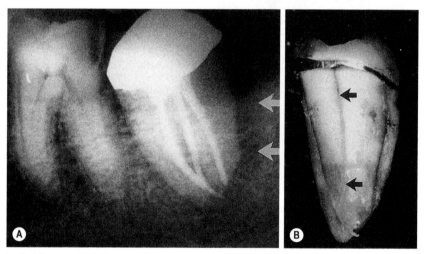

FIGURE 13-11 Longitudinal fracture. (A) A distal pocket (*arrowed*) probable to the apex on a mandibular left second molar persisted after root canal treatment, necessitating extraction. (B) After extraction, a longitudinal fracture on the distal root surface (*arrowed*) extending the length of the tooth was evident. Fused roots prevented 'anatomical redesigning'.

to that of a vertically fractured tooth. A fracture that has exposed the pulp space, with resultant necrosis, may also be labelled a true combined lesion and yet not be amenable to successful treatment. If a sinus tract is present, it may be necessary to raise a flap to determine the aetiology of the lesion (see Figure 13-9).

DIAGNOSIS

The diagnosis of primary endodontic lesion and primary periodontal lesion usually present no clinical difficulty. In a primary endodontic lesion, the pulp is infected and often nonvital. On the other hand, in a tooth with primary periodontal lesion, the pulp is vital and responsive to sensitivity testing. However, primary endodontic lesions with secondary periodontal involvement, primary periodontal lesions with secondary endodontic involvement, or true combined lesions may be clinically and radiographically very similar. If a lesion is provisionally diagnosed and treated as being primarily a result of endodontic

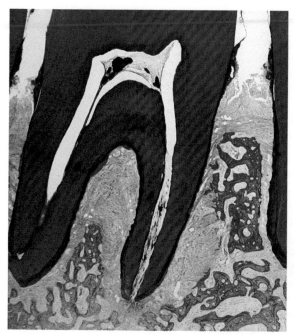

FIGURE 13-12 Histological examination shows that furcation involvement can be severe in advanced marginal periodontitis. The pulp can become affected through lateral or accessory canals.

disease because of a lack of evidence of marginal periodontitis, and there is soft-tissue healing on clinical probing and bony healing on a recall radiograph, a valid retrospective confirmed diagnosis can then be made. The degree of healing that has taken place after root canal treatment will determine the retrospective classification. In the absence of adequate healing, further periodontal treatment is indicated.

PROGNOSIS

The prognosis depends primarily on the diagnosis and degree of the specific endodontic and/or periodontal disease. The main factors to consider, at the time of diagnosis, are pulp vitality and type and extent of the periodontal defect. The prognosis and treatment of each type of endodontic–periodontal lesion varies. Primary endodontic lesion should only be managed by endodontic treatment, and the prognosis is good. Primary periodontal lesions should only be managed by periodontal treatment; in this case the prognosis depends on the severity of the periodontal lesion and

the patient's response. Primary endodontic lesions with secondary periodontal involvement should first be managed with endodontic treatment. The treatment results should be evaluated in 2 to 3 months and only then should periodontal treatment be considered. This sequence of treatment allows sufficient time for initial tissue healing and better assessment of the periodontal condition.[26,72] It also reduces the potential risk of introducing bacteria and their byproducts during the initial healing phase. In this regard, it has been suggested that during interim endodontic treatment, aggressive removal of the periodontal ligament and underlying cementum will adversely affect periodontal healing[1]; areas of the roots that were not aggressively treated showed unremarkable healing. The prognosis of a primary endodontic lesion with secondary periodontal involvement depends primarily on the severity of periodontal involvement, the periodontal treatment and the patient's response.

Primary periodontal lesions with secondary endodontic involvement and true combined endodontic-periodontal lesions require both endodontic and periodontal treatments. It has been demonstrated that intrapulpal infection tends to promote marginal epithelial downgrowth along a denuded dentine surface.[53] Additionally, experimentally induced periodontal defects in infected teeth were associated with 20% more epithelium than noninfected teeth.[35] Noninfected teeth showed 10% more connective tissue coverage than infected teeth.[35] The prognosis of primary periodontal lesions with secondary endodontic involvement and true combined lesions depends primarily on the severity of the periodontal disease and the periodontal tissues response to treatment.

True combined lesions usually have a more guarded prognosis. In general, assuming the endodontic treatment is adequate, the lesion of endodontic origin will heal. Thus, the prognosis of combined diseases is dependent on the efficacy of periodontal treatment. In such cases, periodontal regeneration procedures may be beneficial.[73,74]

The prognosis for each classification can be summarized as in the section that follows.

Primary Endodontic Lesion

Treatment:	Root canal
Prognosis:	Excellent

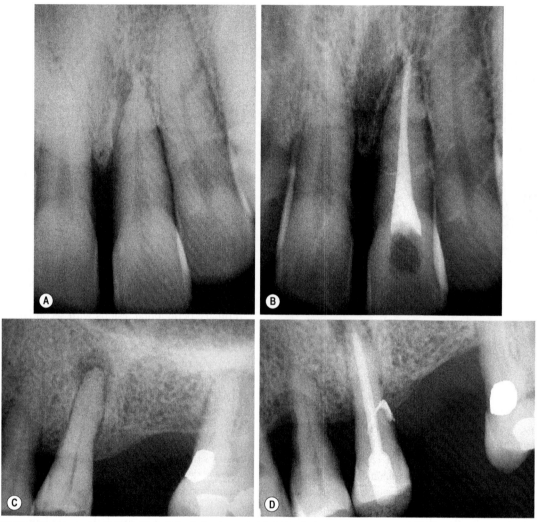

FIGURE 13-13 Marginal periodontitis with endodontic involvement. (A) Radiograph of an unrestored tooth with generalized periodontitis and a necrotic pulp. (B) After endodontic treatment, a communication with the oral environment through a lateral canal was demonstrated. (C) A similar situation on a premolar with generalized periodontitis and a necrotic pulp. (D) Filling material extruding through a lateral canal suggests the aetiology for the pulp necrosis.

Primary Periodontal Lesion

Treatment: Periodontal (root surface debridement, surgery, regeneration)

Prognosis: Dependent on efficacy of periodontal treatment and patient's response

Combined Lesions

Treatment: Endodontic and periodontal

Prognosis: Dependent on periodontal treatment and patient's response; the lesion caused by endodontic disease will usually heal; therefore, prognosis is dependent on periodontal treatment

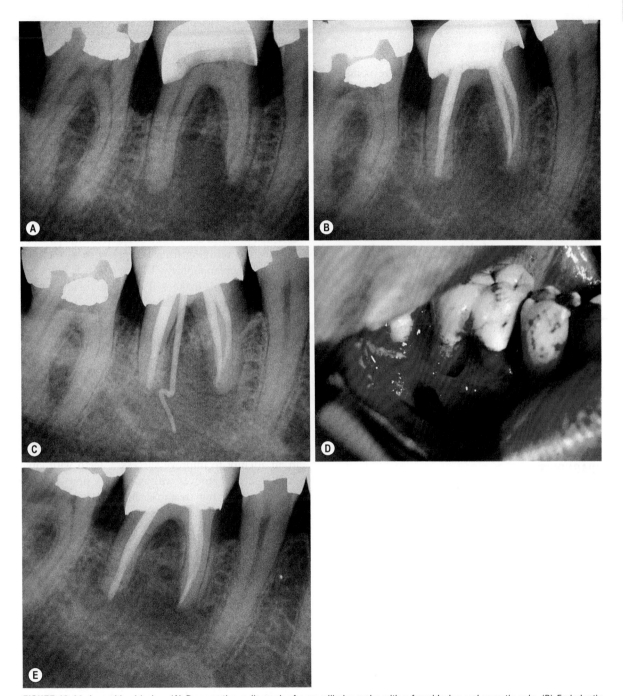

FIGURE 13-14 A combined lesion. (A) Preoperative radiograph of a mandibular molar with a furcal lesion and necrotic pulp. (B) Endodontic treatment was completed. (C) Recall radiograph with a gutta-percha point in the gingival sulcus. (D) Periodontal surgery and treatment were performed on the cervical and furcal areas. (E) One year after both endodontic and periodontal treatment, the lesions healed.

Complications Caused by Radicular Anomalies

A particular group of teeth that fails to respond well to treatment is those associated with an invagination or a longitudinal, developmental radicular groove. Such conditions can lead to untreatable localized marginal periodontitis. These grooves usually begin in the central fossa of maxillary central, or lateral, incisors, over the cingulum, and continue apically down the root for varying distances. Such a groove is apparently the result of an attempt by the tooth germ to form another root. This fissure-like channel may provide a nidus for biofilm formation and infection, and an avenue for the progression of marginal periodontitis.

From the time the tooth develops with this anomalous root defect, the potential for isolated marginal periodontitis exists. As long as the epithelial attachment remains intact, the periodontium remains healthy. However, once the integrity of the attachment is breached and the groove becomes inflamed, a self-sustaining infrabony pocket can be formed along its entire length; radiographically, an area of bone destruction follows the course of the groove (Figure 13-15). In selected cases, radicular grooves can be treated satisfactorily and maintained.[75–77]

DIAGNOSIS

Correct clinical diagnosis of this condition at an early stage is important. The clinician must look for the groove because it may have been altered by a previous restoration on the palatal surface. The use of an operating microscope during clinical examination is advantageous because of enhanced magnification and illumination.

The patient may have symptoms of a periodontal abscess. Endodontic symptoms may vary. If the condition is purely periodontal, it can be diagnosed visually by following the groove to the gingival sulcus and probing the depth of the pocket. This pocket is usually tubular and isolated, as opposed to a more generalized periodontal condition. The tooth is usually responsive to pulp sensitivity testing. If this entity is also associated with pulp infection, the patient may present with endodontic symptoms, and the results of pulp sensitivity testing will not be normal.

Bone destruction that follows the groove longitudinally may be apparent radiographically. The appearance of a teardrop-shaped area on the radiograph should also arouse suspicion. The developmental groove may actually be visible on the radiograph; if so, it will appear as a dark longitudinal line. This condition must be differentiated from a longitudinal fracture, which may give a similar radiographic appearance.

PROGNOSIS

The prognosis for endodontic treatment is guarded, depending on the apical extent of the groove. The essential problem is the need to eliminate the pathway of infection resulting from the presence of the anatomical radicular anomaly. The prognosis is improved if the condition is diagnosed and treated early, but its management remains challenging.

TREATMENT

In essence, since this lesion is a self-sustaining infrabony pocket, root surface debridement alone may be inadequate. Although the acute nature of the problem may be alleviated initially, the reason for the inflammation must be eradicated by cutting out the groove and surgical management of the tissues. This can be combined with placement of a biocompatible material in an attempt to improve success.[75] Teeth with large developmental grooves with advance lesions need to be extracted if not treatable, and implant treatment should then be considered.

Alternatives to Implants

ANATOMICAL REDESIGNING

To assist periodontal treatment and in certain endodontic situations, anatomical redesigning may become necessary. Such redesigning may include root amputation, resection and bicuspidization. It provides a periodontally maintainable environment for the remaining root(s). The reported survival rate is approximately 68%.[78] Generally such cases should be referred to a specialist to assess prognosis and enhance survival rate. Often, the natural tooth can be retained. However, if the prognosis appears poor, early extraction is advisable to avoid compromising future implant treatment.

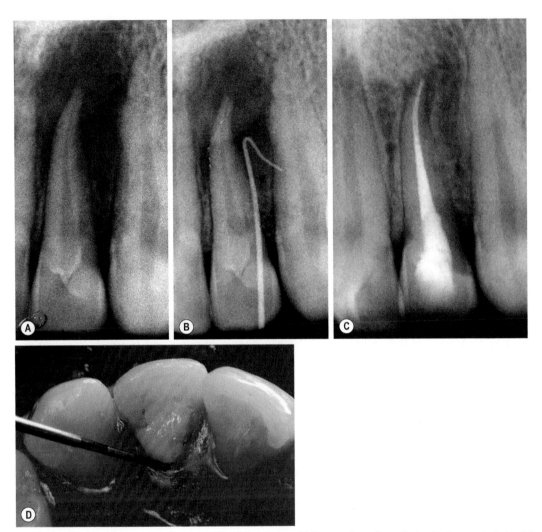

FIGURE 13-15 Developmental radicular anomaly in a maxillary lateral incisor. (A) Preoperative radiograph showing large periapical radiolucency associated with a palatal radicular groove; clinically there was a 13-mm palatal periodontal defect. (B) A gutta-percha point is used to trace the suppurative periodontal pocket. Combined management includes endodontic treatment, atraumatic extraction, groove reduction, Emdogain® application and tooth reimplantation. (C) The 4-year follow-up radiograph shows substantial decrease in size of the periapical radiolucency. (D) Clinically, the tooth is symptom-free and the periodontal probing depth was reduced to 3 mm. (From Al-Hezaimi et al[75] with permission of Elsevier.)

Root amputation is the removal of one or more roots from a multirooted tooth, leaving the majority of the crown and any existing coronal restoration intact. Tooth resection involves the removal of one, or more, roots of a tooth along with their coronal part(s); it is sometimes referred to as hemisection. Bicuspidization is the separation of a multirooted tooth by a vertical cut through the furcation.

Indications for root amputation or tooth resection include:

- Advanced marginal periodontitis. The pattern of alveolar bone loss in marginal periodontitis may affect the different roots of a molar tooth unequally. If left untreated, the adjacent healthier root support could, eventually, become involved by direct extension of the periodontal lesion, resulting in poorer prognosis. Removal of the offending root(s) allows the well-supported part of the tooth to be retained as a functional unit, resulting in healthy tissues and a normal radiographic appearance.

- Close root proximity. The morphology of the distobuccal root of the maxillary first molar and the mesiobuccal root of the second molar often tend to flare toward each other. Marginal periodontitis in these sites may lead to angular bone loss, which is difficult to treat and leaves the patient with a plaque control management problem. Selective root removal will allow the reestablishment of a proper embrasure area.
- Furcation involvement.
- Extensive radicular caries.
- Root resorption.
- Root fracture or perforation.
- Inability to perform root canal treatment because of calcification or other canal obstructions.

Indications for bicuspidization include:

- Gross perforation in the furcation area. However, the length of the remaining roots must be favourable.
- Close root proximity. This makes periodontal treatment and home maintenance by the patient more difficult. It can be improved by root separation.

Contraindications for anatomical redesigning include:

- Poor plaque control and an unmotivated patient. This is particularly important if there was no improvement after initial periodontal treatment.
- Unfavourable bony support. This relates to all remaining roots of the involved tooth, particularly, if it serves as an abutment for fixed prosthodontics.
- Fused roots. These prevent root removal. A special clinical situation with a more favourable prognosis exists when there is only apical fusion and adequate interradicular bone, allowing for surgical root removal.
- Short, thin roots.
- A long root trunk. The furcation area is situated so far apically that considerable supporting bone would need to be sacrificed.

- Surrounding anatomy. This may preclude the formation of a functional band of attached gingiva around the remaining roots.
- Nonnegotiable canals. The canals are sclerosed or blocked and root-end surgery is not feasible.
- Nonrestorable tooth.

ROOT AMPUTATION

This form of treatment relates primarily to maxillary molar teeth. The distobuccal root of the first molar is most commonly affected. Before root removal, whenever possible after root canal treatment, the pulp chamber should be sealed with a permanent restorative material extending into the coronal entrance of the root to be resected (Figure 13-16). Coronal reshaping and buccolingual narrowing to reduce the occlusal table should also be performed to redirect occlusal forces to the remaining solid roots.

The need for root removal may become apparent during diagnosis and treatment planning instead of treating roots with extensive periodontal breakdown. Root canal treatment is completed, and a permanent restorative material placed in the pulp chamber and coronal entrance of the root to be amputated, so that the root end is already sealed when the root is removed. The patient's plaque control needs to reach a satisfactory level, and the inflammatory phase resolved before root amputation. A full-thickness mucoperiosteal flap is reflected to expose the furcation area, which is carefully explored with a periodontal probe to ensure that the furcation has not been exposed on all three surfaces. If so, tooth resection is required, leaving one root *in situ*; otherwise, the tooth would need to be extracted. The cut in the root is made with a long thin bur, long enough to reach from one side of the root to the other. Care must be taken to maintain the correct angulation of the bur, so as not to damage the remaining root(s) or the crown. The bur is held at a 45-degree angle to the tooth at the level of the furcation. Removal of some of the buccal cortical plate of bone may be required so that the separated root can be gently elevated out of its socket, without undue pressure being applied to the adjacent tooth or bone. Once the root has been removed, the area of the stump is reshaped with burs, so that it blends imperceptibly into the remaining tooth structure. Enough clearance

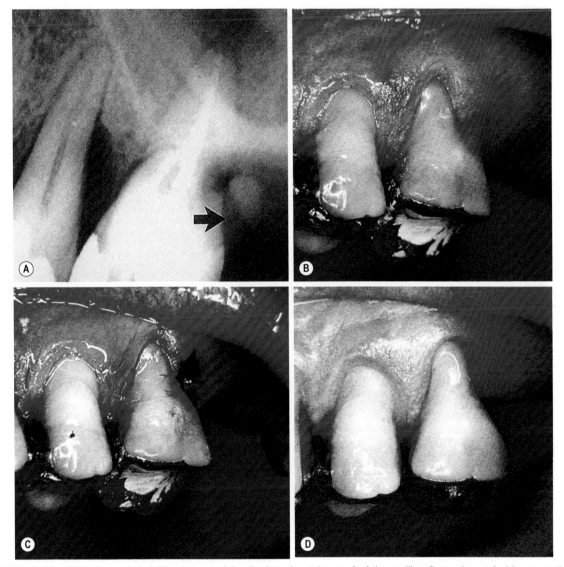

FIGURE 13-16 (A) Marginal periodontal involvement of the distobuccal root (*arrowed*) of the maxillary first molar required its amputation. (B) Before amputation. (C) After amputation. (D) The remaining tooth after polishing and smoothening.

should also be left between the undersurface of the crown and the gingival tissue to allow for adequate plaque control. The tooth surface is finished with fine burs and then polished. The periodontal condition is reevaluated approximately 3 months after root removal. If the mucogingival and osseous deformities still remain, definitive periodontal surgery should be carried out.

An alternative treatment modality allows for root amputation to be performed at the time of periodontal surgery; this has the advantage of combining both stages into only one surgical procedure. The disadvantage is that bony healing has yet to occur, and the extent to which this will progress cannot always be predicted; this may also result in more radical reshaping at the site than might otherwise be required. In

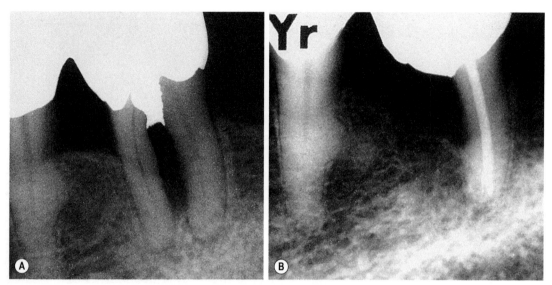

FIGURE 13-17 (A) A perforation with periodontal breakdown in the furcation of a mandibular molar; the tooth was part of a 4-unit splint. The mesial root was amputated, and the coronal restoration recontoured and reduced buccolingually. (B) The 13-year recall demonstrates long-term stability.

this approach, a cavity is cut over the pulp stump with a suitable bur, and an appropriate dressing placed over the exposed pulp. Definitive root canal treatment is carried out at a later stage and after the periodontal dressings had been removed.

There may be situations where it is reasonable to amputate the root of a mandibular molar. If such a tooth presents with a periodontally involved mesial root and it is part of a multiunit bridge, or splinted crowns, amputation should be considered. The buccolingual dimension of the occlusal aspect of the tooth and pontics should be reduced to minimize and redirect the occlusal forces, if possible (Figure 13-17). Another situation in which an amputation could be considered is when the periodontally involved root of a crowned tooth is adjacent to another crowned tooth. They could be firmly splinted to each other to avoid longitudinal fracture of the remaining root (Figure 13-18); for support, broad interproximal contact without splinting is not sufficient. Maxillary molars do not normally present such a problem because of the support provided by the two remaining roots. The remaining coronal portion of the amputated root should be contoured to allow for maintenance of periodontal health. The canal at the amputation site should be prepared and filled with a suitable restorative material to prevent the accumulation of plaque

and development of caries. It is best to place the filling internally before root removal. If this is not feasible, the filling should be placed into the resected root end during the surgical procedure.

TOOTH RESECTION

Tooth resection is often the treatment of choice where there is deep furcation involvement. It is also the treatment of choice in cases in which teeth are to be included in a fixed prosthesis.[61] It is advantageous to complete the initial crown preparation first; this will then serve as a guide when entering the furcation. Full-thickness mucoperiosteal flaps are reflected and the tooth is sectioned using a long, tapered fissure bur. In maxillary molars, depending on the degree of furcation involvement, it may be possible to retain two roots, provided the furcation is not opened between them, such as mesial and palatal, or distal and palatal, or the two buccal roots. If the furcation is opened mesially, buccally and distally, only the best-supported root is retained. Sometimes, this can only be determined after sectioning all three roots and assessing them individually.[6] The bur is positioned in the long axis of the tooth at the most coronal level of the involved furcation. Initial cuts are made in the crown in the direction of the adjacent furcation. The same step is then followed from the adjacent furcation toward the initial cut. The

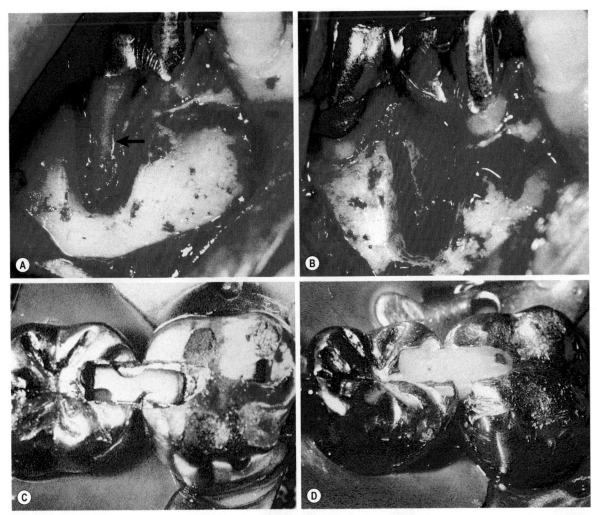

FIGURE 13-18 Splinting of lower molars. (A) The distal root of a mandibular first molar had a longitudinal fracture (*arrowed*) necessitating removal. (B) After amputation of the root and contouring of the remaining structure. (C) An occlusal preparation was made for a metal splint. (D) A restorative filling material was used to keep the splint in place.

bur is then alternated between the two cuts until they are joined. Mandibular molars are sectioned buccolingually into two halves.

As a general rule, it is important to make the cut at the expense of the part that is to be removed (Figure 13-19A). This minimizes the risk of overcutting the retained section. Once sectioning has been completed, the involved part of the tooth is extracted with forceps. When finishing the preparation, it is important to remove the overhang of the crown that may be left at the roof of the furcation and to blend the cut surface into the retained portion of the tooth. This should be

checked radiographically. When the vertical cut to the furcation ends in close proximity to or at the level of bone, it is necessary to remove approximately 1 mm of the bone with a sharp scalpel to expose some intact cementum beyond the cut surface (see Figure 13-19B). It is not advisable to end the restoration within the cut, leaving raw-cut dentine exposed because of the risk of subsequent development of marginal caries (Figure 13-20). The biological width of the periodontium must be maintained. This will facilitate the preparation for the restoration that follows (Figure 13-21). There may be situations where it is necessary to consider occlusal factors as in amputation and reduce the size of the occlusal table. Root fracture is a common cause of failure of root-resected teeth.[67]

BICUSPIDIZATION

This procedure is used on roots of a multirooted tooth, primarily mandibular molars (Figure 13-22). An adequate length and width of the root and clinical crown are primary considerations in case selection and treatment decision-making. The cut should be directed vertically to the middle of the furcation. It is necessary to expose the margin of the cut surface to facilitate crown preparation later. When there is close root proximity, it is necessary to separate the roots orthodontically (Figure 13-23). Both roots are then restored as single units to simulate two premolars.

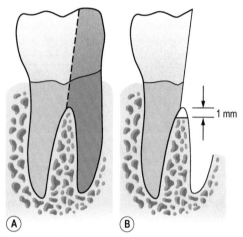

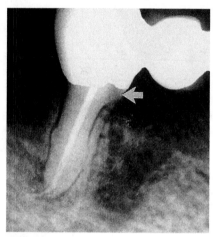

FIGURE 13-19 Resection. (A) The cut should be made at the expense of the part to be removed. (B) The restoration should not leave the raw cut exposed; 1 mm of the bone should be removed to facilitate preparation.

FIGURE 13-20 Lack of the 1-mm space in bone led the restoration to end on raw-cut dentine with long-term adverse consequence of marginal caries (*arrowed*).

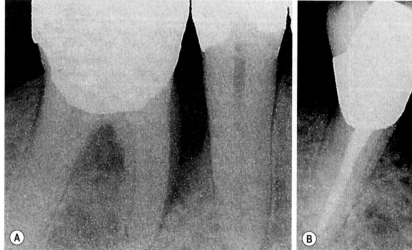

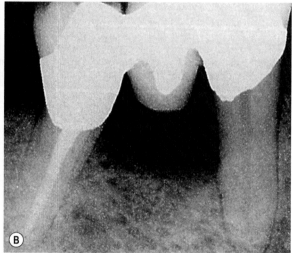

FIGURE 13-21 (A) Angular bone loss extending close to the apex of the mesial root of a mandibular first molar. The widely splayed roots made hemisection suitable. (B) The mesial root was removed. The distal root underwent root canal treatment and surgery and was used as a bridge abutment.

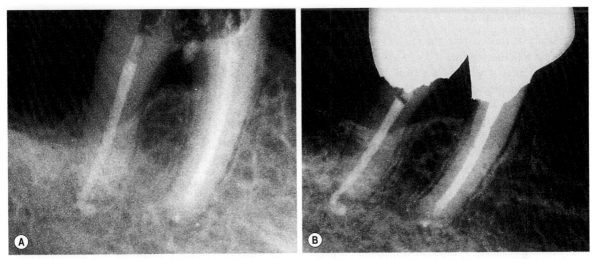

FIGURE 13-22 (A) Perforation into the furcation of a lower molar necessitated bicuspidization. (B) Recall examination after 6 years showing enlarged furcation space permitting effective oral hygiene.

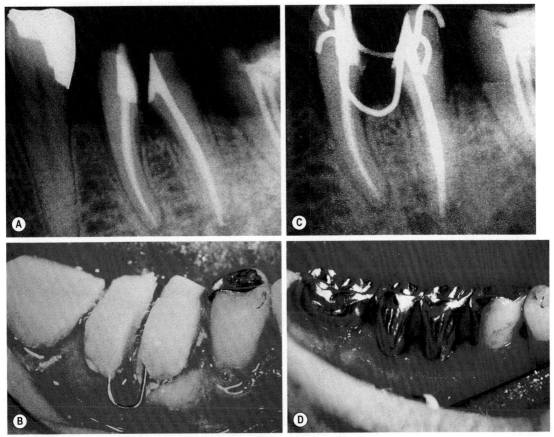

FIGURE 13-23 Bicuspidization achieved by root separation. (A) Radiograph immediately after sectioning. (B) The roots were separated orthodontically. (C) Radiograph after separation. (D) The separate crowns cemented.

Learning Outcomes

After studying this chapter, the reader should be able to explain and discuss the:

- anatomical structures involved in endodontic–periodontal diseases;
- effect of pulpal inflammation on the periodontium;
- effect of marginal periodontitis on the dental pulp;
- classification of endodontic–periodontal diseases;
- treatment modalities for endodontic–periodontal diseases, prognosis and complications.

REFERENCES

1. Blomlöf LB, Lindskog S, Hammarstrom L. Influence of pulpal treatments on cell and tissue reactions in the marginal periodontium. Journal of Periodontology 1988;59:577–83.
2. Burch JG, Hulen S. A study of the presence of accessory foramina and the topography of molar furcations. Oral Surgery, Oral Medicine, Oral Pathology 1974;38:451–5.
3. Czarnecki RT, Schilder H. A histological evaluation of the human pulp in teeth with varying degrees of periodontal disease. Journal of Endodontics 1979;5:242–53.
4. De Deus QD. Frequency, location and direction of the lateral, secondary and accessory canals. Journal of Endodontics 1975;1:361–6.
5. Dongari A, Lambrianidis T. Periodontally derived pulpal lesions. Endodontics and Dental Traumatology 1988;4:49–54.
6. Gutmann JL. Prevalence, location, and patency of accessory canals in the furcation region of permanent molars. Journal of Periodontology 1978;49:21–6.
7. Jansson L, Ehnevid H, Lindskog S, et al. The influence of endodontic infection on progression of marginal bone loss in periodontitis. Journal of Clinical Periodontology 1995;22:729–34.
8. Kirkham DB. The location and incidence of accessory pulpal canals in periodontal pockets. Journal of the American Dental Association 1975;91:353–6.
9. Langeland K, Rodrigues H, Dowden W. Periodontal disease, bacteria, and pulpal histopathology. Oral Surgery, Oral Medicine, Oral Pathology 1994;37:257–70.
10. Lowman JV, Burke RS, Pelleu GB. Patent accessory canals: incidence in molar furcation region. Oral Surgery, Oral Medicine, Oral Pathology 1973;36:580–4.
11. Mandi FA. Histological study of the pulp changes caused by periodontal disease. Journal of the British Endodontic Society 1972;6:80–2.
12. Mazur B, Massler M. Influence of periodontal disease on the dental pulp. Oral Surgery, Oral Medicine, Oral Pathology 1964;17:592–603.
13. Mjör IA, Nordahl I. The density and branching of dentinal tubules in human teeth. Archives of Oral Biology 1996;41:401–12.
14. Rubach WC, Mitchell DF. Periodontal disease, accessory canals and pulp pathosis. Journal of Periodontology 1965;36:34–8.
15. Heasman PA. An endodontic conundrum: the association between pulpal infection and periodontal disease. British Dental Journal 2014;216:275–9.
16. Kambale S, Aspalli N, Munavalli A, et al. A sequential approach in treatment of endo-perio lesion. A case report. Journal of Clinical and Diagnostic Research 2014;8:22–4.
17. Rotstein I, Simon JHS. The endodontic-periodontal continuum. In: Ingle JI, Bakland L, Baumgartner JC, editors. Ingle's endodontics. 6th ed. BC Decker Inc; 2008. p. 638–59.
18. Rotstein I, Simon JHS. The endo-perio lesion: a critical appraisal of the disease condition. Endodontic Topics 2006;13:34–56.
19. Bergenholtz G, Lindhe J. Effect of experimentally induced marginal periodontitis and periodontal scaling on the dental pulp. Journal of Clinical Periodontology 1978;5:59–73.
20. Muller CJ, Van Wyk CW. The amelo-cemental junction. Journal of the Dental Association of South Africa 1984;39:799–803.
21. Schroeder HE, Scherle WF. Cemento-enamel junction-revisited. Journal of Periodontal Research 1988;23:53–9.
22. Ehnevid H, Jansson L, Lindskog S, et al. Endodontic pathogens: propagation of infection through patent dentinal tubules in traumatized monkey teeth. Endodontics and Dental Traumatology 1995;11:229–34.
23. Rotstein I, Friedman S, Mor C, et al. Histological characterization of bleaching-induced external root resorption in dogs. Journal of Endodontics 1991;17:436–41.
24. Rotstein I, Torek Y, Misgav R. Effect of cementum defects on radicular penetration of 30% H_2O_2 during intracoronal bleaching. Journal of Endodontics 1991;17:230–3.
25. Simon JHS, Dogan H, Ceresa LM, et al. The apical radicular groove: its potential clinical significance. Journal of Endodontics 2000;26:295–8.
26. Paul BF, Hutter JW. The endodontic-periodontal continuum revisited: new insights into etiology, diagnosis and treatment. Journal of the American Dental Association 1997;128:1541–8.
27. Goldberg F, Massone EJ, Soares I, et al. Accessory orifices: anatomical relationship between the pulp chamber floor and the furcation. Journal of Endodontics 1987;13:176–81.
28. Seltzer S, Bender IB, Ziontz M. The inter-relationship of pulp and periodontal disease. Oral Surgery, Oral Medicine, Oral Pathology 1963;16:1474–90.
29. Abbott PV, Castro Salgado J. Strategies for the endodontic management of concurrent endodontic and periodontal diseases. Australian Dental Journal 2009;54:S70–85.
30. Aksel H, Serper A. A case series associated with different kinds of endo-perio lesions. Journal of Clinical Experimental Dentistry 2014;6:e91–5.
31. Seltzer S, Bender IB, Nazimov H, et al. Pulpitis-induced inter-radicular periodontal changes in experimental animals. Journal of Periodontology 1967;38:124–9.
32. Baumgartner JC, Falkler WA. Bacteria in the apical 5 mm of infected root canals. Journal of Endodontics 1991;17:380–3.
33. Dahle UR, Tronstad L, Olsen I. Characterization of new periodontal and endodontic isolates of spirochetes. European Journal of Oral Sciences 1996;104:41–7.
34. Haapasalo M, Ranta H, Ranta K, et al. Black-pigmented *Bacteroides* spp. in human apical periodontitis. Infection and Immunity 1986;53:149–53.
35. Jansson L, Ehnevid H, Blomlof L, et al. Endodontic pathogens in periodontal disease augmentation. Journal of Clinical Periodontology 1995;22:598–602.

36. Sundqvist G, Johansson E, Sjogren U. Prevalence of black-pigmented *Bacteroides* species in root canal infections. Journal of Endodontics 1989;15:13–9.

37. Sundqvist G. Associations between microbial species in dental root canal infections. Oral Microbiology and Immunology 1992;7:257–62.

38. Thilo BE, Baehni P, Holz J. Dark-field observation of the bacterial distribution in root canals following pulp necrosis. Journal of Endodontics 1986;12:202–5.

39. Trope M, Tronstad L, Rosenberg ES, et al. Darkfield microscopy as a diagnostic aid in differentiating exudates from endodontic and periodontal abscesses. Journal of Endodontics 1988;14:35–8.

40. Baumgartner JC. Microbiologic aspects of endodontic infections. Journal of the California Dental Association 2004;32:459–68.

41. Egan MW, Spratt DA, Ng YL, et al. Prevalence of yeasts in saliva and root canals of teeth associated with apical periodontitis. International Endodontic Journal 2002;35:321–9.

42. Jung IY, Choi BK, Kum KY, et al. Molecular epidemiology and association of putative pathogens in root canal infection. Journal of Endodontics 2000;26:599–604.

43. Nair PNR. Pathogenesis of apical periodontitis and the causes of endodontic failures. Critical Reviews in Oral Biology and Medicine 2004;15:348–81.

44. Siqueira JF Jr, Sen BH. Fungi in endodontic infections. Oral Surgery, Oral Medicine, Oral Pathology, Oral Radiology, and Endodontics 2004;97:632–41.

45. El-Labban NG. Electron microscopic investigation of hyaline bodies in odontogenic cysts. Journal of Oral Pathology 1979;8:81–93.

46. Nair PNR. Cholesterol as an aetiological agent in endodontic failures: a review. Australian Endodontic Journal 1999;25:19–26.

47. Silver GK, Simon JHS. Charcot-Leyden crystals within a periapical lesion. Journal of Endodontics 2000;26:679–81.

48. Tagger E, Tagger M, Sarnat H. Russell bodies in the pulp of a primary tooth. Oral Surgery, Oral Medicine, Oral Pathology, Oral Radiology, and Endodontics 2000;90:365–8.

49. Nair PNR, Pajarola G, Schroeder HE. Types and incidence of human periapical lesions obtained with extracted teeth. Oral Surgery, Oral Medicine, Oral Pathology 1996;8:93–101.

50. Simon JHS. Incidence of periapical cysts in relation to the root canal. Journal of Endodontics 1980;6:845–8.

51. Blomlof L, Lengheden A, Lindskog S. Endodontic infection and calcium hydroxide-treatment. Effects on periodontal healing in mature and immature replanted monkey teeth. Journal of Clinical Periodontology 1992;19:652–8.

52. Jansson LE, Ehnevid H, Lindskog SF, et al. Radiographic attachment in periodontitis-prone teeth with endodontic infection. Journal of Periodontology 1993;64:947–53.

53. Jansson L, Ehnevid H. The influence of endodontic infection on periodontal status in mandibular molars. Journal of Periodontology 1998;69:1392–6.

54. Rupf S, Kannengiesser S, Merte K, et al. Comparison of profiles of key periodontal pathogens in periodontium and endodontium. Endodontics and Dental Traumatology 2000;16:269–75.

55. Adriaens PA, Deboever JA, Loesche WJ. Bacterial invasion in root cementum and radicular dentin of periodontally diseased teeth in humans. A reservoir of periodontopathic bacteria. Journal of Periodontology 1988;59:222–30.

56. Bender IB, Seltzer S. The effect of periodontal disease on the pulp. Oral Surgery, Oral Medicine, Oral Pathology 1972;33:458–74.

57. Gold SI, Moskow BS. Periodontal repair of periapical lesions: the borderland between pulpal and periodontal disease. Journal of Clinical Periodontology 1987;14:251–6.

58. Solomon C, Chalfin H, Kellert M, et al. The endodontic-periodontal lesion: a rational approach to treatment. Journal of the American Dental Association 1995;126:473–9.

59. Torabinejad M, Kiger RD. A histologic evaluation of dental pulp tissue of a patient with periodontal disease. Oral Surgery, Oral Medicine, Oral Pathology 1985;59:178–200.

60. Wong R, Hirsch RS, Clarke NG. Endodontic effects of root planing in humans. Endodontics and Dental Traumatology 1989;5:193–6.

61. Abbott PV. Endodontic management of combined endodontic-periodontal lesions. Journal of the New Zealand Society of Periodontology 1998;83:15–28.

62. Belk CE, Gutmann JL. Perspectives, controversies and directives on pulpal–periodontal relationships. Journal of the Canadian Dental Association 1990;56:1013–7.

63. Simon JH, Glick DH, Frank AL. The relationship of endodontic-periodontic lesions. Journal of Periodontology 1972;43:202–8.

64. Katsamakis S, Slot DE, Van der Sluis LW, et al. Histological responses of the periodontium to MTA: a systematic review. Journal of Clinical Periodontology 2013;40:334–44.

65. Pitt Ford TR, Torabinejad M, McKendry D, et al. Use of mineral trioxide aggregate for repair of furcal perforations. Oral Surgery, Oral Medicine, Oral Pathology, Oral Radiology, and Endodontics 1995;79:756–63.

66. Schmitt D, Lee J, Bogen G. Multifaceted use of ProRoot™ MTA root canal repair material. Journal of the American Academy of Pediatric Dentistry 2001;23:326–30.

67. Langer B, Stein SD, Wagenberg B. An evaluation of root resections: a ten-year study. Journal of Periodontology 1981;52:719–22.

68. Ross IF, Thompson RH. A long term study of root retention in the treatment of maxillary molars with furcation involvement. Journal of Periodontology 1978;49:238–44.

69. Kipioti A, Nakou M, Legakis N, et al. Microbiological findings of infected root canals and adjacent periodontal pockets in teeth with advanced periodontitis. Oral Surgery, Oral Medicine, Oral Pathology 1984;58:213–20.

70. Kobayashi T, Hayashi A, Yoshikawa R, et al. The microbial flora from root canals and periodontal pockets of nonvital teeth associated with advanced periodontitis. International Endodontic Journal 1990;23:100–6.

71. Adriaens PA, Edwards CA, Deboever JA, et al. Ultrastructural observations on bacterial invasion in cementum and radicular dentin of periodontally diseased human teeth. Journal of Periodontology 1988;59:493–503.

72. Chapple I, Lumley P. The periodontal-endodontic interface. Dental Update 1999;26:331–4.

73. Cortellinni P, Stalpers G, Mollo A, et al. Periodontal regeneration versus extraction and prosthetic replacement of teeth severely compromised by attachment loss to the apex: 5-year results of an ongoing randomized clinical trial. Journal of Clinical Periodontology 2011;38:915–24.

74. Ob SL, Fouad AF, Park SH. Treatment strategy for guided tissue regeneration in combined endodontic-periodontal lesions: case report and review. Journal of Endodontics 2009;35:1331–6.

75. Al-Hezaimi K, Naghshbandi J, Simon JHS, et al. Successful treatment of a radicular groove by intentional replantation and Emdogain treatment: four years follow-up. Oral Surgery, Oral Medicine, Oral Pathology, Oral Radiology, and Endodontics 2009;107:e82–5.

76. Gaund TG, Maze GI. Treatment options for the radicular lingual groove: a review and discussion. Practical Periodontics and Aesthetic Dentistry 1998;10:369–75.

77. Hans MK, Srinivas RS, Shetty SB. Management of lateral incisor with palatal radicular groove. Indian Journal of Dental Research 2010;21:306–8.

78. Buhler H. Evaluation of root-resected teeth. Results after 10 years. Journal of Periodontology 1988;59:805–10.

CHAPTER 14

Problems in Endodontic Treatment

M. Hülsmann and B. S. Chong

Chapter Contents

Summary

Problems may be encountered when carrying out endodontic treatment. A patient in pain will require emergency treatment. Achieving adequate anaesthesia allows endodontic treatment to be carried out painlessly and efficiently. However, failure of anaesthesia may occur in acute inflammation; alternative techniques and supplementary anaesthesia may then be required. There may be problems during primary root canal treatment and nonsurgical retreatment. These include gaining access to the root canal system, which may entail the removal of natural obstructions, previous restorations, root filling material/s and broken instruments; there may also be problems with preparation and filling of the root canal system. Although routine endodontic procedures may be tackled by general dental practitioners, complex problems such as instrument removal and perforation repair are often better attempted by specialists. If a problem is foreseeable, all efforts must be directed at avoiding its occurrence; it is axiomatic that 'Prevention is better than cure!'

Introduction

All procedures in healthcare are not without risk. The benefits must outweigh the risks before any intervention, especially irreversible, is undertaken. When problems are encountered, this may have a negative effect on treatment outcome. However, if it can be successfully managed and resolved, it may have relatively little, to no, impact on treatment outcome. In this chapter, some of the common problems encountered in endodontic treatment are outlined, including the decision-making process and management techniques. For more comprehensive coverage, readers may wish to consult textbooks on this subject.[1-3]

Emergency Treatment

It is important that a patient who is in pain, or has a swelling, is rendered comfortable as soon as possible. Even in an emergency situation where the cause/s of the problem appears to be obvious, an accurate diagnosis must be established before any treatment is provided. This can only be achieved by taking a careful history and conducting a thorough clinical examination, followed by appropriate radiographic examination and special tests. The practice of treating the patient with antibiotics and analgesics without attempting to arrive at a correct diagnosis and effectively treat the cause of the pain or swelling is not recommended. In general, antibiotics should only be prescribed when the diagnosis has been established and there is facial or localized swelling but no possibility of access to dental care within a reasonable period.[4]

If the clinician is unclear as to the precise cause of the pain or swelling after the initial examination, active, especially irreversible, intervention should be delayed. Otherwise, treatment rendered may be incorrect and may cause the patient harm. This should be explained to the patient; in the meantime, the patient should not be discharged but carefully monitored or referred to a specialist for an opinion or management. The subject of diagnosis is covered in Chapter 3.

Although the following three conditions: acute pulpitis, acute apical periodontitis and acute periapical abscess, can cause patients to present as an emergency, it must be remembered that other nonendodontic conditions can also cause pain, e.g. food packing, sinusitis, parafunction, neuropathic pain and temporomandibular joint syndrome. The differential diagnosis of dental pain, in general, is covered in Chapter 2.

In situations where the diagnosis is clearer, the emergency treatment consists of applying one or more of these basic surgical principles:

- remove the cause of pain;
- provide drainage if fluid exudate is present;
- prescribe analgesics if required;
- adjust the occlusion if indicated.

There is suggested guidance, a quick reference guide and a web app on the management of acute dental problems available online.[5]

ACUTE PULPITIS

The causes of pulp injury, its prevention and treatment are discussed in Chapter 5. The question is often asked: At what stage should palliative treatment cease and be replaced by pulp extirpation? Ideally, the treatment should be related to the state of the pulp, but this can only be determined indirectly. The clinician relies on the history given by the patient and a thorough examination. As a rule of thumb, if the pulp of a mature permanent tooth causes severe and prolonged pain even after exciting factors such as thermal stimuli are removed or the patient is woken at night with pain, then it is likely that the pulp has been irreversibly damaged and pulp extirpation is indicated. The pulp may die even when the symptoms are apparently those of reversible pulpitis. In a survey, 20% of cracked teeth without spontaneous pain or short-term response to cold eventually became necrotic.[6] With irreversible pulpitis, if the clinician does not have time to extirpate the entire pulp, emergency pulpotomy, as a temporary measure, can usually achieve pain relief.[7,8] However, it may be difficult to anaesthetize an acutely inflamed pulp; this problem is covered later in this chapter. It should be remembered that antibiotics have no beneficial role in treating irreversible pulpitis.[9,10]

ACUTE APICAL PERIODONTITIS

Acute apical periodontitis may be defined as acute inflammation of the periodontium. It is often a direct result of irritation due to the infection in the root canal system[11] and may be associated with acute pulpitis. A purulent exudate is not present periapically, and treatment consists of removing any pulp remnants from the root canal space, irrigation of the root canal system with sodium hypochlorite, drying the canals, sealing in an antimicrobial dressing such as calcium hydroxide and closure of the access cavity. The importance of cleaning the root canal system thoroughly cannot be overemphasized.[12]

Care must be taken not to irritate the periapical tissues by extruding infected intracanal material through the apical foramen. Likewise, overmedicating the canal with an irritant drug may lead to it diffusing periapically, provoking inflammation, or causing damage to apical tissues; this is covered later in the chapter. When an intracanal medicament is used, there is conflicting evidence that the choice of medicament has any influence on postoperative pain.[13,14]

The tooth may be slightly extruded, and the occlusion can be relieved by selectively trimming either the tooth itself or in exceptional circumstances, the opposing tooth. The guiding principle on occlusal reduction should be to do no permanent harm. However, it has been reported that occlusal reduction made no difference to further postoperative pain reduction for teeth with irreversible pulpitis and mild tenderness to percussion.[15] Clinically, heavily worn or heavily restored teeth that require root canal treatment may need to be protected against fracture by the placement of, for example, an orthodontic band; in these cases, the occlusion should be adjusted. The importance of preventing a tooth from fracturing by placing a band to act as a splint cannot be overemphasized.

ACUTE PERIAPICAL ABSCESS

An acute periapical abscess may develop as a sequel to acute apical periodontitis or present as an acute phase of chronic apical periodontitis. An accurate diagnosis may sometimes be difficult. It is common for adjacent teeth to be tender to pressure. It is essential to carry out sensitivity testing of the adjacent teeth so that the correct tooth is identified and treated. Radiography may not be helpful as acute lesions do not become radiologically visible until bone, including the cortical plates, has been resorbed. It is often useful to take a bitewing, as well as a periapical radiograph for diagnostic purposes as coronal leakage or caries may be more evident.

Where a soft tissue swelling exists, the diagnosis is generally easier, but it is important to confirm which tooth is related to the swelling. Relief of pain can be obtained speedily by draining and adjusting the occlusion of the causative tooth. The practice of prescribing antibiotics without draining is incorrect and unnecessarily prolongs the patient's misery. Opening the pulp chamber may cause considerable discomfort because of instrument vibrations, but this can be minimized by stabilizing the tooth with fingers and obtaining access with a small round bur in a high-speed turbine handpiece.

Ideally, the tooth should be allowed to drain until the discharge stops, and the canals should then be irrigated gently with sodium hypochlorite, cleaned of debris and prepared fully, dressed and sealed as normal. Such a regimen rarely leads to complications[16]; however, this is not always possible either because of a lack of time, the tooth is exceedingly tender or there is copious discharge of exudate. In that case, it is permissible to leave the tooth on open drainage but for no longer than 24 hours. At the end of this period, the patient should be seen again and, if comfortable, the root canal system cleaned of debris, irrigated with sodium hypochlorite and instrumented before closure. It is important that the root canal system is cleaned and sealed as soon as possible so that food debris do not pack into the canal/s and invading microorganisms do not cause a further acute flare-up. The practice of leaving the root canal system opened for weeks, if not months, has not been commended[17] and usually leads to periodic 'flare-ups' caused by reinfection from the oral cavity by microorganisms that may be more difficult to eliminate. Leaving the access cavity open for a long period may also lead to further micobial contamination of the root canal system and caries in the pulp chamber.

If a tooth is symptom free while on open drainage but flares up as soon as it is sealed, the thoroughness of root canal system debridement must be questioned; it is also possible that there may be coronal microleakage. These are probably the commonest causes of postoperative flare-up; for no tooth will settle until the root canal system is thoroughly cleaned and there is no coronal microleakage; the coronal seal must be effective. If the clinical crown contains caries or inadequate restorations, these must be removed and well-sealed restorations placed.

Sometimes, because of anatomical difficulties, or the presence of an immovable obstruction in the root canal, it may not be possible to obtain drainage through the canal. In such instances, emergency treatment will depend on the presence, or absence, of a swelling. If a swelling is present and fluctuant, incision and drainage or aspiration through a large bore needle into a syringe, are advisable and generally relieves acute pain. If there is no swelling, supportive antibiotic therapy may be appropriate, followed by nonsurgical (see Chapter 7) or surgical endodontic treatment (see Chapter 10), after the acute symptoms have subsided.

ACUTE FLARE-UP

After instrumentation of a symptom-free tooth, in the majority of cases, the patient can expect little pain. If there is an established periapical lesion before treatment, the likelihood of severe postoperative pain is higher. In general, if there is pain, its intensity will reduce with time. In the short term, the pain is substantially helped by prescribing analgesics, and its intensity is reduced after 24 to 48 hours. Apart from obtaining drainage, patients who present with pain and swelling during a flare-up are managed by prescribing analgesics and antibiotics. If tolerated, ibuprofen prescribed in 600- to 800-mg doses is one of the most effective nonsteriodal antiinflammatory drugs (NSAIDs) for acute dental pain.[18] If the patient is unable to tolerate ibuprofen or aspirin, then paracetamol (acetaminophen) is the analgesic of choice. Flare-ups are more likely to occur in teeth with a periapical lesion.[19] However, there is also suggestion that gender, genetics and psychological state may be predisposing factors in the patient's response to endodontic intervention and the likelihood of flare-ups.[20]

The incidence of flare-ups has been reported to be low, but a much higher incidence of pain could be expected where treatment is inadequate or infected debris is extruded through the apical foramen.[21] Generally, the incidence of extrusion of debris through the apical foramen is lower when the root canal is prepared using a Crown-down approach.[22]

Failure of Anaesthesia in Acute Inflammation

Profound analgesia is essential for pulpotomy or vital pulp extirpation,[23,24] yet there are occasions where in spite of normally sufficient dosage and satisfactory technique, adequate analgesia is not obtained. Such occasions are distressing for the patient and embarrassing for the dentist.

The term *hot tooth* has been used to describe such a situation.[25] There may be heightened pain when the tooth is stimulated by heat or cold and may be tender to bite; it may be difficult, if not impossible, to achieve analgesia of sufficient depth despite repeated local anaesthetic injections. The reasons for this failure are not entirely clear, although various explanations have been proposed.[20,26]

- Anatomical causes

  Due to the anatomy, the local anaesthetic agent is not deposited or insufficient quantity is distributed in proximity to the targeted nerve supply or there may be accessory nerve innervations. In particular, with nerve block injections, relying on anatomical landmarks to locate a 'blind' target.

- Acute tachyphylaxis of local anaesthetics

  Tachyplaxis is the phenomenon in pharmacology in which there is diminished responsiveness after successive administration of a drug. Since local anaesthetic formulations usually include a vasoconstrictor, it may lead to the anaesthetic drug persisting in the tissue for a sufficient amount of time to produce tachyphylaxis rendering the anaesthetic drug less effective when readministered.

- Effects of inflammation

  Local tissue pH – The pH of inflammatory products in the region of the tooth may be more acidic, thus making the local anaesthetic solution potentially less effective.

  Blood flow – There is usually increased vascularity of the tissues in the region of the inflamed tooth, and hence the local anaesthetic agent may be more rapidly removed by the bloodstream, shortening its duration of action.

  Pain receptors (nociceptors) – Inflamed tissue releases mediators that activate, or sensitize, normally quiescent neurons, resulting in an increase in the resistance of nerves to local anaesthetics.

- Central sensitization

  Inflammation induces increased excitability of pain processing neurons in the central nervous system so that normal inputs produce abnormal responses, resulting in difficulties in achieving adequate analgesia.

ALTERNATIVE ANAESTHETIC TECHNIQUES

In endodontic practice, the failure to obtain analgesia is not an infrequent occurrence, and when it does occur, it is more likely to be with a mandibular molar tooth.[20] It must be noted that an acutely inflamed pulp can remain very painful in spite of what appears to be an otherwise satisfactory inferior alveolar nerve (IAN) block injection.[27-29] It has been found that a single IAN block injection of local anaesthetic was ineffective in 30% to 80% of patients diagnosed with irreversible pulpitis.[26] In such instances, an initial option is to repeat the inferior dental nerve block injection and/or the addition of buccal or lingual infiltration injections. If adequate analgesia is still not achieved, several alternatives, including supplementary local anaesthetic techniques and agents, are available[25,30]:

- application of a sedative dressing to the pulp;
- intrapulpal anaesthesia;
- intraosseous anaesthesia;
- sedation.

Application of a Sedative Dressing to the Pulp

Occasionally, the kindest approach is to accept the failure of local anaesthesia, dress the tooth to reduce pulpal inflammation and attempt pulpal extirpation on a subsequent occasion. The pulp may be sedated with a zinc oxide-eugenol dressing[31] or with a corticosteroid–antibiotic dressing.[32,33]

If the pulp has been exposed and is inflamed, it bleeds copiously and should be allowed to do so for 2 to 3 minutes to wash out inflammatory mediators. The exposure is then covered with a pledget of cotton wool dampened with a medicament such as a corticosteroid–antibiotic combination (Ledermix, Haupt Pharma GmbH, Wolfratshausen, Germany, or Odontopaste, Australian Dental Manufacturing, Kenmore Hills, Brisbane, Queensland, Australia). The cotton wool is then covered by a fortified zinc oxide-eugenol cement such as intermediate restorative material (IRM; Dentsply, Milford, DE, USA). On the subsequent visit, a local anaesthetic should again be administered and when considered effective, the pulp should be extirpated. It is usually possible to achieve sufficient anaesthesia for pulp extirpation when it had not been possible on the previous occasion.

Intrapulpal Anaesthesia

Intrapulpal anaesthesia may be used to supplement existing inadequate anaesthesia. The technique consists of injecting local anaesthetic solution into the pulp. The needle is advanced into the pulp chamber, and the solution injected under pressure. Initial pain when the anaesthetic solution is injected under pressure may be reduced by placing topical anaesthetic gel

on the exposed pulp before injection; the patient should also be warned to expect pain. Most topical anaesthetic gels contain either benzocaine or lignocaine (lidocaine) at concentrations of 20% to 30%. Intracanal use of a topical anaesthetic may also helpful when 'hot' vital pulp tissue is encountered apically.

Intraosseous Anaesthesia

Intraosseous injections of anaesthetic may be delivered either via the periodontal ligament, or through the cortical plate. They may be used to supplement existing inadequate anaesthesia,[34] reportedly achieving a higher rate of successful anaesthesia than an IAN block alone in cases with irreversible pulpitis.[25]

In the case of periodontal ligament injections, special syringes allow small, preset increments of anaesthetic solution to be injected intraosseously through the periodontal ligament. The anaesthetic capsule is inserted into a protective sleeve to guard against breakage, and a 30-gauge ultrashort needle is used to inject the solution into the ligament. Before injection, the gingival sulcus must be disinfected and the soft tissues anaesthetized to reduce discomfort during injection. The primary injection is given on the distal aspect of the tooth, and the needle with the bevel toward the root face is inserted into the periodontal ligament space until it is stopped by alveolar bone. The lever is squeezed extremely slowly, and about 0.2 mL of anaesthetic solution deposited. The procedure may be repeated on the mesial aspect of the tooth and in the case of molars, on other surfaces.

Intraosseous anaesthetic techniques, such as the Stabident system (Fairfax Dental, Miami, FL, USA), uses a small, disposable 'perforator' to create a hole in the cortical plate of bone through the attached gingiva. The soft tissues must be adequately anaesthetized first. Anaesthetic is then delivered into the cancellous bone, within the mandible or maxilla, with a matching needle.

Both periodontal ligament injection and injection through the cortical plate produce effective and rapid intraosseous anaesthesia. However, clinicians should be aware of some of the following disadvantages:

- Infection may be introduced into the tissues unless the soft tissues have been disinfected beforehand.

- The injections are painful unless surface anaesthetic and/or conventional anaesthetic have been administered first. Alternative local anaesthetic delivery systems, devices and aids are available to help minimize painful injections.[35]
- Adrenaline (epinephrine) injected intraosseously is rapidly absorbed intravenously. This may result in a noticeable tachycardia. It may therefore be wise to use non-adrenaline containing anaesthetics for these injections in patients with cardiac conditions.
- Periodontal ligament injections alter the occlusion of the tooth very slightly by raising it out of its socket, and a careful check of the occlusion, especially the temporary restoration, must be made.
- During delivery of an intraosseous anaesthetic solution through the cortical plate, the needle may accidentally come into contact and damage the root surface.[36]
- Depending on the agent, the duration of anaesthesia may be shorter. However, there are a number of recent advances in local anaesthesia, including the availability of newer local anaesthetic agents.[37,38]
- It may be difficult to locate the entrance created with the perforator with the injection needle. The X-Tip system (Dentsply, Addlestone, Surrey, UK), for example, overcomes this problem by using a hollow perforator through which the injection needle can be inserted.

Sedation

There are rare cases in which the use of relative analgesia or intravenous sedation is the only way that a vital pulp can be extirpated, or an abscess drained. Generally, the reasons are not related to the effectiveness of local anaesthesia but to the attitude of the patient, for example, someone that is anxious and has a fear, or phobia, of dentists.[20] In such instances, before embarking on such a course, the clinician must be satisfied that the patient is fit, the tooth is of sufficient importance to the patient's well-being and that the patient will accept subsequent, routine treatment without recourse to further intravenous sedation. For further information on sedation, the reader is referred elsewhere.[39]

Problems with Preparation of the Root Canal System

ACCESS CAVITY PREPARATION

The preoperative radiograph must be examined carefully before commencing root canal treatment in order to detect the likely position of the coronal pulp chamber, the root canals and any obstructions that may prevent canal negotiation and instrumentation. Newer, three-dimensional imaging techniques such as Cone beam computed tomography (CBCT) may be useful in selected cases of difficult diagnosis, complex tooth or root canal morphology provided there is sufficient justification, so that the benefits to the patient outweigh the potential risks.[40–42]

In the case of a tooth that has been occlusally 'misaligned' or 'realigned' with a cast restoration, the position of the access cavity may have to be adjusted. It is essential to prepare an access cavity of adequate size so that there are no visual or physical restrictions; the entire roof of the pulp chamber should be removed. If the tooth has been restored with a crown with a satisfactory marginal seal, it may be left in place during endodontic treatment. Removal of the crown with a crown and bridge remover (see later) may improve access but may hinder dental dam placement. Use of magnification and axial light will eliminate most access problems when working through a crown. If the crown is technically deficient, or secondary caries is present, it should be removed along with any caries and a well-sealed temporary restoration placed, before commencing endodontic treatment. Pulp space anatomy and access cavities are covered in Chapter 4.

PROBLEMS WITH PRIMARY PREPARATION OF THE ROOT CANAL SYSTEM

During primary (nonretreatment) preparation of the root canal, the clinician may encounter various natural problems, which may hamper biomechanical debridement of the entire root canal system. These include intracanal hard tissue formation and acute canal curvature.

Intracanal Hard Tissue Formation

Pulp Stones. Pulp stones are not uncommon and may be identified from preoperative radiographs; they are normally not too difficult to remove when ultrasonic instrumentation is utilized. Piezo-electric-powered ultrasonic devices are far more efficient for this purpose than magnetostrictive units. The ultrasonic instrument should be worked around the edge of the stone until it becomes loose. However, it is more difficult to remove a stone from a root canal, particularly if it is attached to the canal wall. In such an instance, if a file can be passed alongside the stone, it may be removed or dislodged by careful filing.

Irritation Dentine. Irritation dentine is formed as a sequel to microbial influence or physical trauma. Careful examination of the preoperative radiograph will show the size of pulp space and the extent of any irritation dentine; hence, it is essential to have an undistorted image. The depth of the floor of the pulp chamber from the occlusal surface of the tooth should also be assessed from the preoperative radiograph. This should help prevent damage to the floor of the pulp chamber when preparing the access cavity. Irritation dentine in the original pulp space should be removed carefully with an ultrasonic instrument or a long-shank bur in the slow-speed handpiece. Diamond-coated ultrasonic tips (CPR tips, SybronEndo, Orange, CA, USA) or periodontal scaling tips (PS tips, EMS, Nyon, Switzerland; See Chapter 6) are particularly well suited to removing irritation dentine. These are designed for piezo-electric ultrasonic units and should be used with copious water coolant; inadequate cooling may cause burning of the dentine.

Good lighting and magnification is helpful as this dentine is normally very different in colour and texture to primary dentine; it may vary from being porous and yellow in colour to hard, dense and dark in colour. The use of an endodontic explorer (DG16) is highly recommended to help detect the canal orifices. Periodically, the operator should stop and assess whether the access cavity is prepared in the correct position. Where the pulp chamber is only partially obliterated, the patent canal orifices are useful landmarks for orientation. If a canal orifice remains elusive, a radiograph should be taken to check that the access cavity is not deviating off course in a mesiodistal direction. Once the endodontic explorer will stick in the canal orifice, it is usually possible to negotiate the canal with a fine file (e.g. ISO size 06).

Calcification normally begins in the pulp chamber and continues in an apical direction as a result of mild pulpal inflammation. Canals that are completely calcified from the pulp chamber to the apical foramen are very rare. Sometimes, canals that look completely calcified on a radiograph can be instrumented because a very fine pathway remains within the calcified material. This may not be visible on the radiograph because of inadequate contrast or resolution. For this reason, where endodontic treatment is indicated, despite the appearance that the root canal is calcified, in the first instance an attempt should be made to negotiate the fine canal using a small file (e.g. ISO size 06) rather than opting for surgery (Figure 14-1). The irritation dentine, which occludes the canal, should be removed with an ultrasonic instrument or a long-shank bur in a slow-speed handpiece. Intracanal irritation dentine, is usually much darker than primary dentine; therefore, magnification and illumination are once again of great help. Once the canal is patent, canal preparation is relatively simple. A lubricant with chelating properties such as Slickgel ES (SybronEndo, Orange, CA, USA), or File-Eze (Ultradent Products, South Jordan, UT, USA), will help to reduce the resistance to passage of a file in a fine canal. It should be made clear that a symptom-free tooth with a calcified canal but no periapical radiolucency does not necessarily require root canal treatment; pulp canal obliteration is often observed, and is not an unusual healing consequence, in teeth with a history of trauma.[43,44]

Acute Canal Curvature

Canals with acute curvature, including S-shaped canals, are more demanding to prepare and the instruments used are subjected to greater mechanical stress. As well as the degree, the more coronal the position of the curvature, the harder it is to instrument the canal. Some preparation techniques and the inherent inflexibility of some endodontic instruments mean that is a tendency to straighten the root canal causing procedural errors such as stripping, ledging, zipping and blockages. Canal transportation is less likely when a Crown-down preparation technique is used. If possible, the coronal third of the canal should be opened sufficiently to allow straight-line access to the middle third of the canal (Figure 14-2). This should not be performed at the expense

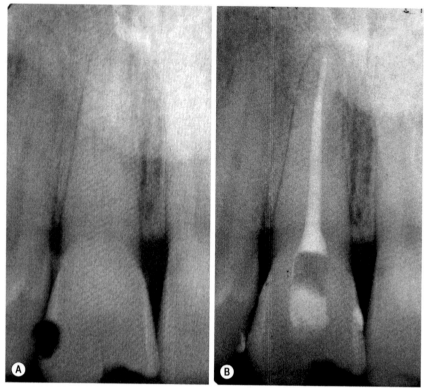

FIGURE 14-1 A maxillary central incisor with a sclerosed root canal. (A) Preoperative radiograph. (B) Removal of irritation dentine coronally enabled access to the root canal, which was then cleaned, shaped and filled.

of unnecessary tooth tissue removal and risking perforating the canal wall. With S-shaped canals, preparing the coronal curve first and then the apical curve has been suggested.[45]

If the canal is to be prepared with hand instruments, better results are achieved with a reciprocal technique, such as the Balanced-force technique, rather than with a filing action.[46] The cross-sectional design and material of manufacture of the instrument are of importance to ensure maximum flexibility. In general, stainless steel files with a triangular cross-sectional design (e.g. Flexofiles, Dentsply Maillefer) and nickel–titanium (NiTi) files are more effective because of better flexibility. Instruments should have a noncutting tip to reduce the likelihood of ledge formation; they should not be overused but discarded as cyclical fatigue has been shown to be associated with instrument failure. Recapitulation is essential to prevent debris build-up in the apical portion of the

canal and resultant blockage. Lubricants such as Slick-gel ES (SybronEndo) or File-Eze (Ultradent Products) help to maintain cutting efficiency and reduce instrument damage caused by clogging of debris.

If engine-driven, especially rotary NiTi instruments are used for canal preparation, then a glide path should first be prepared with either hand or rotary (e.g. Pathfinder or ProGlider, Dentsply Maillefer; ScoutRace, FKG, La Chaux-de-Fonds, Switzerland; G-Files, Micro-Mega, Besançon, France) NiTi pathfinding instruments.[47] It has been reported that when used to prepare severely curved root canals, both engine-driven rotary and reciprocating instruments maintained the original canal curvature well and were safe to use.[48] Although it has also been reported that with S-shaped canals, preparation could be completed faster and canal curvature was better maintained, especially in the apical part, with engine-driven reciprocating compared with rotary NiTi instruments.[49]

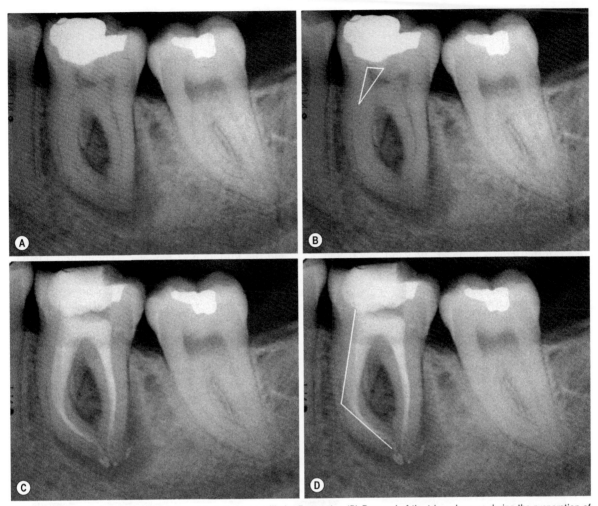

FIGURE 14-2 (A) Acute curvature of the mesial root of a mandibular first molar. (B) Removal of the triangular area during the preparation of the coronal part of the canal reduces the overall canal curvature and the stress on instruments. (C) Completed root canal treatment. (D) Overall canal curvature was reduced.

There is further coverage on canal preparation, including the use of engine-driven NiTi instruments in Chapter 7.

PROBLEMS WITH PREPARATION OF THE PREVIOUSLY TREATED ROOT CANAL (ROOT CANAL RETREATMENT)

Compared with primary root canal treatment, teeth that had been previously root treated requiring retreatment present different challenges.[50] Obstructions encountered during root canal retreatment include extracoronal restorations, posts, ledges, blocked

canals, root filling materials and broken root canal instruments.

Extracoronal Restorations

The decision to remove a satisfactory fitting crown before root canal retreatment may be made to improve access, or prevent damage to the crown, during access cavity preparation. Improved access may be required for locating additional canals and removing broken root canal instruments, or other canal obstructions. However, crown removal also risks damage to the restoration and underlying tooth structure.

There are various devices currently available, which may help remove a crown with minimum damage or intact. In general, a cast alloy crown is easier to remove than a metal–ceramic crown, which may fracture. Removal of crown and bridgework intact is at best an unpredictable process. With careful case selection, a crown may be removed with minimum damage by making a small buccal entrance and inserting a suitable sized instrument, for example, a WAMKey (WAM, Aix-en-Provence, France) to elevate and loosen the crown; the cavity is repaired with restorative material when the crown is re-cemented. Most devices for removing a crown intact rely on the application of a sharp axial force on the crown margin to dislodge the crown. The force may be provided by a sliding weight (e.g. Morrell crown remover, JR Rand, NY, USA), a spring-loaded system (e.g. S-U Crown Butler, Schuler-Dental, Ulm, Germany) or by compressed air (e.g. CORONAflex crown and bridge remover, Kavo, Biberach/Riss, Germany).

Posts

A post that obstructs root canal retreatment will have to be removed.[51] The method of removal will depend on the type of post present.

Metal Posts. The removal of parallel or tapered, passively retained posts may be facilitated by ultrasonic vibration, a post puller, or a Masserann (Micro-Mega, Besançon, France) trepan. Ultrasonic energy may be imparted to the post, or its cement lute via an ultrasonic scaler in order to loosen and aid post removal (Figure 14-3). In general, piezo-electric-driven ultrasonic units are more efficient than magnetostrictive units for this purpose. They should be operated at higher power with waterspray coolant; lack of adequate cooling will cause heat build-up, which may damage the tooth and the supporting tissues. If cement remains at the bottom of the post hole after post removal, it may be loosened and removed with the aid of an ultrasonic tip.

Post pullers such as the Gonon (Thomas) post remover (FFDM Pneumat, Bourges Cedex, France) and the Ruddle post remover (SybronEndo, Orange, CA, USA) work by tapping onto the head of the post and extracting it axially using special forceps; the root face is used as an anchorage point. These devices are efficient at removing both posts that extend above the canal, and posts that have fractured within the canal. However, it is inappropriate to try to remove screw or threaded posts with axial loading devices as it will lead to root fracture.

The Masserann trepan, which is available in different diameters, fits over the post and aims to cut away the cement lute; it works best on parallel-sided posts and least satisfactorily on oval and tapered cast posts.

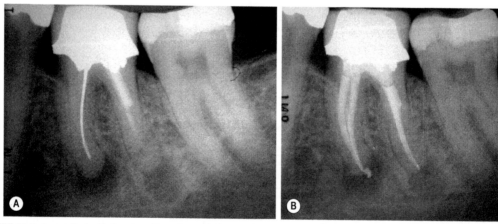

FIGURE 14-3 A mandibular first molar with a silver point and a post requiring root canal retreatment. (A) Preoperative radiograph. (B) The silver point was removed with Steiglitz forceps and the post with ultrasonic instruments. All the canals were prepared and filled with vertical compaction of gutta-percha.

The Masserann trepan has the potential disadvantage of being destructive as circumferential dentine may be removed together with the cement lute.

If a screw post is present, the cement around the head of the post should initially be removed with an ultrasonic instrument. If possible, the type of post should be ascertained, and the relevant spanner, which was used for screw post placement, may be used for its removal. Otherwise, once the post is loosened, it may be rotated using fine forceps. Alternatively, the tapping component of the Ruddle post removal system is designed to screw on to the post end in an anticlockwise direction; this can be used with a torque bar to facilitate the application of force to unscrew the post.

Posts Made from Other Materials. Posts made of materials containing glass, or carbon, fibres are designed to be cemented with adhesive luting agents. This method of luting, allied with the fact that these materials are less rigid than metal alloys, means that they are not suitable for removal with ultrasonic instruments or post pullers. Carbon fibre posts can often be split vertically by drilling through with a small Gates-Glidden bur; the remnants within the root canal should then be removed with an ultrasonic file. Some glass fibre posts may prove impossible to remove; therefore, apical surgery may be indicated.[42]

Ledges and Blocked Canals. Ledges and blockages within canals often occur simultaneously. Inadequate use of irrigant and lack of attention to the preparation of a glide path, or recapitulation, lead to a build-up of debris within the canal. The constrained file, having lost its natural passage to the working length, will then create a ledge within the root canal wall. Once created, ledges are very difficult to bypass. If patency to full working length is to be reestablished, the canal should first be filled with a lubricant with chelating properties, such as Slickgel ES (SybronEndo), or File-Eze (Ultradent Products). A small curve is placed in the last 3 mm of a small file, for example, ISO size 10, and it is manipulated circumferentially around the canal in a watch-winding motion. The file should be of a design with a noncutting tip, such as a Flexofile (Dentsply Maillefer). Eventually, the file should encounter 'tight resistance'; the file is now no longer loose in the canal and is engaging the canal beyond

the ledge. The file should then be worked up and down in a watch-winding action until loose. The canal should be flushed with copious amounts of a suitable irrigant such as sodium hypochlorite. The next file should pass the ledge more easily, and root canal retreatment can then proceed as normal.

Ledging can be avoided in the first instance with the use of more flexible NiTi instruments,[52] generous and frequent irrigation, and if close attention is paid to recapitulation. The causes, recognition, prevention and management of ledging[53] and canal blockage have been reviewed.[54]

Root Filling Materials

A variety of materials may be used to fill the root canal system and will have to be removed as part of root canal retreatment.[55,56]

Gutta-Percha. Gutta-percha may be removed mechanically, thermomechanically, or chemically.[55,56] If the existing gutta-percha points have been poorly condensed, it is often possible to negotiate a file (e.g. Hedstrom) alongside, engage the gutta-percha with a quarter-turn clockwise action and remove it when the file is withdrawn. With well-condensed gutta-percha, the coronal portion should first be removed with Gates-Glidden burs, or engine-driven NiTi instruments; this creates a coronal 'well' for placement of a small amount of solvent (e.g. chloroform, methyl chloroform or xylol) so that the remaining, softened, gutta-percha can then be removed efficiently again with engine-driven NiTi instruments.[55,56] Increasing the speed of the instrument to 300 to 600 rpm may facilitate quicker removal of gutta-percha. Care should be taken to use an instrument with a small tip size so that it does not engage dentine; cutting of dentine at such high speeds is likely to cause NiTi instrument separation. Alternatively, the remaining gutta-percha may be removed with hand files in conjunction with a solvent; care should be taken not to allow the solvent to contact the dental dam as it will be damaged. A file will then pass easily into the mass of gutta-percha, which clings to the file as it is withdrawn; this should be cleaned off before the file is reinserted and the process repeated.

Carrier-Based Systems. The use of engine-driven NiTi files in conjunction with a solvent such as chloroform works particularly well for removing carrier-based systems such as Thermafil (Dentsply).[55] The gutta-percha around the coronal portion of the carrier should be removed to a depth of approximately 4 to 5 mm. Once loosened, an ISO size 35 to 40 Flexofile (Dentsply Maillefer) should be carefully 'screwed' in alongside to engage the carrier. If the file is then gripped with silver point forceps (e.g. Steiglitz), or artery forceps and axial force is applied in a coronal direction, the carrier and remaining gutta-percha can, normally, be removed in one piece. With chloroform in the canal, any last traces of dissolved gutta-percha may be removed with a paper point; this is known as 'wicking'. After all the gutta-percha has been removed, canal preparation proceeds as for initial treatment.

Silver Points. Silver points are rarely used as a root filling material today as they do not fill the canal well and corrode easily. They are easy to remove if loosely placed, if the head of the point protrudes into the pulp chamber and it is possible to gain purchase. Sometimes, an excavator may be used to elevate and remove a very loose silver point. Corroded silver points, or those that are tightly jammed-in, are challenging to remove.

If a silver point is embedded in restorative material, great care should be taken not to cause damage when trying to free the head from the surrounding material; an ultrasonic scaler should be used to remove the last remnants of material. Once the head of the silver point is freed, the point may be gripped with either a pair of Steiglitz forceps, or a Masserann extractor, and removed. Gentle and even pressure should be applied as silver points are very soft and may otherwise break.

If the silver point is entirely within the root canal, removal is more difficult; one Hedstrom file may be inserted, or two Hedstrom files may be passed around the point and braided together in order to engage it to facilitate removal. Occasionally, a silver point may have been cemented with resin-based sealers such as AH 26 (Dentsply); it may prove very difficult to remove and require long periods of careful ultrasonic vibration. Unfortunately, because of the softness of the metal, this often causes the silver point to disintegrate within the canal. For further information on silver point removal, the reader is referred to other information sources.[55,57]

Cement/Paste Root Fillings. Soft pastes such as Endomethasone (Septodont, St. Maur, France) rarely prove difficult to remove (Figure 14-4); endodontic instruments tend to pass straight through them relatively easily. Hard-setting materials, for example, AH

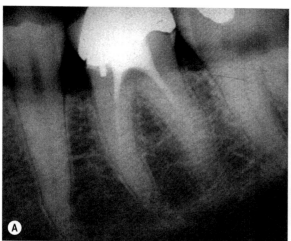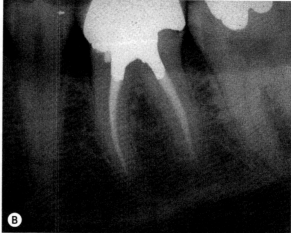

FIGURE 14-4 Paste/cement root fillings that are soft do not normally present problems when it comes to removal. (A) Preoperative radiograph of a mandibular molar; the canals were filled with a soft paste/cement. (B) Postoperative radiograph showing completed root canal retreatment using gutta-percha and placement of an amalgam intraradicular core.

26 (Dentsply) and SPAD (Quetigny, France), are very difficult to remove. In a straight canal, it may be possible to remove such a material with an ultrasonically energized file.[55] Occasionally, voids in the material may allow the passage of a small file. Once the canal is patent, root canal retreatment is relatively straightforward. If a hard-setting paste proves impossible to bypass, surgical retreatment may be indicated. As for root canal sealers, generally, and dependent on the sealer type, a suitable solvent may be used to facilitate removal.[58]

Broken Root Canal Instruments

The use of engine-driven NiTi canal preparation systems is popular; instrument separation can occur and is more common in the hands of inexperienced practitioners.[59] The likelihood of removal of the separated instrument depends on a number of factors[60,61] including its position or whether it is visible and accessible; it is aided by good illumination and magnification. Management of separated instruments may be considered according to whether the instrument has separated in the straight part of the canal, or beyond the curve. However, given the equipment and expertise needed, it is often preferable to refer the case to a specialist.[62,63]

Within the Straight Part of the Canal. If an instrument is present in the pulp chamber, it may be possible, provided access is sufficient, to grip and remove it using Steiglitz forceps, a Masserann extractor (Figure 14-5), or the IRS system (Dentsply).

If the instrument is entirely within the canal, removal is more difficult; these cases are best managed by specialists. A most conservative and efficient way of retrieving such an instrument is by using ultrasonic instrumentation if the fragment is small, or with a Masserann extractor or IRS if the fragment is large (Figure 14-6). The instrument should be vibrated using slender ultrasonic tips, e.g. ProUltra titanium tips (Dentsply) or an ultrasonic file. As most separated endodontic files and burs have flutes which are wound in a clockwise direction, the ultrasonic tip should be applied in a counterclockwise direction around the instrument until it is worked loose (Figure 14-7). In the case of spiral fillers, however, the reverse is true. Care should be taken not to work in a completely dry

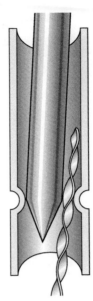

FIGURE 14-5 Diagram of a Masserann extractor which consists of a tube with a constriction; into this a stylet is inserted to trap the broken instrument against the constriction. The broken instrument is removed when the whole assembly is withdrawn.

field as ultrasonic energy can create significant heat build-up, which may potentially damage the tooth and periodontium.[64,65]

Sometimes, if removal is impossible, an instrument may be bypassed, in which case preparation should then proceed as normal. In carefully selected cases, there is no evidence that this recourse will adversely affect the prognosis.[66]

Beyond the Curve. If an instrument is not visible because it has separated within the curved part of a canal (Figure 14-8), removal is more challenging[67] and unpredictable; sometimes it may be possible with the aid of ultrasonic instrumentation.[68] Great care should be taken as significant damage to the root may occur from attempted removal.[69] If it is not possible to remove the instrument, attempts should be made to bypass and incorporate it into the root canal filling. In some cases, it may only be possible to clean, shape and fill the canal to the fractured end of the instrument; in teeth without periapical radiolucencies, this does not seem to adversely affect the prognosis.[70–72]

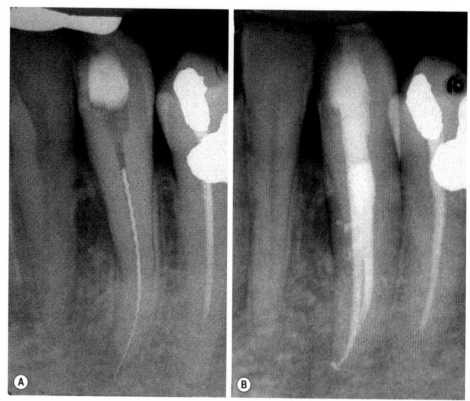

FIGURE 14-6 A long section of a broken Hedstrom file is lodged in this mandibular canine. (A) Preoperative radiograph. (B) Postoperative radiograph; the instrument was removed with a Masserann extractor, and a second canal was also treated.

If removal is unsuccessful and the patient continues to experience pain, swelling or a discharging sinus tract after root canal retreatment, then assessment for endodontic surgery is needed. The presence of a broken instrument in itself is not a problem as it is made of a noncorrodible alloy (e.g. stainless steel, or NiTi); however, it causes a blockage and prevents decontamination of the remaining canal apical to the level of the obstruction, leaving residual infection which will negatively impact on outcome.[70,71,73]

Prevention of Instrument Fracture

Engine-driven NiTi instruments may break because of cyclic fatigue,[74] i.e. they have been used too many times, or torsional failure caused by using too much apical force.[75] Existing UK guidelines, in line with those issued by the Department of Health (England), advised dentists to ensure that endodontic files and reamers are treated as single-patient use[76]; this should mean that instrument fracture through fatigue is significantly reduced.

The angle of canal curvature is a major factor influencing the risk of intrument fracture.[77] Torsional failures may still occur with new instruments in canals with abrupt curvature, a great angle of curvature, or curvature in the coronal portion of the root canal; this may be mitigated by regular disposal of instruments and greater use of hand files beforehand. Coronal curvatures tend to place greater stress on the thicker sections of an engine-driven instrument and increased the likelihood of fracture.[78] If a file is bent, it should not be straightened and reused but discarded. All instruments should be regularly inspected during root canal preparation for signs of distortion, or damage. The breaking of an instrument in a root canal is distressing to the operator and may alarm the patient; its retrieval is also very time-consuming. For these reasons, the use of damaged instruments is a false economy. A number of

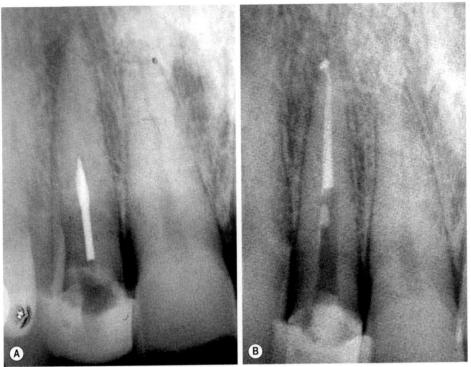

FIGURE 14-7 A Gates-Glidden drill fractured in this maxillary lateral incisor. (A) Preoperative radiograph. (B) Postoperative radiograph; the instrument was removed using ultrasound, the root canal treatment was completed and post space prepared.

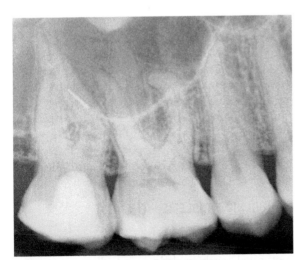

FIGURE 14-8 An endodontic instrument separated beyond the curve in the mesiobuccal canal of a maxillary second molar; successful removal is unlikely possible.

ways of reducing the risk of rotary NiTi instrument fracture have been suggested.[79]

Hypochlorite Accidents. The consequences of unintentional extrusion of sodium hypochlorite into the periapical tissues have been extensively reported in the literature.[80–84] Factors that can contribute to this happening[85,86] include overpreparation of the apical foramen, a preexisting open apex, poor working length control, not using a dedicated endodontic irrigation needle and syringe, and even poor access cavity design.[87] Irrigating syringes should never be jammed into the apical part of the canal, and irrigation should always be performed relatively passively without excessive hydraulic pressure. In addition, it is imperative that sodium hypochlorite is not dispensed in such a way that it may be confused with local anaesthetic solution[88]; severe pain, necrosis and swelling will occur if sodium hypochlorite is injected into the soft tissues.

Sodium hypochlorite is a tissue solvent and is highly caustic to soft tissues at therapeutic concentrations. Contact with tissues may cause acute pain, swelling and bruising, soft tissue necrosis[89] and neurological complications.[90] A case of life-threatening airway obstruction has also been reported.[91]

The treatment of sodium hypochlorite accidents is mostly based on severity of the injury and includes further irrigation with sterile saline, or water, antibiotics and painkillers.[92] Other treatment modalities that have been suggested include local anaesthesia, cold compresses and antihistamines,[93] extraction of the tooth,[94] or surgical intervention.[91] An exhaustive review on complications during root canal irrigation has been published.[95]

In general, extrusion of calcium hydroxide does not appear to cause similar problems as extrusion of sodium hypochlorite, and healing does not appear to be delayed.[96] The exception to this is when calcium hydroxide is extruded into the inferior alveolar canal; this may cause permanent nerve damage so advice should be sought from a maxillofacial surgeon as soon as possible. For this reason, caution should be exercised with the use of spiral fillers to prevent overfilling of calcium hydroxide, especially in mandibular premolars and molars.

Problems with Filling of the Root Canal System

Complications during treatment and retreatment can create particular problems when it comes to filling the root canal system. Noniatrogenic problems as a result of inflammatory processes or the death of the pulp in an immature tooth may also pose a challenge.

NONIATROGENIC PROBLEMS WITH ROOT CANAL FILLING

Chronic inflammatory processes within the pulp may lead to internal hard tissue resorption (internal resorption); this process ceases after pulpectomy. The root canal shape following preparation, however, is irregular and difficult to fill. Warm gutta-percha filling techniques lend themselves better to this type of problem (Figure 14-9).

Resorption of dental hard tissue is common in the presence of chronic apical periodontitis; this is known

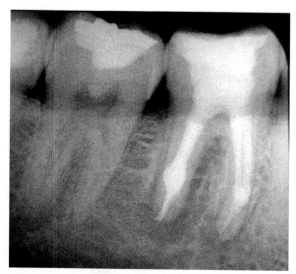

FIGURE 14-9 A mandibular molar with internal resorptive defects; this was filled with gutta-percha using warm vertical condensation.

as external inflammatory resorption. In severe cases of external inflammatory resorption, the apical constriction may be lost. This leads to difficulty in creating a sufficiently robust 'end-point' at the apex that will prevent extrusion of root filling material. Overfilling and a poor apical seal are likely to occur. Traditionally, the problem may be overcome by employing a root-end closure technique such as that used in immature teeth but Mineral Trioxide Aggregate (MTA) is gaining wider acceptance as an apical barrier (see Chapter 12). MTA may be used to fill the canal apically (Figure 14-10) to avoid the laborious process of inducing apical closure. MTA is biocompatible, creates a good seal and stimulates hard tissue formation. The MTA should be placed in the canal using a specially designed carrier such as an MTA gun (Dentsply) and condensed with vertical pluggers such as Machtou pluggers (Dentsply); see Chapter 6. The MTA can be condensed further using an ultrasonically aided file without water spray.[97]

IATROGENIC PROBLEMS WITH ROOT CANAL FILLING

During root canal retreatment, irregularities within the root canal, such as ledges and elbows, are often encountered. An evenly tapered root canal space is easiest to fill with most techniques.[98] The use of a warm gutta-percha technique enables three-dimensional

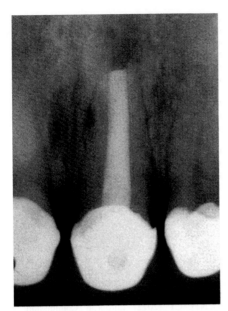

FIGURE 14-10 A maxillary central incisor with an immature apex; the root canal has been filled with mineral trioxide aggregate using pluggers and an ultrasonically activated file.

filling of irregular canals where cold lateral condensation would not be effective.

Dealing with perforations within the root canal system are challenging for the operator. Traditionally, materials such as amalgam and gutta-percha have been used to repair these defects; these materials have been associated with high rates of failure, probably because of microleakage. Modern perforation repair materials such as MTA have been reported to give good results[99,100] in the absence of infection and if there was no communication between the perforation and the oral cavity.[100] Therefore, coronally sited perforations should be cleaned well with sodium hypochlorite to disinfect the dentine and sealed as early as possible; this prevents extrusion of infected material through the defect during preparation of the root canal and will reduce interappointment microleakage. Deeper perforations may be created by stripping the inner wall of a curved canal (strip perforations), or injudicious post space preparation. These are often extremely difficult to manage and should be referred to a specialist. Magnification and good illumination are essential in deep perforation repair. Deeper perforations may have to be repaired at the time of root canal filling.

Learning Outcomes

At the end of this chapter, the reader should be able to recognize and describe the:

- problems commonly encountered in endodontic treatment;
- prevention and avoidance of problems commonly encountered;
- techniques available to deal with these problems;
- effect of commonly encountered problems on prognosis;
- necessity of referral to a specialist.

REFERENCES

1. Chong BS. Managing endodontic failure in practice. London, UK: Quintessence Publishing Co. Ltd.; 2004.
2. Gutmann JL, Lovdahl PE. Problem solving in endodontics: prevention, identification, and management. 5th ed. St. Louis, MO, USA: Elsevier Mosby; 2010.
3. Hülsmann M, Schäfer E. Problems in endodontics: etiology, diagnosis and treatment. London, UK: Quintessence Publishing Co. Ltd; 2013.
4. Robertson DP, Keys W, Rautemaa-Richardson R, et al. Management of severe acute dental infections. British Medical Journal 2015;350:h1300.
5. Scottish Dental Clinical Effectiveness Programme (2013) Management of Acute Dental Problems. Online: <http://www.sdcep.org.uk/wp-content/uploads/2013/03/SDCEP+MADP+Guidance+March+2013.pdf>.
6. Krell KV, Rivera EM. A six-year evaluation of cracked teeth diagnosed with reversible pulpitis: treatment and prognosis. Journal of Endodontics 2007;33:1405–7.
7. Hasselgren G, Reit C. Emergency pulpotomy: pain relieving effect with and without the use of sedative dressings. Journal of Endodontics 1989;15:254–6.
8. McDougal RA, Delano EO, Caplan D, et al. Success of an alternative for interim management of irreversible pulpitis. Journal of the American Dental Association 2004;135:1707–12.
9. Fedorowicz Z, van Zuuren EJ, Farman AG, et al. Antibiotic use for irreversible pulpitis. Cochrane Database of Systematic Reviews 2013;(12):Art. No.: CD004969.
10. Keenan JV, Farman AG, Fedorowicz Z, et al. Antibiotic use for irreversible pulpitis. Cochrane Database of Systematic Reviews 2005;(2):Art. No.: CD004969, doi:10.1002/14651858.CD004969.pub2.
11. Siqueira JF Jr, Rôças IN. Distinctive features of the microbiota associated with different forms of apical periodontitis. Journal of Oral Microbiology 2009;doi:10.3402/jom.v3401i3400.2009.
12. Haapasalo M, Endal U, Zandi H, et al. Eradication of endodontic infection by instrumentation and irrigation solutions. Endodontic Topics 2005;10:77–102.
13. Ehrmann EH, Messer HH, Adams GG. The relationship of intracanal medicaments to postoperative pain in endodontics. International Endodontic Journal 2003;36:868–75.

14. Torabinejad M, Cymerman JJ, Frankson M, et al. Effectiveness of various medications on postoperative pain following complete instrumentation. Journal of Endodontics 1994;20: 345–54.

15. Parirokh M, Rekabi AR, Ashouri R, et al. Effect of occlusal reduction on postoperative pain in teeth with irreversible pulpitis and mild tenderness to percussion. Journal of Endodontics 2013;39:1–5.

16. August DS. Managing the abscessed tooth: instrument or close? Journal of Endodontics 1977;3:316–8.

17. Bence R, Meyers RD, Knoff RV. Evaluation of 5000 endodontic treatments: incidence of the opened tooth. Oral Surgery, Oral Pathology, Oral Medicine 1980;49:82–4.

18. Oxford league table of analgesic efficiency. 2007. Online: <http://www.medicine.ox.ac.uk/badolier/booth/painpag/acutrev/analgesics/lftab>.

19. Iqbal M, Kurtz E, Kohli M. Incidence and factors related to flare-ups in a graduate endodontic programme. International Endodontic Journal 2009;42:99–104.

20. Rosenberg PA. Endodontic pain. Endodontic Topics 2014;30: 75–98.

21. Tsesis I, Faivishevsky V, Fuss Z, et al. Flare-ups after endodontic treatment: a meta-analysis of literature. Journal of Endodontics 2008;34:1177–81.

22. Tanalp J, Gungör T. Apical extrusion of debris: a literature review of an inherent occurrence during root canal treatment. International Endodontic Journal 2014;47:211–21.

23. Malamed SF. Handbook of local anesthesia. 6th ed. St. Louis, MO, USA: Elsevier-Mosby; 2012.

24. Reader A, Nusstein J, Drum M. Successful local anesthesia. Chicago, IL. USA: Quintessence; 2012.

25. Nusstein JM, Reader A, Drum M. Local anesthesia strategies for the patient with a "hot" tooth. Dental Clinics of North America 2010;54:237–47.

26. Hargreaves KM, Keiser K. Local anesthetic failure in endodontics. Endodontic Topics 2002;1:26–39.

27. Kanaa MD, Whitworth JM, Meechan JG. A prospective randomized trial of different supplementary local anesthetic techniques after failure of inferior alveolar nerve block in patients with irreversible pulpitis in mandibular teeth. Journal of Endodontics 2012;38:421–5.

28. Parirokh M, Sadr S, Nakhaee N, et al. Efficacy of supplementary buccal infiltrations and intraligamentary injections to inferior alveolar nerve blocks in mandibular first molars with asymptomatic irreversible pulpitis: a randomized controlled trial. International Endodontic Journal 2014;47: 926–33.

29. Singla M, Subbiya A, Aggarwal V, et al. Comparison of the anaesthetic efficacy of different volumes of 4% articaine (1.8 and 3.6 mL) as supplemental buccal infiltration after failed inferior alveolar nerve block. International Endodontic Journal 2015;48:103–8.

30. Meechan JG. Supplementary routes to local anaesthesia. International Endodontic Journal 2002;35:885–96.

31. Hume WR. In vitro studies on the local pharmacodynamics, pharmacology and toxicology of eugenol and zinc oxide–eugenol. International Endodontic Journal 1988;21: 130–4.

32. Ehrmann EH. The effect of triamcinolone with tetracycline on the dental pulp and apical periodontium. Journal of Prosthetic Dentistry 1965;15:144–52.

33. Schroeder A. Cortisone in dental surgery. International Dental Journal 1962;12:356–73.

34. Bangerter C, Mines P, Sweet M. The use of intraosseous anesthesia among endodontists: results of a questionnaire. Journal of Endodontics 2009;35:15–8.

35. Chong BS, Miller JE, Sidhu SK. Alternative local anaesthetic delivery systems, devices and aids designed to minimise painful injections – a review. ENDO (Lond Engl) 2014;8: 7–22.

36. Graetz C, Fawzy-El-Sayed KM, Graetz N, et al. Root damage induced by intraosseous anesthesia. An in vitro investigation. Medicina Oral, Patologia Oral y Cirugia Bucal 2013;1: e130–4.

37. Ramacciato JG, Meechan JG. Recent advances in local anaesthesia. Dental Update 2005;32:8–10.

38. Ogle OE, Mahjoubi G. Advances in local anesthesia in dentistry. Dental Clinics of North America 2011;55:481–99.

39. Craig D, Skelly AM. Practical conscious sedation. London, England: Quintessence Publishing Co Ltd; 2004.

40. AAE & AAOMR (2015) Use of Cone Beam-Computed Tomography in Endodontics 2015 Update. Joint position statement of the American Association of Endodontists and the American Academy of Oral and Maxillofacial Radiology; <http://www.aae.org/uploadedfiles/clinical_resources/guidelines_and_position_statements/cbctstatement_2015 update.pdf>.

41. SEDENTEXCT (2012) European Commission. Radiation Protection No 172 Cone Beam CT for Dental and Maxillofacial Radiology (Evidence-Based Guidelines); <http://www.sedentexct.eu/files/radiation_protection_172.pdf>.

42. Patel S, Durack C, Abella F, et al. European Society of Endodontology position statement: the use of CBCT in endodontics. International Endodontic Journal 2014;47:502–4.

43. McCabe PS, Dummer PMH. Pulp canal obliteration: an endodontic diagnosis and treatment challenge. International Endodontic Journal 2012;45:177–97.

44. Abd-Elmeguid A, El Salhy M, Yu DC. Pulp canal obliteration after replantation of avulsed immature teeth: a systematic review. Dental Traumatology 2015;doi:10.1111/edt.12199.

45. Lopez-Ampudia N, Gutmann J. Management of S-shaped root canals – technique and case report. ENDO (London Engl) 2011;7–15.

46. Sepic AO, Pantera EA, Neaverth EJ, et al. A comparison of Flex-R files and K-type files for enlargement of severely curved molar root canals. Journal of Endodontics 1989;15:240–5.

47. Ajuz NC, Armada L, Gonçalves LS, et al. Glide path preparation in S-shaped canals with rotary pathfinding nickel-titanium instruments. Journal of Endodontics 2013;39:534–7.

48. Bürklein S, Hinschitza K, Dammaschke T, et al. Shaping ability and cleaning effectiveness of two single-file systems in severely curved root canals of extracted teeth: Reciproc and WaveOne versus Mtwo and ProTaper. International Endodontic Journal 2012;45:449–61.

49. Shao T, Hou X, Hou B. Comparison of the shaping ability of reciprocating instruments in simulated S-shaped canals. Zhonghua Kou Qiang Yi Xue Za Zhi 2014;49:279–83.

50. Hülsmann M, Drebenstedt S, Holscher C. Shaping and filling root canals during root canal re-treatment. Endodontic Topics 2008;19:74–124.

51. Rhodes JS. Disassembly techniques to gain access to pulp chambers and root canals during non-surgical root canal re-treatment. Endodontic Topics 2008;19:22–32.

52. Hülsmann M, Peters O, Dummer P. Mechanical preparation of root canals: shaping goals, techniques and means. Endodontic Topics 2005;10:30–76.

53. Jafarzadeh H, Abbott PV. Ledge formation: review of a great challenge in endodontics. Journal of Endodontics 2007;33: 1155–62.

54. Lambrianidis T. Ledging and blocking of root canals during canal preparation: causes, recognition, prevention, management and outcomes. Endodontic Topics 2006;15:56–74.

55. Duncan HF, Chong BS. Removal of root filling materials. Endodontic Topics 2008;19:33–57.

56. Duncan HF, Chong BS. Non-surgical retreatment: experimental studies on the removal of root filling materials. ENDO (Lond Engl) 2010;2:111–26.

57. Hülsmann M. The retrieval of silver cones using different techniques. International Endodontic Journal 1990;23: 298–303.

58. Martos J, Bassotto APS, González-Rodríguez MP, et al. Dissolving efficacy of eucalyptus and orange oil, xylol and chloroform solvents on different root canal sealers. International Endodontic Journal 2011;44:1024–8.

59. Mandel E, Adib-Yazdi M, Benhamou LM, et al. Rotary Ni-Ti Profile systems for preparing curved canals in resin blocks: influence of operator on instrument breakage. International Endodontic Journal 1999;32:436–43.

60. Alomairy KH. Evaluating two techniques on removal of fractured rotary nickel-titanium endodontic instruments from root canals: an in vitro study. Journal of Endodontics 2009; 35:559–62.

61. Shen Y, Peng B, Cheung GS. Factors associated with the removal of fractured NiTi instruments from root canal systems. Oral Surgery Oral Medicine Oral Pathology Oral Radiology Endodontics 2004;98:605–10.

62. Hülsmann M. Methods for removing metal obstructions from the root canal. Endodontics and Dental Traumatology 1993;9: 223–7.

63. Madarati AA, Hunter MJ, Dummer PMH. Management of intracanal separated instruments. Journal of Endodontics 2013;39:569–81.

64. Hashem AA. Ultrasonic vibration: temperature rise on external root surface during broken instrument removal. Journal of Endodontics 2007;33:1070–3.

65. Madarati AA, Qualtrough AJ, Watts DC. Factors affecting temperature rise on the external root surface during ultrasonic retrieval of intracanal separated files. Journal of Endodontics 2008;34:1089–92.

66. Crump MC, Natkin E. Relationship of broken root canal instruments to endodontic case prognosis: a clinical investigation. Journal of the American Dental Association 1970;80: 1341–7.

67. Cujé J, Bargholz C, Hülsmann M. The outcome of retained instrument removal in a specialist practice. International Endodontic Journal 2010;43:545–54.

68. Suter B, Lussi A, Sequeira P. Probability of removing fractured instruments from root canals. International Endodontic Journal 2005;38:112–23.

69. Madarati AA, Qualtrough AJ, Watts DC. Vertical fracture resistance of roots after ultrasonic removal of fractured instruments. International Endodontic Journal 2010;43: 424–9.

70. Spili P, Parashos P, Messer HH. The impact of instrument fracture on outcome of endodontic treatment. Journal of Endodontics 2005;31:845–50.

71. Panitvisai P, Parunnit P, Sathorn C, et al. Impact of a retained instrument on treatment outcome: a systematic review and meta-analysis. Journal of Endodontics 2010;36:775–80.

72. Ungerechts C, Bardsen A, Fristad I. Instrument fracture in root canals – where, why, when and what? A study from a student clinic. International Endodontic Journal 2014;47:183–90.

73. Cheung GS. Instrument fracture: mechanisms, removal of fragments, and clinical outcomes. Endodontic Topics 2007; 16:1–26.

74. Plotino G, Grande NM, Cordaro M, et al. A review of cyclic fatigue testing of nickel-titanium rotary instruments. Journal of Endodontics 2009;35:1469–76.

75. Sattapan B, Nervo GJ, Palamara JE, et al. Defects in rotary nickel-titanium files after clinical use. Journal of Endodontics 2000;26:161–5.

76. Cockcroft B. Letter from Chief Dental Officer. Department of Health. April 2008. <www.library.nhs.uk/SpecialistLibrary Search/Download.aspx?resID=260319>.

77. Martín B, Zelada G, Varela P, et al. Factors influencing the fracture of nickel-titanium rotary instruments. International Endodontic Journal 2003;36:262–6.

78. Inan U, Aydin C, Tunca YM. Cyclic fatigue of ProTaper rotary nickel-titanium instruments in artificial canals with 2 different radii of curvature. Oral Surgery, Oral Medicine, Oral Pathology, Oral Radiology, and Endodontics 2007;104: 837–40.

79. Di Fiore PM. A dozen ways to prevent nickel-titanium rotary instrument fracture. Journal of American Dental Association 2007;138:196–201.

80. Baldwin VE, Jarad FD, Balmer C, et al. Inadvertent injection of sodium hypochlorite into the periradicular tissues during root canal treatment. Dental Update 2009;36:14–9.

81. Chaudhry H, Wildan TM, Popat S, et al. Before you reach for the bleach … British Dental Journal 2011;210:157–60.

82. de Sermeño RF, da Silva LA, Herrera H, et al. Tissue damage after sodium hypochlorite extrusion during root canal treatment. Oral Surgery Oral Medicine Oral Pathology Oral Radiology Endodontics 2009;108:e46–9.

83. Gursoy UK, Bostanci V, Kosger HH. Palatal mucosa necrosis because of accidental sodium hypochlorite injection instead of anaesthetic solution. International Endodontic Journal 2006;39:157–61.

84. Spencer HR, Ike V, Brennan PA. Review: the use of sodium hypochlorite in endodontics – potential complications and their management. British Dental Journal 2007;202:555–9.

85. Boutsioukis C, Psimma Z, van der Sluis LWM. Factors affecting irrigant extrusion during root canal irrigation: a systematic review. International Endodontic Journal 2013;46: 599–618.

86. Mehdipour O, Kleier DJ, Averbach RE. Anatomy of sodium hypochlorite accidents. Compendium of Continuing Education in Dentistry 2007;28:544–50.

87. Doherty MA, Thomas MB, Dummer PMH. Sodium hypochlorite accident – a complication of poor access cavity design. Dental Update 2009;36:7–12.

88. Pontes F, Pontes H, Adachi P, et al. Gingival and bone necrosis caused by accidental sodium hypochlorite injection instead of anaesthetic solution. International Endodontic Journal 2008;41:267–70.

89. Lee J, Lorenzo D, Rawlins T, et al. Sodium hypochlorite extrusion: an atypical case of massive soft tissue necrosis. Journal of Oral Maxillofacial Surgery 2011;69:1776–81.

90. Witton R, Henthorn K, Ethunandan M, et al. Neurological complications following extrusion of sodium hypochlorite solution during root canal treatment. International Endodontic Journal 2005;38:843–8.

91. Bowden JR, Ethunandan M, Brennan PA. Life-threatening airway obstruction secondary to hypochlorite extrusion during root canal treatment. Oral Surgery, Oral Medicine, Oral Pathology, Oral Radiology, and Endodontics 2006;101: 402–4.

92. Farook SA, Shah V, Lenouvel D, et al. Guidelines for management of sodium hypochlorite extrusion injuries. British Dental Journal 2014;217:679–84.

93. Hülsmann M, Hahn W. Complications during root canal irrigation – literature review and case reports. International Endodontic Journal 2000;33:186–93.

94. Neaverth EJ, Swindle R. A serious complication following the inadvertent injection of sodium hypochlorite outside the root canal system. Compendium of Continuing Education in Dentistry 1990;11:474, 476, 478–81.

95. Hülsmann M, Rödig T, Nordmeyer S. Complications during root canal irrigation. Endodontic Topics 2007;16:27–63.

96. De Moor RJ, De Witt AM. Periapical lesions accidentally filled with calcium hydroxide. International Endodontic Journal 2002;35:946–58.

97. Lawley GR, Schindler WG, Walker WA III, et al. Evaluation of ultrasonically placed MTA and fracture resistance with intracanal composite resin in a model of apexification. Journal of Endodontics 2004;30:167–72.

98. Schilder H. Cleaning and shaping the root canal. Dental Clinics of North America 1974;18:269–96.

99. Krupp C, Bargholz C, Brüsehaber M, et al. Treatment outcome after repair of root perforations with mineral trioxide aggregate: a retrospective evaluation of 90 teeth. Journal of Endodontics 2013;39:1364–8.

100. Mente J, Leo M, Panagidis D, et al. Treatment outcome of mineral trioxide aggregate: repair of root perforations – long-term results. Journal of Endodontics 2014;40:790–6.

CHAPTER 15

Restoration of Endodontically Treated Teeth

F. Mannocci and M. Giovarruscio

Chapter Contents

Summary

There have been many recent advances in the methods available for restoring endodontically treated teeth. Most are related to adhesive techniques, and as a result, composite resin/ceramic materials and nonmetallic posts have become popular. These techniques, including the choice of restoration, are discussed in this chapter. However, regardless of the technique, or the type of restoration, the survival of endodontically treated teeth may be improved by preserving as much useful tooth structure as possible and ensuring that the stress within the tooth and restoration is kept to a minimum.

Introduction

The completion of root canal treatment does not signal the end of patient management. The endodontically treated tooth has to be restored to both form and function. In addition, there is now a greater appreciation that coronal leakage may cause failure. Therefore, the quality of the coronal restoration has an influence on treatment outcome.

The restoration of endodontically treated teeth has changed considerably in recent years. The availability of adhesive techniques has expanded treatment modalities. Amalgam cores and cast metal posts are being replaced by adhesive techniques and fibre posts; all-ceramic and composite resin crowns may be chosen for better aesthetics. Nonadhesive techniques and restorations remain valid treatment options. However, in this chapter, the emphasis will be on adhesive restorations for endodontically treated teeth. Consequently, other restorative techniques have not been covered in

307

any detail. The techniques suggested in this chapter are a matter of preference for the authors.

Effects of Endodontic Treatment on the Tooth

The fracture of endodontically treated teeth can have dire consequences,[1] and in some cases, extraction is the only possible treatment option. The loss of tooth substance as a result of endodontic and restorative procedures may be one of the reasons for the increased number of crown/root fractures that have been observed in endodontically treated teeth compared with vital teeth with similar restorations.[2] The loss of the marginal ridge/s in particular has been found to increase cuspal flexure in vitro.[3] The physical properties of the remaining dentine may also be altered by the effect of medicaments and irrigants.[4] In addition, there is loss of proprioception when the pulp tissue is removed; nonvital teeth have a higher load perception and can withstand up to twice the amount of loading compared with vital teeth before registering discomfort.[5] Other potential reasons for the increased susceptibility to fracture of endodontically treated teeth include changes in the chemical composition of coronal and root dentine as a result of moisture loss and alterations in collagen alignment.[2] However, apart from perhaps a very small increase in the modulus of elasticity,[6] which could be interpreted to be consistent with making the tooth more brittle, most other research has failed to show any change in the inherent physical properties of dentine.[7]

In a study on the impact of endodontic treatment on tooth rigidity,[8] access cavity and post space preparations resulted in a significant reduction in tooth rigidity. In a microcomputed tomographic study on extracted premolar teeth, the amount of hard tooth tissue structure lost as a result of caries removal, access cavity preparation, root canal preparation and post (fibre and cast) space preparation were investigated.[9] Access cavity and post space preparation caused the greatest loss of hard tooth tissue; the loss of coronal tooth structure caused by cast post space preparation was greater than that caused by fibre post preparation.[9] From the available evidence, mostly related to premolar teeth, the loss of tooth structure is the most

significant factor in the weakening of endodontically treated teeth. Since adhesive restorative techniques do not require the creation of macromechanical retention, there is consequently a reduction in hard tooth structure loss.

Survival of the Endodontically Treated Tooth

The survival of endodontically treated[10,11] and of retreated teeth[10] have been found to be between 8% and 97% respectively, in large epidemiological studies, involving a large number of teeth, in subjects followed between 3 and 8 years. This compares favourably with implant-supported crowns.[12] The failure rate of endodontically treated teeth restored with metal–ceramic crowns has been reported to be significantly higher than that of vital teeth.[13] However, a systematic review[14] showed that endodontically treated teeth restored with crowns have a higher long-term survival rate (81 ± 12% after 10 years) compared with teeth without crown coverage (63 ± 15% after 10 years). Interestingly, in the first 3 years, the survival rate of teeth without crown coverage was found to be satisfactory (84 ± 9%), but there was a significant decrease in survival rate after this period.[14] These results are in agreement with those of two randomized clinical trials on endodontically treated premolars restored without crown coverage.[15,16] Teeth restored with fibre posts and direct composite resin were found to be more effective than amalgam in preventing root fractures but less effective in preventing secondary caries.[16] Therefore, an adequate assessment of the tooth prognosis is essential[17] (see Chapter 3). It was shown that endodontically treated teeth are more often extracted as a result of restorative, rather than endodontic, failures. It is generally acknowledged that such failures are the result of errors made in the treatment planning phase.[18]

Timing the Restorative Procedure

Some patients are willing to go to almost any length to try and hold on to a tooth, even if the prognosis is acknowledged to be guarded. Others may be unmotivated to embark on any complex treatment or may wish only to invest in options they consider entirely predictable. Therefore, it is essential that endodontic treatment is part of an overall strategic patient management plan. It would be better to consider extraction and construction of a fixed prosthodontics supported by a tooth, or implant, if the restorability is questionable (see Chapter 3). Although finance should never dictate treatment planning, in reality, it remains a factor to consider when decision-making. In certain circumstances, after considering the costs of endodontic treatment and restoration and the prognosis for the tooth, extraction and replacement may be preferable to preservation. If tooth retention is desired, often a combination of endodontic, periodontal and restorative treatment may be necessary to rescue a tooth (Figure 15-1). However, once the decision to root treat and restore has been taken, the next decision will be how long to wait after root canal treatment before placing the final restoration. There is no set answer but the following factors should be considered:

- preexisting endodontic status;
- quality of the root canal filling;
- position of the tooth in the mouth;
- type of restoration planned.

After completion of root canal treatment, if the result is technically satisfactory and the tooth is free of symptoms, it would be reasonable to proceed immediately to placement of the final restoration, especially when dealing with a previously vital, uninfected tooth. Although previously vital, if the tooth is tender to biting, or lateral pressure after satisfactory completion of root canal treatment, it should be put on probation for 2 to 3 weeks. Hopefully, at the end of this period, the tooth is more comfortable and the final restoration can then proceed. If not, then an extended period of monitoring, or a review of the possible causes, for continuing symptoms including the need for retreatment should be considered.

If there was apical periodontitis before treatment but the periapical radiolucency is less than 2 mm in diameter and the root filling is satisfactory, then if symptom free, the tooth should be treated in the same way as for vital teeth and restored without delay. In contrast, if the periapical radiolucency is greater than 2 mm in diameter, the root filling is technically satisfactory, and the tooth is symptom free, a short probationary period may be necessary. Regardless of whether a tooth is vital or nonvital, if the quality of the root filling is unsatisfactory, root canal retreatment should be considered before placement of the final restoration. Similarly, in cases where the prognosis is in doubt for whatever reason, it is prudent to delay the final restoration until there is clinical evidence and in some cases, radiological evidence of healing. If the decision is taken to wait for evidence of healing, it is imperative that the remaining tooth structure is protected by an adequate interim restoration, which also prevents coronal leakage. If adequate cusp coverage is difficult to achieve with interim plastic restorations, the placement of, for example, an orthodontic band is indicated to prevent tooth/root fracture.

Restoration Choice

The choice of restoration for an endodontically treated tooth is dependent on the amount of coronal tooth tissue left. In fact, this single most important factor will dictate the retention of the restoration and the fracture susceptibility of the tooth.

Most randomized clinical trials on the restoration of endodontically treated teeth are focused on posterior teeth. The data on the survival of anterior teeth are only available from studies in which both anterior and posterior teeth have been included.[19,20] The suggestion from the existing literature is that there is a relationship between the fracture resistance of endodontically treated teeth and the residual amount of tooth structure. Hence, the life expectancy of endodontically treated teeth may not necessarily be increased by the choice of restoration but rather by the amount of tooth structure preserved.

Anterior and posterior endodontically treated teeth present differing restorative demands. Anterior teeth may be less prone to fracture, but compared with posterior teeth, aesthetics is a major consideration.

ANTERIOR TEETH

Composite Resin Restoration

In anterior teeth where there has been little previous restoration, a combination of composite resin placed over a base of glass ionomer cement may suffice. Composite resin is the most appropriate material for restoring the access cavity given its physical properties,

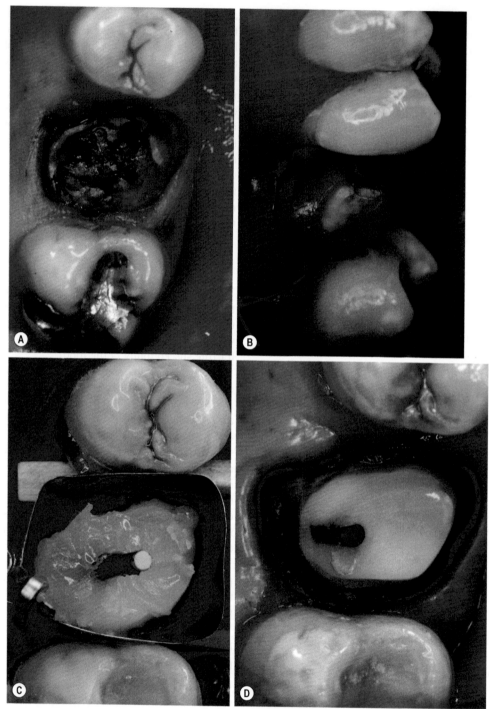

FIGURE 15-1 A badly broken-down maxillary left first molar (A) requiring crown lengthening (B) before being restored with a fibre post and composite resin core (C, D), followed by a metal–ceramic crown (E, F). (From Mannocci et al 2008, with permission of Quintessence Publishing Co., Ltd.)

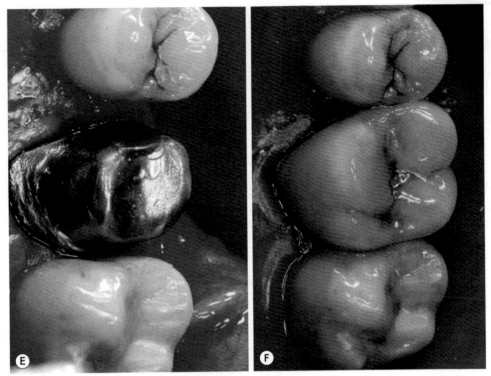

FIGURE 15-1, cont'd

high-quality surface finish and the good seal achieved with bonding. Where a eugenol-containing root canal sealer has been used, care should be taken to ensure that the root canal filling is removed to the level of the cervical neck of the tooth if potential discoloration of the dentine is to be avoided.

If the tooth is discoloured, bleaching techniques may be used, particularly if the discolouration is mild (Figure 15-2). Internal and external bleaching techniques may be applied.

Ceramic or Composite Resin Veneers

If the coronal tooth tissue loss is less than one-third, the palatal aspect of the tooth can be preserved, but it is impossible to obtain a good aesthetic result using a direct restoration; therefore, a ceramic, or composite resin, veneer may be placed. Veneers normally cover the entire labial surface of the tooth, including the incisal edge and through to the proximal contacts (Figure 15-3). Ceramic, or composite resin, veneers are seldom recommended for endodontically treated

anterior teeth as it is not easy to incorporate the access cavity within such restorations.

Metal–Ceramic Crowns

Among nonadhesive techniques, metal–ceramic crowns have become the most commonly prescribed indirect restoration for endodontically treated anterior teeth. A reduction in the labial surface of approximately 1.8 to 2 mm is necessary. The extent of tooth reduction may compromise the strength of the remaining tooth tissue; therefore, caution should be exercised before prescribing such a restoration. Far from preserving residual tooth structure, it may actually promote its loss. In general, crowning of anterior teeth is indicated if the amount of tooth structure left is not sufficient for a direct restoration and for aesthetic reasons.

Gold–Porcelain Infusion Crowns

Gold–porcelain infusion crowns offer two main advantages. The labial tooth reduction required (1.0–1.2 mm) is less extensive compared with that for a

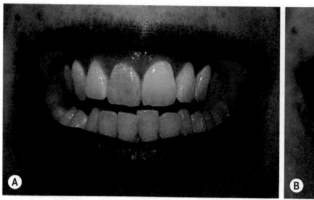
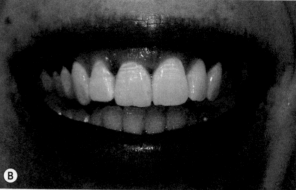

FIGURE 15-2 A root-treated maxillary right central incisor, discoloured resulting from trauma (A); after internal bleaching, an aesthetically improved result was obtained (B) without the need for a cosmetic restoration. (Reproduced courtesy of C. Jones.)

metal–ceramic crown; this is of potential benefit in terms of strength and tooth preservation. In addition, the colour of the underlying gold allows for a better aesthetic result, especially at the cervical area (Figure 15-4).

All-Ceramic Crowns

All-ceramic crowns are more fragile than metal–ceramic crowns. However, the advantages of all-ceramic crowns are:

- labial tooth reduction required is less than that for metal–ceramic crowns;
- absence of a metallic substructure allows a better aesthetic result, especially in areas close to the soft tissues.

Endodontically treated teeth are often dischromic, and therefore, opaque ceramic cores are indicated. As abutments for bridges, all ceramic crowns are only indicated for three-unit bridges in cases of high aesthetic requirement; in such cases, a zirconium construction is indicated.

Resin Crowns

Resin crowns require less tooth tissue reduction (typically 0.8–1.0 mm), and the aesthetics are good. However, they are just as expensive as metal–ceramic and all-ceramic crowns, yet they are not as durable. They may be considered as interim rather than final restorations.

POSTERIOR TEETH

Amalgam Restoration

A conventional amalgam restoration, including interproximal extension but no cuspal coverage, is largely contraindicated because of the high risk of cuspal or root fracture.[21] Amalgam restorations providing a minimum of 2 mm of cuspal coverage were regarded as particularly suitable for mandibular molars, but aesthetic concerns have diminished its popularity. In a study on the long-term survival of extensive amalgam restorations that involve the rebuilding of cusps and the provision of auxiliary retention, it was reported that clinical survival was independent of retention method, operator, tooth type and the extent of the restoration[22]; the cumulative survival rate was 88% at 100 months.

In maxillary molars, the coverage of the functional palatal cusp is mandatory; the coverage of the buccal cusps may not be necessary if there is no contact in lateral movements. However, in mandibular molars, all the cusps should be covered and protected.

Amalgam restorations are also used as core build-ups before crowning of posterior teeth; there are no clinical studies on the performance of amalgam as a core material. The amalgam is packed into the pulp chamber, and if necessary, the root canal space to provide intraradicular retention. If the pulp chamber is less than 4-mm deep, a metal post is necessary to help retain the amalgam core. For intraradicular

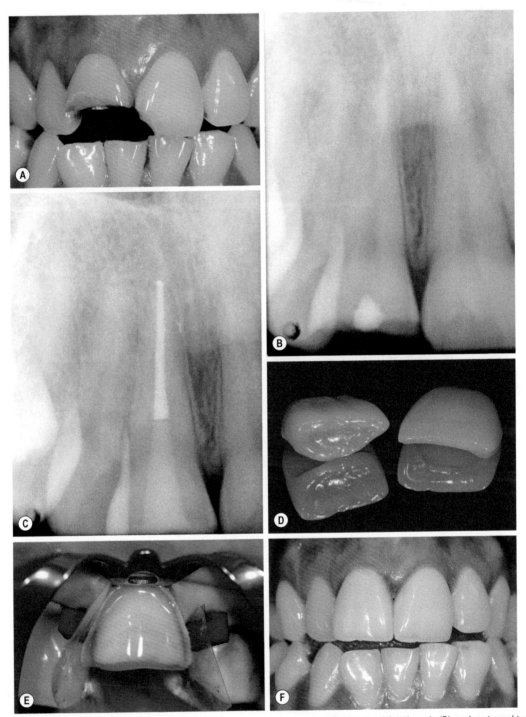

FIGURE 15-3 Traumatized maxillary central incisors (A). Radiograph showing a crown fracture involving the pulp (B), and root canal treatment was needed (C). Ceramic veneers were then made for both teeth (D). These were cemented with composite resin under dental dam isolation (E). An excellent aesthetic result was achieved (F), and the supragingival margins ensure good periodontal health.

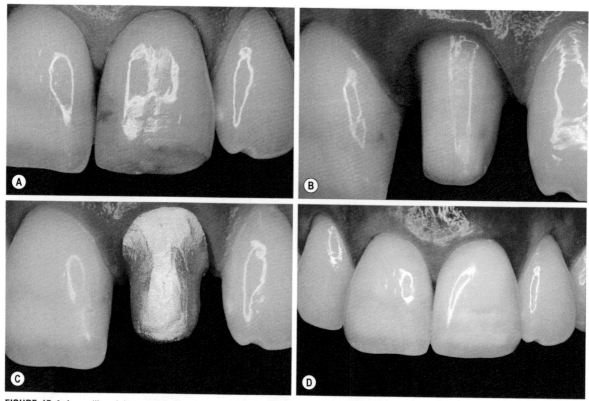

FIGURE 15-4 A maxillary left central incisor is restored with a gold–porcelain infusion crown. (From Mannocci et al 2008, with permission of Quintessence Publishing Co., Ltd.)

retention, a minimum of 3 mm of amalgam should be packed into the root canal space.

Composite Resin Restoration

In general, composite resin restorations cannot be regarded as definitive restorations in posterior teeth except in cases where there has been very limited loss of tooth structure, for example, small interproximal boxes and little or no cuspal overlay (Figure 15-5).

There is no consensus on the minimum thickness of composite resin required to protect cusps from fracture. Coverage of all cusps with less than 2.5-mm thickness of composite resin has been suggested. In most cases, the loss of tooth structure caused by proximal caries and the resultant large and deep access cavity makes the placement, shaping and finishing of a direct composite resin restoration difficult to perform. The problem may be compounded if cuspal coverage has to be provided. In such cases, a direct composite filling may result in a poor reconstruction of the coronal anatomy, and deficient contact points will not be capable of preventing food impaction.

Composite resin restorations are also used as core build-ups before provision of crowns. They may be used in conjunction with posts if radicular retention is required.

Gold Onlays

Gold onlays may be an excellent option for the restoration of endodontically treated teeth, but they have largely been abandoned because of poor aesthetics. They have the advantage of allowing for the preservation of sound tooth structure. The impression procedure is relatively simple because the margins are supragingival, and periodontal health is easy to maintain.

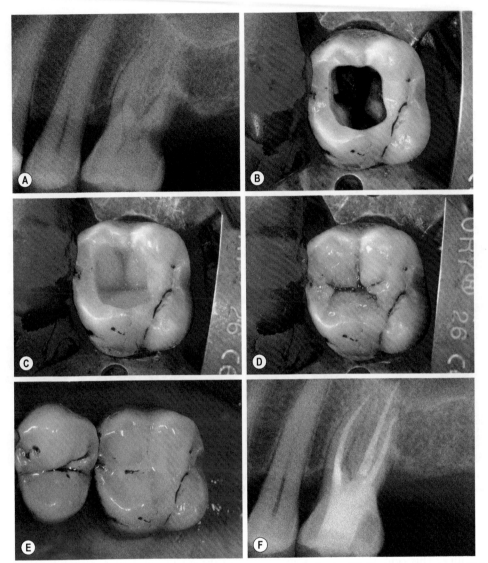

FIGURE 15-5 A maxillary left first molar with distal root caries penetrating into the pulp chamber (A). The tooth was restored with two separate composite resin fillings after completion of the root canal treatment (B–E); this restoration will form an ideal core should a crown be needed in the future. Radiograph after completion of endodontic and restorative treatment (F).

Gold onlays are still appropriate in cases where aesthetics are not a major concern. If this type of restoration is planned, coverage of all cusps is advisable.

Gold Crowns

Like gold onlays, this type of restoration is still appropriate in teeth where aesthetics are not of paramount importance, such as the maxillary second molar (Figure 15-6) or where there is limited interocclusal

space and as bridge abutments. Gold crowns permit the preservation of a greater amount of sound tooth structure compared with metal–ceramic crowns as the required tooth reduction is comparatively less.

Composite Resin and Ceramic Onlays/Crowns

Such restorations are contraindicated in teeth that are meant as bridge abutments. An initial direct, self-curing composite resin core build-up is generally

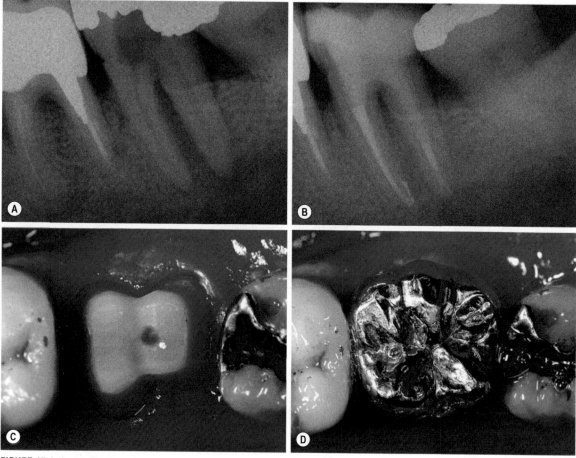

FIGURE 15-6 A mandibular left second molar with a significant interradicular endodontic lesion (A). After completion of root canal treatment, the tooth was restored with a fibre post and composite resin core (B, C), and a gold crown placed (D).

indicated; the colour should be a shade different from that of dentine in order to differentiate the composite from the dentine. This core will serve as a guide in designing a cavity for optimal material thickness. Posts are not normally used for retention of the core.

The onlay preparation is similar to that used for vital teeth. A minimum thickness of 1.5 to 2.0 mm is required for the composite resin or ceramic material. The margins are normally a 90-degree shoulder finish, and the internal line angles of the cavity are rounded. Proximal boxes should only be extended above the contact points, and internal walls should be divergent. Coverage of all the cusps with a thickness of no more than 2.5 to 3.0 mm is usually recommended. Glass ionomer cement, or flowable composite resin, may be

placed over the root filling and in the pulp chamber to achieve the required thicknesses and internal form of the cavity preparation. Ceramic onlay/crowns are normally cemented with adhesive resins.

All ceramic crowns are not indicated in posterior teeth because of the risk of fracture; although they are sometimes used for aesthetic reasons. Zirconia-based crowns (Figure 15-7), in particular, have become very popular because of their good midterm survival rates, which were found to be 89% after 2 to 6 years in a recent retrospective study.[23] However, the available evidence on the long-term survival of such restorations is still inconclusive despite the robust nature of zirconia as a coping for crowns; the plane of weakness of these crowns is at the interface between this coping

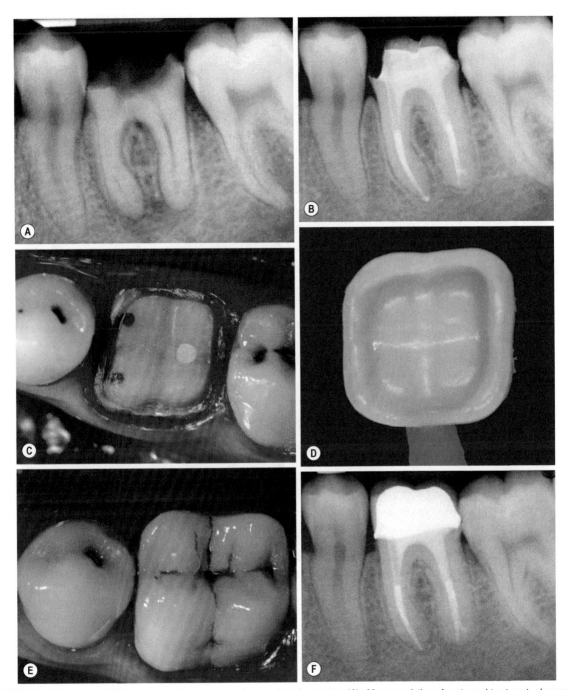

FIGURE 15-7 Mandibular left first molar with severe loss of coronal tooth structure (A). After completion of root canal treatment, placement of fibre posts and composite resin core (B, C), the tooth was restored with a zirconia crown (D, E). The review radiograph after 3 years shows evidence of healing (F).

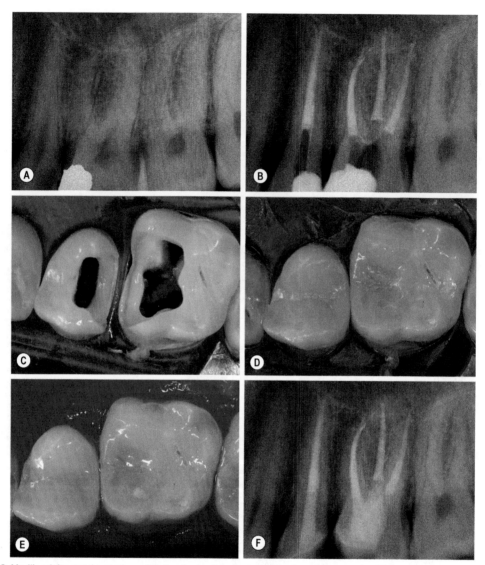

FIGURE 15-8 Maxillary left second premolar and first molar requiring root canal treatment. Preoperative (A) and postoperative radiographs (B). Since there is still a considerable amount of residual tooth structure left (C), both teeth were restored with composite onlays (D,E). Radiograph after the completion of endodontic and restorative treatment (F); the composite resin onlays are radiolucent, hence not obvious radiologically.

and the laminated porcelain.[24] There is no clear evidence to favour ceramic, or composite resin, onlays/crowns, but composite resin onlays/crowns are generally less expensive and easier to repair (Figure 15-8).

Metal–Ceramic Crowns

Cuspal coverage is required where tooth structure loss is more than that associated with an access cavity. Metal–ceramic crowns are most extensively used for restoring posterior teeth (see Figure 15-1) and as bridge abutments. Unfortunately, a disadvantage is that heavy tooth reduction is necessary to create sufficient room for provision of metal–ceramic crowns. A recent clinical trial[25] showed a 94% survival rate of metal–ceramic crowns at 8 years.

Posts

INDICATIONS FOR POSTS

In the restoration of endodontically treated teeth, the placement of a post is generally suggested if the amount of residual tooth structure is not sufficient to support a core made of a plastic material (amalgam or composite). Composite resin as a core material has been tested extensively in clinical trials. In a controlled clinical study of up to 17 years,[20] and another after 5 to 10 years,[26] teeth restored with crowns and composite resin cores performed similarly to those restored with prefabricated metal and cast posts.

The idea that the placement of a post does not reinforce a tooth is indeed very popular and remains debatable. However, this concept was challenged in two studies; a 2-year[27] and a 3-year[28] randomized clinical trial on endodontically treated premolars restored with crowns and fibre posts reported the increased probability of survival. In other words, there were more teeth not restored with a fibre post lost because of crown or root fractures.

Clearly, there are many clinical cases in which the use of a post is not indicated. The classical example being the restoration of a mandibular molar with a ceramic or composite onlay where there is a wide and deep pulp chamber, and a considerable amount of tooth structure left (see Figure 15-5). In these cases, the preparation of a post space will not only result in a significant loss of tooth structure but also in an increased risk of root perforation.

A systematic review of the literature[29] on root canal posts for the restoration of root-filled teeth; only one randomized clinical trial was found comparing fibre and cast posts, providing evidence of a longer survival rate for fibre post restored teeth, but the evidence was regarded as weak. In a microcomputed tomographic study on the restoration of teeth with three residual coronal walls, the modification of the post space for a fibre post into that required for a cast post of the same size and shape more than doubled the loss of hard tooth tissue.[9]

A literature review[30] on clinical studies of fibre posts reported that fibre-reinforced composite posts outperform metal posts in the restoration of endodontically treated teeth; however, the evidence cannot be considered as conclusive. The placement of a fibre-reinforced composite post would seem to protect against failure, especially under conditions of extensive coronal destruction; the most common type of failure with fibre-reinforced composite posts is debonding.[30]

The number of variables involved in designing clinical studies on the restoration of endodontically treated teeth does not allow for its application to all teeth. For example, both the aforementioned clinical studies were carried out on premolar teeth, and clearly the clinical context may be very different, for instance, with anterior teeth, or with molars.

The available evidence does not rule out the use of cast posts; however, since the use of cast posts may result in a significantly greater loss of tooth structure compared with fibre posts,[9] their use should be limited to those cases in which no additional dentine has to be removed to allow for their cementation.

LENGTH OF POSTS

The rules regarding the length, diameter and root/post ratio are based on laboratory studies,[31] or anecdotal evidence. The length of the post classically assumed to be ideal is when it reaches two-thirds the length of the root. Unfortunately, most roots have curvatures that begin far more coronally; therefore, this rule cannot be applied in many cases (Figure 15-9). However, in a finite element analysis, it was shown that the extension of posts to the apical third of the root allowed for ideal stress distribution to the alveolar bone.[32] It was also shown that the tensile strength of the dentine in the apical third of the root was far higher than that of the coronal third.[33] In conclusion, a post that is longer than the clinical crown of the tooth is advisable to limit the chance of decementation and root fracture. Longer posts will ensure an even better distribution of stresses; however, particularly in long roots, posts that reach, for example, three-quarters of the length of the canal may be extremely difficult or impossible to remove if nonsurgical retreatment is necessary. In such cases, apical surgery is the only option left to address endodontic failure.

Post length cannot be considered in isolation without reviewing the length of the root canal filling that must remain if the apical seal is to be preserved.[34] There does not appear to be a satisfactory answer to this question. The minimum acceptable length of root

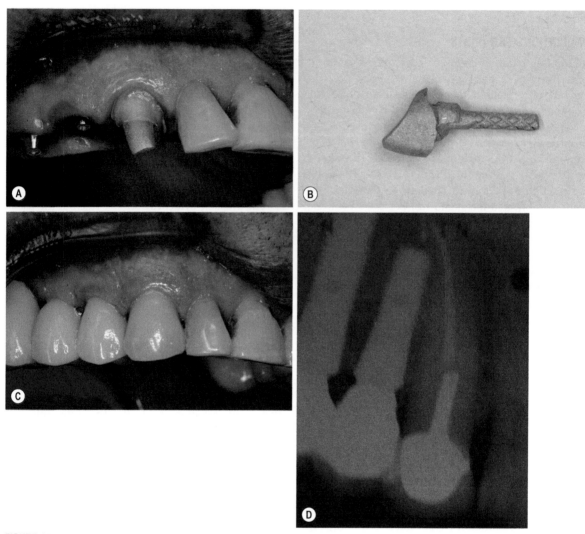

FIGURE 15-9 A maxillary right canine that looks easy to restore with a cast post and core (A–B), followed by a metal–ceramic crown (C). However, the canal curvature in the coronal third is such that an ideal length of post cannot be achieved (D). (Reproduced courtesy of L. Howe.)

filling is 5 mm,[35] but it is based on the use of traditional root canal sealers and luting cement for posts. With more modern materials, a minimum of 4 mm of root filling should be acceptable to ensure the preservation of an adequate apical seal. If this is not possible, it is a restorative dilemma deciding on whether to compromise the length of root canal filling or the length of the post. If the length of root canal filling falls shorter 3 mm, the relative frequency of periapical lesions increases significantly.[36]

DIAMETER OF POSTS

In most cases, if the canal is adequately shaped during root canal treatment, the enlargement that is necessary to obtain a correct post space preparation is minimal; again, it is impossible to define rules that are valid for all root types. To avoid root perforations, or the excessive removal and weakening of root structure, post space preparation is best carried out by the clinician that root-treated the tooth, who is best placed to appreciate the inherent root morphology of the tooth concerned.

THE FERRULE EFFECT

A ferrule effect may be defined as the envelopment of the tooth structure by a crown. The ability to obtain a ferrule effect is regarded as pivotal to the success of any extracoronal restoration, irrelevant of the core that has been placed. Evidences in favour of this concept are limited to laboratory studies.[37] The ideal extent of a ferrule remains contentious, with the complete envelopment of, at least, 2.0 mm of coronal tooth tissue regarded as optimal.[37] This should provide adequate resistance to the lateral forces imparted on the restored tooth. Ideally, this ferrule should be continuous around the entire circumference of the tooth.

A randomized clinical trial[27] found that in premolar teeth with almost complete loss of coronal tooth structure restored with fibre posts and composite, the presence of a ferrule did not improve tooth survival. Therefore, any ferrule should be considered in the context of the individual case, with respect to the occlusion and the quality and nature of the post and core in that particular case. Adhesive techniques may allow thinner sections of coronal tissue to be preserved in ways which are not possible with traditional methods.

IDEAL PROPERTIES OF POST/CORES

The ideal properties of post/cores include:
- adequate compressive strength;
- strong enough to prevent flexion of the core during parafunctional movement;
- resistance to leakage of oral fluids at the core/tooth interface;
- ease of manipulation;
- ability to bond to the remaining tooth structure;
- thermal coefficient of expansion and contraction similar to tooth tissue;
- minimal potential for water absorption and inhibition of dental caries.

Although not ideal, composite resins have the majority of these properties and are the material of choice as both post and core materials. As a core build-up material, composite resin may be bonded to the remaining tooth structure using dentine adhesives.

PROPERTIES OF FIBRE POSTS

Studies have shown that the mechanical properties of carbon, glass and quartz fibre posts are substantially similar; for this reason, the more aesthetic glass and quartz fibre posts have now replaced carbon fibre posts.[38] The modulus of elasticity of fibre posts is generally lower than that of metal posts; nonetheless, it is three to four times higher than that of dentine.[38] The main difference, in terms of mechanical properties between fibre and metal posts, is the loss of flexural strength that affects fibre posts that are exposed to cyclic loading in a wet environment, or are thermocycled.[38] As a result of this, the mode of failure of fibre post-restored teeth is unlikely to be root fracture but normally, decementation that may, or may not, be associated with the development of caries at the interface between the tooth and the restoration.

The adhesion of fibre posts to the composite core is mainly micromechanical. The irregularities on the surface of the post provide the retention for the bonding resin. It has been reported that silanization of fibre posts may increase the retention of the composite cores,[39] but these results have not been confirmed by others.[40]

CLINICAL AND TECHNICAL ASPECTS OF FIBRE POST RESTORATIONS

Tooth Isolation

As with all clinical procedures that involve adhesive dentistry, the use of the dental dam is preferred.

Removal of the Gutta-Percha and Canal Enlargement

This is easily carried out using Gates-Glidden or Largo drills (Figure 15-10A). Heated instruments such as System B (SybronEndo, Orange, CA, USA) may also be used to remove gutta-percha root filling. If a drill is used, overenlargement of the canal should be avoided; it is preferable to fill any potential gaps between the post and the canal with composite resin rather than risk root perforation. The need for a bur matching the post is usually not necessary, but if desired, it should be used with caution to reduce the risk of root perforation.

Removal of Temporary Cement and Sealer Remnants

The removal of temporary cement and any sealer remnants is easily accomplished with the use of ultrasonic

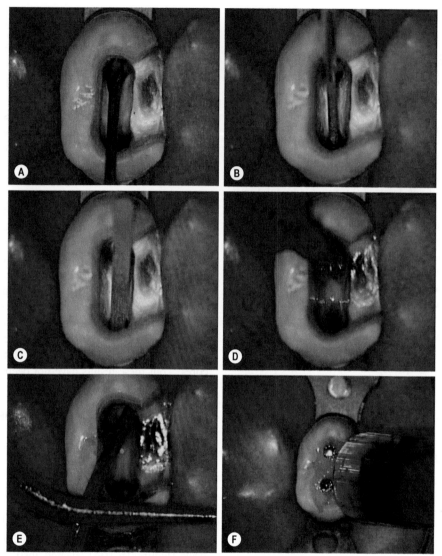

FIGURE 15-10 Fibre post placement and composite resin core build-up. Post space preparation; the gutta-percha root filling is removed with a Gates-Glidden drill (A). Sealer and temporary cement remnants are removed with an ultrasonic tip with magnification (B). The root canals are dried with paper points, and the chosen fibre post is tried in the root canal (C). The primer is placed into the root canal using a microbrush (D); a specially designed tip is used to introduce the composite resin into the root canal and with the help of ultrasound (E). The composite resin core is light cured (F).

tips and preferably, aided by magnification with an operating microscope (Figure 15-10B).

Drying of the Root Canal

The canal needs to be dried before the application of the bonding system. Paper points, or a controlled stream of air from a Stropko irrigator (SybronEndo),

may be used for this purpose. Once the required size of post has been selected, it is advisable to try the post in the root canal (Figure 15-10C).

Bonding Systems

Both three-step bonding systems and self-etching primers can be used for the cementation of fibre posts as the bond strength to root dentine achieved with these two types of bonding agents is similar. The primer is applied on both the root dentine and the post. It is advisable to use a self- or dual-curing resin. Microbrushes are needed to ensure a uniform distribution of the bonding agent into the depth of the root canal (Figure 15-10D).

Composite Resin Cement

Conventional core, or dual-cured, composite resins are also preferred for the cementation of the post. These materials have mechanical properties closer to that of dentine. Light-cured composite resins are too thick to be inserted properly into the root canal, whereas flowable composite and composite resin cements have a much lower modulus of elasticity and may, therefore, be the weakest part of the restoration.

Insertion of Composite Resin

To minimize void formation within the composite resin in the canal, it should be injected using a syringe with a special tip specifically designed for this purpose. The composite resin is injected into the canal starting from the bottom of the post space until it is completely filled. Ultrasound transmitted via a tip placed in contact with the syringe may help ensure a more uniform distribution of the composite resin into the root canal (Figure 15-10E).

Insertion of the Post

The post is simply inserted into the root canal. There is no need to place composite resin onto the post itself.

Composite Resin Core Build-Up

The composite resin core is created immediately using the same self-curing material. A light-cured composite resin may also be used to complete the core build-up (Figure 15-10F). Crown preparation can be carried out at the same visit.

Learning Outcomes

After completion of this chapter, the reader should be able to recognize and describe the:
- effects of endodontic treatment on teeth;
- factors influencing the survival of endodontically treated teeth, including the preservation of tooth

structure and ensuring that the stress within the tooth and restoration is minimized;
- timing of the restoration for endodontically treated teeth;
- choice of restoration for both anterior and posterior teeth, and the different restorative requirements;
- adhesive techniques for the restoration of endodontically treated teeth including fibre post and composite resin cores;
- importance of the ferrule effect for the success of any extracoronal restoration.

REFERENCES

1. Eckerbom M, Magnusson T, Martinsson T. Reasons for and incidence of tooth mortality in a Swedish population. Endodontics and Dental Traumatology 1992;8:230–4.
2. Gutmann JL. The dentin-root complex: anatomic and biologic considerations in restoring endodontically treated teeth. Journal of Prosthetic Dentistry 1992;67:458–67.
3. Reeh ES, Messer HH, Douglas WH. Reduction in tooth stiffness as a result of endodontic and restorative procedures. Journal of Endodontics 1989;15:512–6.
4. Grigoratos D, Knowles J, Ng YL, et al. Effect of exposing dentine to sodium hypochlorite and calcium hydroxide on its flexural strength and elastic modulus. International Endodontic Journal 2001;34:113–9.
5. Randow K, Glantz PO. On cantilever loading of vital and non vital teeth. Acta Odontologica Scandinavica 1986;44:271–7.
6. Huang TJG, Schilder H, Nathanson D. Effects of moisture content and endodontic treatment on some mechanical properties of human dentin. Journal of Endodontics 1991;18: 209–15.
7. Sedgley CM, Messer HH. Are endodontically treated teeth more brittle? Journal of Endodontics 1992;18:332–5.
8. Lang H, Korkmaz Y, Schneider K, et al. Impact of endodontic treatments on the rigidity of the root. Journal of Dental Research 2006;85:364–8.
9. Ikram O, Patel S, Sauro S, et al. The loss of hard tissue volume following root canal preparation and fiber post space preparation: A Micro Computed Tomography investigation. International Endodontic Journal 2009;42:1071–6.
10. Salehrabi R, Rotstein I. Endodontic treatment outcomes in a large patient population in the USA: an epidemiological study. Journal of Endodontics 2004;30:846–50.
11. Raedel M, Hartmann A, Bohm S, et al. Three-year outcomes of root canal treatment: Mining an insurance database. Journal of Dentistry 2015;43:412–7.
12. Pabst AM, Walter C, Ehbauer S, et al. Analysis of implant-failure predictors in the posterior maxilla: A retrospective study of 1395 implants. Journal of Cranio-Maxillo-Facial Surgery 2015;43:414–20.
13. Walton TR. An up to 15-year longitudinal study of 515 metal-ceramic FPDs: Part 1. Outcome. International Journal of Prosthodontics. 2002;15:439–45.
14. Stavropoulou A, Koidis P. A systematic review of single crowns on endodontically treated teeth. Journal of Dentistry 2007;35: 761–7.

15. Mannocci F, Bertelli E, Sherriff M, et al. Three year clinical comparison of survival of endodontically treated teeth restored with either full cast coverage or direct composite restoration. Journal of Prosthetic Dentistry 2002;88:297–301.

16. Mannocci F, Qualtrough AJ, Worthington H, et al. Randomized clinical comparison of endodontically treated teeth restored with amalgam or with fiber posts and resin composite: five year results. Operative Dentistry 2005;30:9–15.

17. Mannocci F, Gagliani M, Cavalli G. Adhesive restorations of endodontically treated teeth. Berlin: Quintessence; 2008.

18. Salvi GE, Siegrist Guldener BE, Amstad T, et al. Clinical evaluation of root filled teeth restored with or without post-and-core systems in a specialist practice setting. International Endodontic Journal 2007;40:209–15.

19. Creugers NH, Mentink AG, Fokkinga WA, et al. Five-year follow-up of a prospective clinical study on various core restorations. International Journal of Prosthodontics 2005;18:34–9.

20. Fokkinga WA, Kreulen CM, Bronkhorst EM, et al. Composite resin core-crown reconstructions: an up to 17-year follow-up of a controlled clinical trial. International Journal of Prosthodontics 2008;21:109–15.

21. Hansen EK, Asmussen E, Christansen NC. In vivo fractures of endodontically treated posterior teeth restored with amalgam. Endodontics and Dental Traumatology 1990;6:49–55.

22. Plasmans PJ, Creugers NH, Mulder J. Long-term survival of extensive amalgam restorations. Journal of Dental Research 1998;77:453–60.

23. Näpänkangas R, Pihlaja J, Raustia A. Outcome of zirconia single crowns made by predoctoral dental students: A clinical retrospective study after 2 to 6 years of clinical service. Journal of Prosthetic Dentistry 2015;113:289–94.

24. Mannocci F, Cowie J. Restoration of endodontically treated teeth. British Dental Journal 2014;216:341–6.

25. Reitemeier B, Hänsel K, Kastner C, et al. A prospective 10-year study of metal ceramic single crowns and fixed dental prosthesis retainers in private practice settings. Journal of Prosthetic Dentistry 2013;109:149–55.

26. Jung RE, Kalkstein O, Sailer I, et al. A comparison of composite post buildups and cast gold post-and-core buildups for the restoration of nonvital teeth after 5 to 10 years. International Journal of Prosthodontics 2007;20:63–99.

27. Ferrari M, Cagidiaco MC, Grandini S, et al. Post placement affects survival of endodontically treated premolars. Journal of Dental Research 2007;86:729–34.

28. Cagidiaco MC, García-Godoy F, Vichi A, et al. Placement of fiber prefabricated or custom made posts affects the 3-year survival of endodontically treated premolars. American Journal of Dentistry 2008;21:179–84.

29. Bolla M, Muller-Bolla M, Borg C, et al. Root canal posts for the restoration of root filled teeth. Cochrane Database of Systematic Reviews 2007;1:CD004623.

30. Cagidiaco MC, Goracci C, Garcia-Godoy F, et al. Clinical studies of fiber posts: a literature review. International Journal of Prosthodontics 2008;21:328–36.

31. Standlee JP, Caputo M, Hanson EC. Retention of endodontic dowels: effect of cement, dowel length, diameter and design. Journal of Prosthetic Dentistry 1978;39:400–5.

32. Lanza A, Aversa R, Rengo S, et al. 3-D FEA of cemented steel, glass and carbon posts in a maxillary incisor. Dental Materials 2005;21:709–15.

33. Mannocci F, Pilecki P, Bertelli E, et al. Density of dentinal tubules affects the tensile strength of root dentin. Dental Materials 2004;20:293–6.

34. DeCleen MJ. The relationship between the root canal filling and post space preparation. International Endodontic Journal 1993;26:53–8.

35. Mattison GD, Delivanis PD, Thacker RW, et al. Effect of post preparation on the apical seal. Journal of Prosthetic Dentistry 1984;51:785–9.

36. Kvist T, Rydin E, Reit C. The relative frequency of periapical lesions in teeth with root canal-retained posts. Journal of Endodontics 1989;15:578–80.

37. Tan PL, Aquilino SA, Gratton DG, et al. In vitro fracture resistance of endodontically treated central incisors with varying ferrule heights and configurations. Journal of Prosthetic Dentistry 2005;93:331–6.

38. Mannocci F, Sherriff M, Watson TF. Three point bending test of fiber posts. Journal of Endodontics 2001;27:758–61.

39. Vano M, Goracci C, Monticelli F, et al. The adhesion between fibre posts and composite resin cores: the evaluation of microtensile bond strength following various surface chemical treatments to posts. International Endodontic Journal 2006;39:31–9.

40. Aksornmuang J, Foxton RM, Nakajima M, et al. Microtensile bond strength of a dual-cure resin core material to glass and quartz fibre posts. Journal of Dentistry 2004;32:443–50.

Index

Page numbers followed by 'f' indicate figures, and 't' indicate tables.

Printed and bound by CPI Group (UK) Ltd, Croydon, CR0 4YY

03/10/2024

01040349-0006